# Evidence-Based Podiatry

Dyane E. Tower
Editor

# Evidence-Based Podiatry

## A Clinical Guide to Diagnosis and Management

Springer

*Editor*
Dyane E. Tower
American Podiatric Medical Association
Bethesda, MD
USA

ISBN 978-3-030-50855-5 ISBN 978-3-030-50853-1 (eBook)
https://doi.org/10.1007/978-3-030-50853-1



This Springer imprint is published by the registered company Springer Nature Switzerland AG
The registered company address is: Gewerbestrasse 11, 6330 Cham, Switzerland

# Preface

Thanks for picking up *Evidence-Based Podiatry: A Clinical Guide to Diagnosis and Management.* You are a busy student, resident, fellow, or practicing provider and you might not have time to cull through the most recent literature to find out the latest information on diagnosis and treatment for conditions you treat. You are in luck; we have done the heaving lifting for you.

I was asked to speak at the American Podiatric Medical Association's Annual Scientific Meeting in Philadelphia in 2016 on evidence-based medicine as an introduction to oral abstract presentations being given by my colleagues who are doing research in podiatric medicine and surgery. This book, *Evidence-Based Podiatry: A Clinical Guide to Diagnosis and Management,* was a result of my involvement at that meeting. A representative from Springer Publishing Company reached out to me to ask if I was interested in putting a book together that had evidence for conditions and treatments in one place. This book represents my attempt to provide a compilation of information on common conditions in podiatric medicine and surgery in one place, for easy access.

In order to practice evidence-based medicine, you must integrate clinical experience and patient values with the best available research. This book provides information and tips based on current evidence in an easy format to save you time.

The chapters, organized from toe to ankle, were written by extremely experienced podiatric physicians and surgeons and researchers who are experts in the field. With all its strengths and flaws, I hope *Evidence-Based Podiatry: A Clinical Guide to Diagnosis and Management* inspires you to engage in evidence-based research of your own.

This book would not exist without the dedication and hard work of the authors and subject matter experts; I am extremely grateful for your contributions. I'd also like to thank Kristopher Spring and Dhanapal Palanisamy from Springer Publishing Company for their perseverance and support throughout this multi-year project.

Bethesda, MD, USA Dyane E. Tower, DPM, MPH, MS, FACFAS

# Contents

# Contributors

**Rachel H. Albright, DPM, MPH** Department of Surgery, Stamford Health, Foot & Ankle, Darien, CT, USA

**Philip Basile, DPM, FACFAS** Department of Surgery, Mount Auburn Hospital, Cambridge, MA, USA

**Emily A. Cook, DPM, MPH, FACFAS** Department of Surgery, Mount Auburn Hospital, Cambridge, MA, USA

**Jeremy J. Cook, DPM, MPH, FACFAS** Department of Surgery, Mount Auburn Hospital, Cambridge, MA, USA

**Adam E. Fleischer, DPM, MPH** Department of Podiatric Medicine & Radiology, Dr. William M. Scholl College of Podiatric Medicine at Rosalind Franklin University of Medicine & Science, North Chicago, IL, USA

**Daniel J. Hatch, DPM, FACFAS** Clinical Instructor: Scholl College of Podiatric Medicine, North Chicago, IL, USA

Director of Surgery: North Colorado Podiatric Surgical Residency, Greeley, CO, USA

Private Practice: Foot and Ankle Center of the Rockies, Denver, CO, USA

**Christopher R. Hood** Hunterdon Podiatric Medicine, Hunterdon Healthcare System, Flemington, NJ, USA

**Erin E. Klein, DPM, MS** Weil Foot and Ankle Institute, Mount Prospect, IL, USA

**Kwasi Y. Kwaadu, DPM, MPH** Department of Surgery, Temple University School of Podiatric Medicine, Philadelphia, PA, USA

**Jeffrey D. Lehrman, DPM, FASPS, MAPWCA, CPC** A Step Ahead Foot & Ankle Center, Fort Collins, CO, USA

**Elena Manning, DPM** Department of Surgery, Mount Auburn Hospital, Cambridge, MA, USA

**Stephen A. Mariash, DPM, FACFAS** International Foot and Ankle Foundation for Education and Research, Everett, WA, USA

Practice: St Cloud Orthopedic Associates, St Cloud, MN, USA

**Bryon McKenna, DPM** Department of Surgery, Mount Auburn Hospital, Cambridge, MA, USA

**Andrew J. Meyr, DPM** Department of Surgery, Temple University School of Podiatric Medicine, Philadelphia, PA, USA

**Samantha Miner, DPM** Department of Surgery, Mount Auburn Hospital, Cambridge, MA, USA

**Roya Mirmiran, DPM, FACFAS** Department of Podiatry, Sutter Medical Group, Sacramento, CA, USA

**Laura E. Sansosti, DPM** Departments of Surgery and Biomechanics, Temple University School of Podiatric Medicine, Philadelphia, PA, USA

**Tracey C. Vlahovic, DPM, FFPM, RCPS (Glasg)** Department of Podiatric Medicine, Temple University School of Podiatric Medicine, Philadelphia, PA, USA

**Lowell Weil Jr, DPM, MBA, FACFAS** Weil Foot and Ankle Institute, Mount Prospect, IL, USA

# Introduction – Overview of Topics and What to Expect

*Evidence-Based Podiatry: A Clinical Guide to Diagnosis and Management* provides useful tips and information on common topics in podiatric medicine and surgery based on recent published literature.

The book starts with four chapters related to the toes, moves into three chapters related to the midfoot, and rounds out with six chapters related to hindfoot and ankle pathology, including wound care. The first two chapters are specific to toenails and discuss several options to treat ingrown and fungal toenails. The next chapter goes through fixation options for hammertoes and the final toe-related chapter is focused on 2nd MPJ pathology. The midfoot chapters focus on the first ray (Lapidus), generalized midfoot arthritis, and flatfoot. The final six chapters highlight complex rearfoot and ankle pathologies and treatments, including ankle arthroscopy, Achilles tendon ruptures, Charcot, clubfoot, and total ankle replacements. The management of chronic wounds is also discussed in a broad manner.

# Chapter 1
# Permanent Ingrown Toenails: Chemical and Surgical Procedures

Tracey C. Vlahovic

## Introduction

An ingrown toenail, also known as unguis incarnatus, can cause significant pain and disability to the patient [1]. It presents as a painful onychocryptosis or incurvation of the lateral edge of the nail plate with or without lateral nail fold edema, redness, or drainage (Fig. 1.1) and is more commonly seen in teenagers and young adults. It is widely accepted that the nail border edge, often in the form of a spicule, invades the lateral nail fold and creates an inflammatory response [2]. Ingrown toenails most often occur in the hallux nail and are attributed to a combination of poor nail trimming, shoe gear pressure, presence of nail disease like onychomycosis, and biomechanical considerations [2]. One theory is that the nail itself is the issue as is seen in pincer nails (Fig. 1.2), whereas another theory attributes the soft tissue surrounding the nail as the causative factor. Patients with diabetes have been found to have a higher rate of ingrown nails compared with those who are nondiabetic [2]. Medications such as indinavir, retinoids, docetaxel, cyclosporine, oral terbinafine, and topical efinaconazole have reported ingrown nails as adverse events. Whatever the prevailing source, it may cause significant quality of life issues due to the associated pain affecting gait and shoe gear wear which can affect sports, school, and work. When focal erythema, swelling, drainage, granulation tissue, and/or hypertrophy of the periungual tissue is present, the ingrown nail becomes known as a paronychia of the toenail.

Before delving into the various treatment options, it is helpful to determine when examining a patient with an ingrown toenail if there is an underlying biomechanical cause as is often the case in the hallux nail of a patient with a bunion

T. C. Vlahovic (✉)
Department of Podiatric Medicine, Temple University School of Podiatric Medicine, Philadelphia, PA, USA
e-mail: traceyv@temple.edu



D. E. Tower (ed.), *Evidence-Based Podiatry*,
https://doi.org/10.1007/978-3-030-50853-1_1

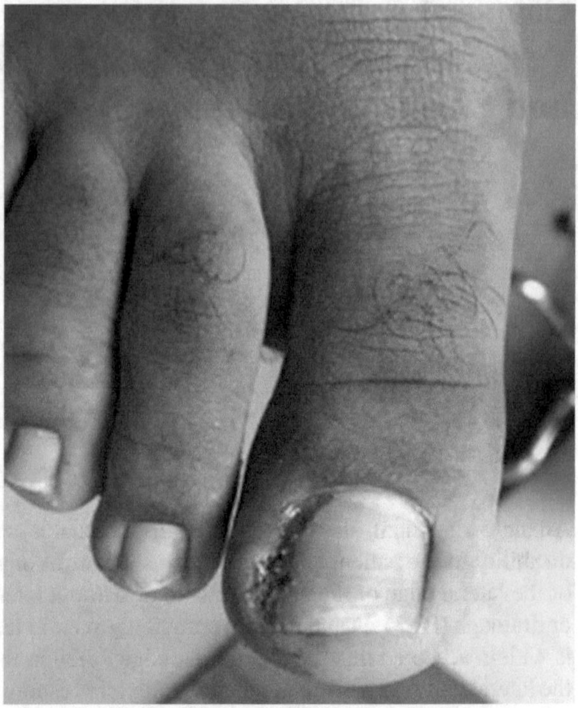

**Fig. 1.1** Incurvation of the lateral edge of the nail plate

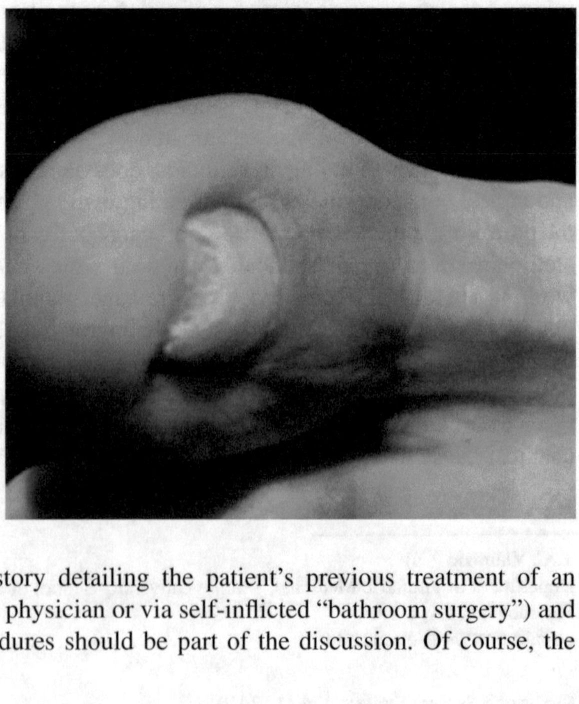

**Fig. 1.2** Typical appearance of pincer nail

deformity. A thorough history detailing the patient's previous treatment of an ingrown nail (whether by a physician or via self-inflicted "bathroom surgery") and the outcome of said procedures should be part of the discussion. Of course, the patient's medical history and vascular status (including any relevant history of Raynaud's phenomenon and pernio) are imperative in determining if the patient can have nail surgery. Nails should be free of nail polish or other adornments on the affected foot. When it comes to ingrown toenails, the physician should note the level of pain as well as the presence of infection, erythema, edema, granulation tissue, and drainage.

Differential diagnoses of an ingrown toenail, especially one with granulation tissue, include pyogenic granuloma, amelanotic melanoma, basal cell carcinoma, squamous cell carcinoma, and subungual exostosis. In cases where a nail procedure with removal of granulation tissue was performed and "granulation tissue" is present at a post-operative visit, one of the skin tumor diagnoses should be considered, and a biopsy of the tissue should be performed.

## Conservative Therapies

Conservative therapies may be considered in certain situations where there is vascular compromise, various issues surrounding an office-based surgical procedure, or a temporary solution until a surgical procedure can be performed. Suggestion of a wider toe box or an open-toed shoe may be useful to some patients. Treatment of an underlying cause such as onychomycosis or hyperhidrosis should be initiated. Patients should be educated on trimming of the nail straight across and not curving in the nail borders which often perpetuates ingrown nails both iatrogenically and organically [2]. The "slant back" procedure of trimming the nail edge as far proximally as possible, which is often done in podiatric physician's offices, offers temporary pain relief but necessitates periodic visits to continue the brief respite it provides.

Other modalities such as gutter splinting, taping the lateral nail fold, and massaging of the nail fold have been described. These methods require patience and time on the patient's part. The gutter splint technique involves length-wise splitting of a plastic intravenous tube and inserting it under local anesthesia as far proximally as possible, thus creating a barrier between the nail spicule and the lateral nail fold [2]. The tubing is then secured and left on the nail for 3–4 weeks to allow the nail spicule to grow distally without injuring the surrounding skin. A similar method utilizing cotton wisps inserted under the nail plate edge is an older method but may be useful for those who can't undergo nail surgery. Taping of the skin surrounding the painful nail corner with a band-aid or another type of medical tape encourages the skin and nail to grow away from each other, relieve pressure, and allow drainage if present. Tape placed at the corner of the offending nail which is then pulled proximally and plantarly on the affected digit often provides instant relief, but no randomized, controlled studies have been done on this technique, and it requires daily use for several months to have a long-term effect.

## Partial Nail Avulsions and Adjunctive Procedures

For those patients whom conservative therapy has failed or whom the presentation is too severe for a non-surgical intervention, a partial nail avulsion of the affected nail edge is indicated. The purpose of this procedure is to decrease the width of the nail plate of the offending border to relieve pain and pressure. This certainly can extend to include removal/destruction of the nail matrix either surgically or chemically to cause long-term narrowing of the nail plate. Prior to performing any toenail procedure, it is imperative to obtain the consent of the patient and document risks, benefits, and consequences of the planned procedure in the chart.

A partial nail avulsion narrows the nail width and removes the offending lateral nail border but is considered a temporary procedure as the nail matrix is typically not destroyed, thus leading to regrowth of the nail plate in the avulsed area. The general technique is as follows: the area is swabbed with 70% alcohol, and local anesthesia is either injected in a digital block or wing block technique (Fig. 1.3). Either lidocaine or bupivacaine without epinephrine is administered, typically between 3 and 5 mL. The surgeon may elect to perform the procedure with or without a digital tourniquet. If there is granulation tissue present, it may be excised to better visualize the nail plate. This tissue may be discarded or sent for pathology depending on the history and clinical presentation. Some surgeons utilize a Freer elevator to lyse the nail plate from the nail bed distal to proximal to have a cleaner and easier removal of the nail plate border. This is an ancillary step based on the surgeon's choice. Then, using an English anvil (nail splitter), small scissors, or a nail nipper, the nail plate border is split from the rest of the nail starting from the hyponychium to the nail matrix (under the proximal nail fold) being careful not to damage the nail bed or the proximal nail fold (Fig. 1.4). The sliver of nail plate is

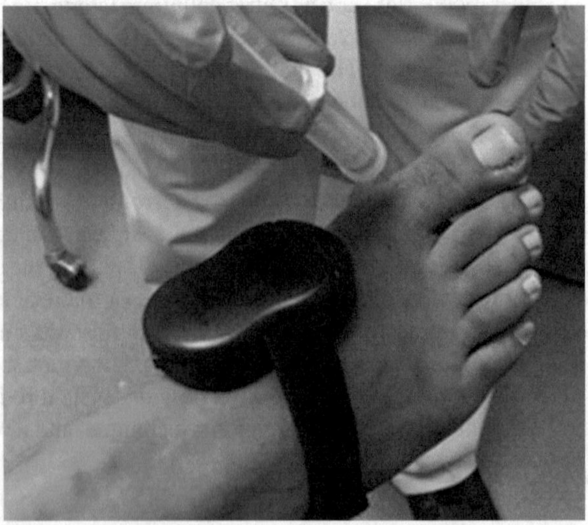

**Fig. 1.3** Needle placement for digital nerve block

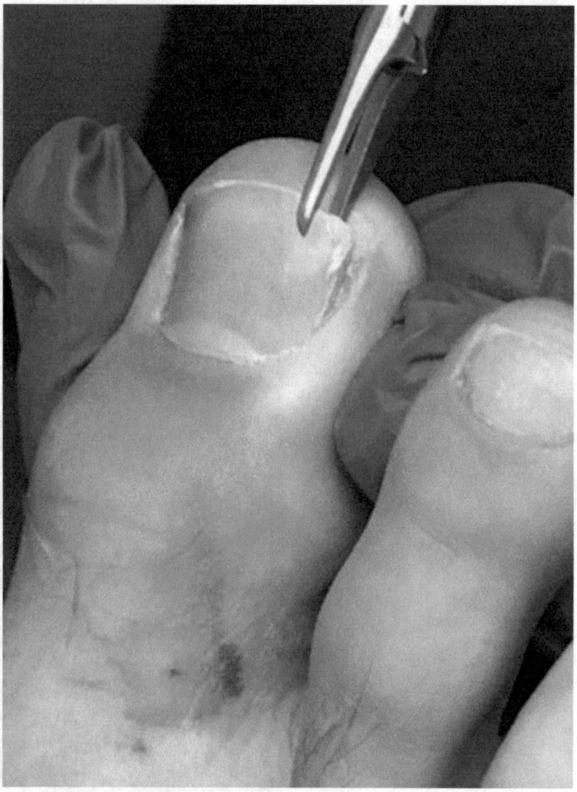

**Fig. 1.4** Splitting of the nail plate with English anvil

then removed with a straight hemostat (Fig. 1.5). A curette may be used to assess if any nail plate remains under the proximal nail fold, but also may be utilized to clean the tissue of any debris [1].

While there are many variations of performing a partial nail avulsion, originally described by Ross, adjunctive interventions are the mainstay to this day [3].

Since a simple partial nail avulsion's recurrence rate is about 70%, one can perform a chemical matrixectomy post-partial nail avulsion utilizing either application of phenol (Fig. 1.6) or sodium hydroxide in the area of the nail matrix at the removed offending nail border [2]. In 1945, Boll was the first to describe the use of phenol following a partial nail avulsion [4]. Phenol, a weak organic acid, is both lipophilic and hydrophilic. It is highly soluble in organic solvents like isopropyl alcohol, which ultimately is the best treatment for phenol burns. Many practitioners will follow the phenol application with a lavage of alcohol. However, irrigating the newly "phenolized" area with alcohol, a weak acid, to "neutralize" the phenol is under debate in the literature. Recent studies have shown that the amount of phenol recovered (i.e., removal of phenol) when one irrigates the area with either polyhexanide (PHMB) or sterile saline solution is greater than irrigation with alcohol [5, 6]. Ultimately, alcohol and the other solutions observed in these studies do not neutralize phenol; they simply serve to dilute it and aid in its removal [6].

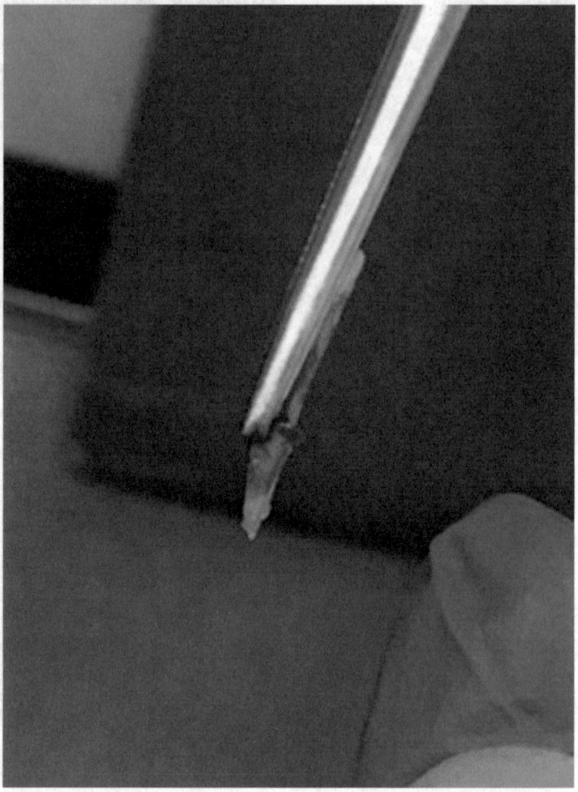

**Fig. 1.5** Offending nail border removed in jaws of hemostat

Researchers have described nail phenolization following a partial nail avulsion as the definitive method of decreasing the width of the nail plate with less recurrence in comparison to partial nail avulsion alone [7]. In addition, there is no significant difference in recurrence when using phenol versus sodium hydroxide to perform a chemical matrixectomy following a partial nail avulsion [7].

The suggested time and amount of phenol varies from practitioner to practitioner depending on training and experience. Two studies focused on determining the amount of time and number of applications that will effectively destroy matrix cells. Boberg et al. utilized nail specimens obtained from patients who had ingrown toenails [4]. Physicians applied an 89% phenol solution for 30 seconds, 1 minute, 90 seconds, and 2 minutes to the nail matrix. After 30 seconds, the basal layer was intact, which would imply recurrence is likely to occur. The 1-minute application of 89% phenol showed complete destruction of the basal layer, while the 90-second and 2-minute applications not only showed basal layer ablation but also necrosis of the dermis.

However, when Becerro de Bengoa Vallejo et al. examined the application of 88% phenol to fresh cadaveric hallux nail samples, they found that a 1-minute application left the basal layer of the epithelium intact [8]. After studying up to 6 minutes

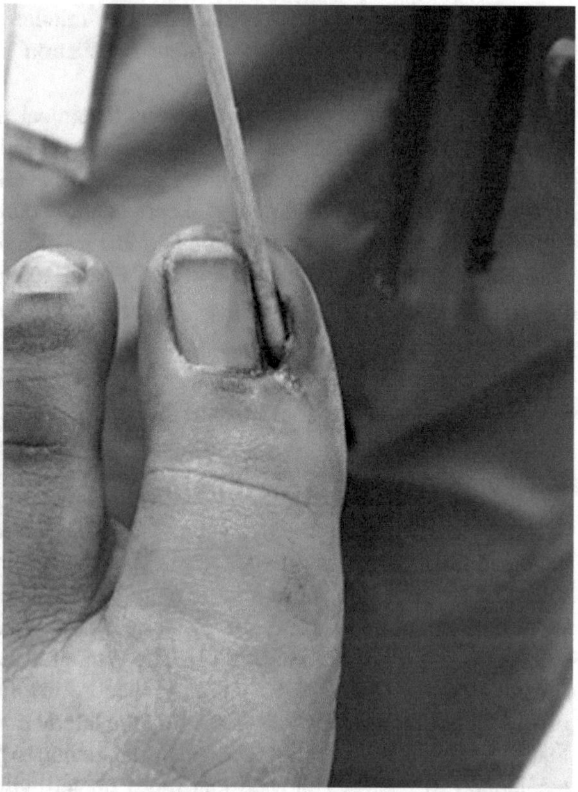

**Fig. 1.6** Application of phenol with cotton tipped applicator after offending nail border was removed

of application, researchers determined that 4 minutes of application destroyed the nail matrix. The Boberg study supports the wide podiatric use of the prepackaged phenol-soaked cotton tip applicators which is 89% phenol intended for a single dose, 1-minute application [4]. Ultimately, further studies are needed not only to determine the amount of exposure required to destroy nail matrix cells but the rate of recurrence and recurrence in the presence of infection as well.

Since phenolization of the nail matrix has side effects of post-operative drainage for days to weeks and pain, two studies examined the use of sodium hydroxide and its potential side effects. Bostanci et al. described three patients who developed allodynia, nail dystrophy, and hyperalgesia after having a 10% sodium hydroxide chemical matrixectomy [9]. However, there are limited reports in the literature of post-operative complications from the use of sodium hydroxide, and these complications shouldn't be considered rare until a larger study or case series demonstrates otherwise.

Recently, Chander et al. compared 88% phenol to 10% sodium hydroxide following partial nail avulsion [10]. Due to phenol causing coagulation necrosis versus the liquefaction necrosis visible with the base amount of sodium hydroxide, the side effect profile with sodium hydroxide in theory should be of a lesser nature. The patients in this study had less recovery time than those in the Bostanci study [9].

However, Chander and colleagues used a 1-minute application time of sodium hydroxide in comparison to a 3-minute application time of phenol, which could lessen side effects [10].

Regarding specific patient populations, chemical matrixectomies may be performed in patients with well-controlled diabetes and patients on anti-coagulant therapy [11]. Any patient undergoing a partial nail avulsion with a chemical matrixectomy should be educated on home care of the wound since phenol may cause a burn to the surrounding skin. Various topical medications and dressings are available for the physician to utilize in office and recommend the patient use for home care.

## Surgical Matrixectomy and Soft Tissue Debulking

Following a partial nail avulsion, a surgical matrixectomy can be performed instead of a chemical matrixectomy in certain cases. This is often reserved for patients who have had failed chemical matrixectomies, have significant hypertrophy of the surrounding tissue, and/or have a large amount of granulation tissue. The procedure involves a partial nail avulsion followed by a partial matrixectomy and wedge excision of the hypertrophic nail fold [2]. The Winograd technique is typically utilized for this purpose [12]. The Winograd procedure involves a wedge excision of the offending border with focus on removing the lateral matrix horn surgically. A study that compared the Winograd technique (50 patients) to the conservative gutter splint technique (50 patients) showed that those treated with the gutter splint had 10% recurrence versus 12% with the Winograd [13]. Workdays lost with the Winograd post-operatively were 2 weeks versus 1.1 weeks with the gutter-split method. Based on these results, the gutter-splint method achieved very similar results recurrence-wise, preserved the matrix, was more economical, created immediate pain relief, and achieved a better cosmetic result [13].

Alternate techniques to excising the nail matrix include $CO_2$ laser, radiofrequency, and electrocautery to destroy the matrix cells [2]. The $CO_2$ laser has a success rate of 50–100% and boasts less bleeding, less pain, and more focused direction of the matrix tissue to be ablated [14]. The downside of this technique is cost (if the practitioner doesn't own this laser or doesn't have access to a hospital that provides this laser), and re-epithelialization of the tissue may create significant downtime post-operatively.

Partial nail avulsion followed by a surgical matrixectomy is certainly an option, but researchers have described debulking of the periungual soft tissue when the hypertrophy of the nail fold contributes to the lateral nail pain [6].

There are two techniques for periungual debulking: the Howard-Dubois procedure and the super U procedure [15–17]. The Howard-Dubois procedure is considered for mild to moderate cases, while the super U procedure is indicated for severe presentations that will involve more tissue removal [1]. Both describe incisions encompassing the distal, lateral, and medial aspects of the nail unit to debulk the soft tissue effectively. When performing the Howard-Dubois procedure, one would make a fish-mouth incision parallel to the distal nail and running medial and lateral to the distal interphalangeal joint. A second incision creates a wedge to further remove excess soft tissue. This technique can also reduce the bulk for an embedded distal toenail edge, which will ultimately allow the nail plate to progress forward. Both procedures will require appropriate post-operative care and some downtime, especially if one performs the super U procedure.

## Summary

Ingrown toenails are a source of pain, disability, and morbidity. After assessing if the nail or the skin folds are the basic source, it is important to look at other causative factors such as hyperhidrosis, biomechanics, or medications. Conservative methods may be useful for mild presentations, but for many patients an office-based surgical procedure to remove the offending nail border is necessary. This can be followed by a chemical matrixectomy which has a lower recurrence rate than a simple partial nail avulsion alone, and in certain situations, a surgical matrixectomy may be indicated. For hypertrophied nail folds, debulking procedures that do not disturb the nail matrix are indicated. Overall, the surgical procedure should match the deformity and clinical presentation. While recurrence is always a concern, it is important to educate the patient on the procedure, post-operative care, and long-term sequelae of narrowing the nail plate or debulking the periungual tissue.

## References

1. Di Chiacchio N, Di Chiacchio NG. Best way to treat an ingrown toenail. Dermatol Clin. 2015;33(2):277–82.
2. Khunger N, Kandhari R. Ingrown toenails. Indian J Dermatol Venereol Leprol. 2012;78:279–89.
3. Ross WR. Treatment of the ingrown toenail and a new anesthetic method. Surg Clin North Am. 1969;49(6):1499–504.
4. Boberg JS, Frederiksen MS, Harton FM. Scientific analysis of phenol nail surgery. J Am Podiatr Med Assoc. 2002;92(10):575–9.
5. Cordoba Diaz D, Becerro de Bengoa Vallejo R, Losa Iglesias ME, Cordoba Diaz M. Polihexanide solution is more efficient than alcohol to remove phenol in chemical matricectomy: an in vitro study. Dermatol Ther. 2014;27(6):369–72.
6. Cordoba Diaz D, Losa Iglesias ME, Cordoba Diaz M, Becerro de Bengoa Vallejo R. Enhanced removal of phenol with saline solution over alcohol: an in vitro study. Dermatol Surg. 2012;38(8):1296–301.
7. Eekhof JA, Van Wijk B, Knuistingh Neven A, et al. Interventions for ingrowing toenails. Cochrane Database Syst Rev. 2012;4:CD001541.
8. Becerro de Bengoa Vallejo R, Cordoba Diaz D, Cordoba Diaz M, Losa Iglesias ME. Alcohol irrigation after phenol chemical matricectomy: an in vivo study. Eur J Dermatol. 2013;23(3):319–23.

9. Bostanci S, Koçyiğit P, Güngör HK, Parlak N. Complications of sodium hydroxide chemical matrixectomy: nail dystrophy, allodynia, hyperalgesia. J Am Podiatr Med Assoc. 2014;104(6):649–51.
10. Chander G, Ananta K, Bhattacharya SN, Sharma A. Controlled trial comparing the efficacy of 88% phenol versus 10% sodium hydroxide for chemical matricectomy in the management of ingrown toenail. Indian J Dermatol Venereol Leprol. 2015;81(5):472–7.
11. Felton PM, Weaver TD. Phenol and alcohol chemical matrixectomy in diabetic versus nondiabetic patients. A retrospective study. J Am Podiatr Med Assoc. 1999;89(8):410.
12. Winograd AM. Modification in the technique of operation for ingrown toe-nail. 1929. J Am Podiatric Med Assoc. 2007;97:274–7.
13. Peyvandi H, Robati RM, Yegane RA, Hajinasrollah E, Toossi P, Peyvandi AA, et al. Comparison of two surgical methods (winograd and sleeve method) in the treatment of ingrown toenail. Dermatol Surg. 2011;37:331–5.
14. Andre P. Ingrowing nails and carbon dioxide laser surgery. J Eur Acad Dermatol Venereol. 2003;17:288–90.
15. Tian J, Li J, Wang F, Chen Z. A new perspective on the nail plate for treatment of ingrown toenail. Dermatol Pract Concept. 2018;8(1):22–7.
16. Richert B. Surgery of the lateral nail folds. In: Richert B, Di Chiacchio N, Haneke E, editors. Nail surgery. 1st ed. London: Healthcare; 2010. p. 89.
17. Rosa IP. Hipercurvatura transversa da lamina ungueal e lamina ungueal que na˜o cresce. Remoc¸a˜o do "U" largo de pele, osteocorrec¸a˜o do leito e cicatrizaca˜o por segund intenc¸a˜o (Tese). Sa˜o Paulo: Universidade Federal de Sa˜o Paulo, Escola Paulista de Medicina; 2005. p. 156.

# Chapter 2
# The Fungal Toenail: Topical, Oral, and Laser Treatments

Tracey C. Vlahovic

## Introduction

Onychomycosis is a common, superficial fungal infection of the nails leading to discoloration, nail plate thickening, and onycholysis. Mycotic nail disease is the most common nail pathology worldwide, reaching all cultures and ethnicities. Onychomycosis is increasing, accounting for up to 90% of toenail and at least 50% of fingernail infections [1]. The most common etiology in the United States is owing to dermatophytes, typically *Trichophyton rubrum* and *Trichophyton mentagrophytes* [2]. In Europe, *T. rubrum* is the chief agent followed by *T. mentagrophytes* and *T. interdigitale* [3, 4]. Non-dermatophyte molds and yeasts also play a role with varying frequency.

Because the initial diagnosis is based on the nail's appearance, the diagnostic gold standard is direct microscopy with potassium hydroxide [KOH] and fungal culture. However, visual nail plate changes are used to classify onychomycosis including distal subungual (also known as distal subungual onychomycosis, the most common form), proximal subungual, superficial white, and total dystrophic [5, 6].

Onychomycosis occurs in 10% of the general population, 20% of individuals 60 years of age and older, and 50% of individuals over 70 years of age [6]. The risk of onychomycosis is 1.9–2.8 times greater in persons with diabetes mellitus, and in patients with HIV infection, the prevalence of onychomycosis ranges from 15% to 40% [6]. Other predisposing factors include older age, sex (male > female), genetic predisposition, tinea pedis (interdigital or moccasin types), peripheral arterial disease, smoking, nail trauma, inappropriate nail hygiene, and family background of onychomycosis and hyperhidrosis [6, 7].

T. C. Vlahovic (✉)
Department of Podiatric Medicine, Temple University School of Podiatric Medicine, Philadelphia, PA, USA
e-mail: traceyv@temple.edu


D. E. Tower (ed.), *Evidence-Based Podiatry*,
https://doi.org/10.1007/978-3-030-50853-1_2

## Clinical Evaluation

To evaluate a patient presenting with nail dystrophy, the practitioner should begin by completing a thorough history and physical evaluation. With treatment options ranging from systemic to surgical, knowledge of medical history, current medications, and family history will aid in the differential diagnosis and formulating the treatment plan. Key questions include the following: how long have you had the nail changes (or when was your nail last normal?), is it painful, and has it affected your quality of life? Daily shoe gear choices, work and athletic/leisure activities, and the home and work environments will all assist treatment plan selection. Level of immunosuppression, vascular status, and the ability to take oral or apply topical medication should be considered. Discussion and examination of any other skin rashes or conditions should be completed, since psoriasis and eczema can mimic mycotic nails.

Visual assessment is imperative. Since the Zaias classification was proposed in 1972, modifications have been published to reflect the wide array of dermatophytes, non-dermatophyte molds, and yeasts as well as the complications of various patterns occurring in the same nail or other inflammatory diseases also presenting with mycosis [8]. Nail plate changes include the distal subungual type where the invasion begins at the hyponychium and disturbs the distal nail bed; proximal subungual, where invasion begins proximally; superficial white, where the upper surface of the nail plate is first attacked; total dystrophic, which describes total nail plate involvement and surrounding periungual tissue; and endonyx, which describes distal nail plate attack resulting in a deeper penetration of hyphae [8].

In addition, the physician should determine how many toenails are involved on one or both feet, percent involvement of the nail, any biomechanically aggravating factors that could contribute to nail dystrophy (adductovarus fifth digit, hammertoe, or hallux valgus) and the presence of tinea pedis interdigitally or plantarly.

Approximately 50% of nail disease is caused by onychomycosis; the remainder is caused by conditions that mimic onychomycosis, having similar signs and symptoms, including psoriasis, lichen planus, reactive arthritis, allergic/irritant contact dermatitis, and eczema [9]. Other differential diagnoses include alopecia, nail changes secondary to biomechanical issues, melanoma (and other skin cancers), traumatic onycholysis, 20-nail dystrophy, and pachyonychia [10–12].

Because not all presenting nail disease is mycotic, it is important to confirm with laboratory diagnosis if the treatment plan includes oral antifungal therapy, if there is concomitant skin disease difficult to distinguish in the nails, and if the patient has been on antifungal therapy previously and the disease has recurred. Laboratory diagnostic methods include direct microscopy (KOH test), nail plate biopsy for periodic acid-Schiff (PAS) stain, and fungal culture. Generally, KOH and fungal culture are done together; KOH shows the presence of hyphae, where culture shows the specific species present. Unfortunately, fungal cultivation is a slow process (4 weeks) and may generate false-negative results in 40% of the cases that are microscopically positive [13]. As an alternative, PAS stain involves sending nail plate (commonly referred to as, but not a true, "biopsy") for staining to determine presence of dermatophytes. PAS staining provides quicker results and is more sensitive, whereas culture is more specific (regarding dermatophyte or non-dermatophyte species) [14–16].

Standard mycological tests, KOH, and fungal culture may yield false-negative or false-positive results and require time to verify the pathogens [17]. Accurate diagnoses are often delayed owing to lack of both specific and rapid methods of pathogen identification. When the mycological analyses are negative and the clinical picture is highly suggestive of onychomycosis, polymerase chain reaction (PCR) testing may be an option [18]. Antifungal drug efficacy and dosages may differ for different causative pathogens, and it has been hypothesized that mixed and non-dermatophyte onychomycosis may be a cause for high rate of treatment failures [19]. A rapidly sensitive method for detection and identification will better guide an appropriate treatment strategy. PCR detects a specific DNA sequence; moreover, fungi species-specific PCR diagnostic methods are available [20, 21], deepening our understanding and treatment of onychomycosis [22]. Because DNA is extremely resistant and can persist even in the absence of viable hyphae, DNA amplification techniques such as PCR may represent a useful addition to standard procedure [23]. Time will tell how truly beneficial PCR will be both in the physician office and in clinical trials.

## Pharmacologic Treatment Options: Topical Therapy

Once confirmatory testing has been completed, onychomycosis can be managed with topical or systemic agents. The current standard of care is an oral antifungal agent (either terbinafine or itraconazole) because they are more effective than topical agents, owing to issues of penetrance into the nail apparatus with topical agents. Drug interactions and the risk of hepatic injury may limit their desirability, especially in the elderly where the disease is most prevalent.

Guidelines suggesting monotherapy with topical antifungals is limited to superficial white, except in transverse or striate infections, and distal subungual types, except in the presence of longitudinal streaks, when less than 80% of the nail plate is affected with lack of involvement of the lunula, or when systemic antifungals are contraindicated [24].

Developing effective topical treatments for onychomycosis has been complicated by low permeation rates through the nail plate to the site of infection [25–28]. The nail may be more permeable to agents formulated in an aqueous vehicle [29]. Unlike ciclopirox and amorolfine nail lacquers, the newer topical agents, efinaconazole and tavaborole, are available as alcohol-based solutions.

Studied in separate trials with similar, but not identical inclusion criteria, reported complete cure rates of tavaborole were 6.5–9.1% [30], while efinaconazole results were 15.2–17.8% [31]. Mycologic cure rates were 31.1–35.9% for tavaborole, whereas the mycologic cure rate for efinaconazole was 53.4–55.2%. Although much emphasis has been placed on the need for active ingredient to pass through the nail plate, recent data suggest that efinaconazole may reach the infection site after transungual and subungual application; subungual delivery data with tavaborole is pending [32, 33].

Lacquer-based topical therapies are applied primarily to the exterior nail plate, with the drug reaching the infection site mostly through nail permeation [34–36]. Efinaconazole and tavaborole are applied to the clean, dry nail plate surface, lateral and proximal nail folds, hyponychium, and undersurface of the nail plate [37]. Application to the hyponychium and ventral aspect of the nail plate may be important in patients wishing to continue to use nail polish [32]. Although nail polish does not seem to influence efinaconazole penetration into the nail, it can become tacky with repeated application [38]. Up to four layers of nail polish do not seem to inhibit penetration of tavaborole either [39]. In neither case has the impact of nail polish on efficacy been assessed, nor is it contraindicated.

Because toenail growth progresses from proximal to distal, newly formed nail plate replaces diseased nail, a process that can take 12–18 months [39]. Clinical trial data suggest that tavaborole and efinaconazole must be applied daily to the toenails for at least 48 weeks. Some patients may require treatment considerably longer because of slow toenail growth, disease severity, or for other reasons. It is not known whether longer treatment regimens with tavaborole or efinaconazole would produce better efficacy results; however, higher cure rates after longer follow-up periods have been reported with other agents [40–42].

It is important that patients recognize that cure may not translate to a completely clear nail [43]. Poor adherence with any long-term chronic therapy is well documented [44]. Several post hoc analyses with efinaconazole have been carried out to identify prognostic factors for treatment success. Gender and disease severity were significant influencers of complete cure over the duration of the studies; female patients and those with milder disease may see results much quicker in clinical practice, whereas male patients and those with moderately severe disease may require a longer treatment course, or combination therapy with oral antifungals [45, 46]. Although male patients are more difficult to treat, reasons are unclear. They tend to seek help for more advanced disease and suffer more nail trauma, and their toenails tend to be thicker. The reduced rate of growth and thickness of the nail may be factors in more severe disease, although it may be that these patients just require longer treatment courses.

Tinea pedis is an important causative factor for onychomycosis, and better results are seen when any coexisting tinea pedis is also treated [47]. In addition, managing tinea pedis is critical to minimizing disease recurrence [48].

## Pharmacological Treatment Options: Oral Agents

Systemic antifungals are currently assumed to be the most effective treatment for onychomycosis according to meta-analyses. Terbinafine achieved a 76% mycotic cure rate; 63% for itraconazole with pulse dosing, 59% for itraconazole with continuous dosing, and 48% for fluconazole [49]. Moreover, modalities such as accompanying nail debridement further increase cure rates [49].

Oral antifungal agents (e.g., terbinafine and itraconazole) are considered treatments of choice for onychomycosis because they can effectively reach the nail bed through systemic circulation [50]. However, these agents have limitations. Confirmatory fungal studies and blood work (specifically liver function testing) should be completed prior to initiation of therapy. Other limitations include drug-drug interactions with agents that are metabolized by specific cytochrome P450 (CYP) enzymes (more often itraconazole), potential inhibition of certain CYP subtypes, and adverse effects such as hepatotoxicity and congestive heart failure [50–52]. Itraconazole has boxed warnings of rare cases of serious hepatotoxicity with treatment, including liver failure and death. Even patients with no pre-existing liver disease or serious underlying medical condition are at risk for hepatotoxicity as well as congestive heart failure [51].

That said, in patients who have a moderate to severe presentation, have several nails involved, and have a past medical history/current medication history that is vetted, oral antifungals can be an excellent treatment option. Patients should be monitored clinically during therapy for adverse events and for healthy nail growth. Ultimately, regardless of which route, oral or topical, is prescribed for onychomycosis, the nail may take 12–18 months to grow out from cuticle to hyponychium.

## Nonpharmacologic Treatment Options

Debridement, the mechanical reduction of toenail length and thickness using nail nipper or rotating burr, may provide a valuable adjunct for patients experiencing pain upon ambulation and in shoe gear [53]. Although debridement alone improves quality of life and nail thickness, it does not result in mycological cure [54]. It may offer benefits through reduced fungal load and enhanced penetration of topical drugs into the nail unit. Topical ciclopirox and debridement improved patient's quality of life and resulted in mycologic cure [54]. However, debridement added to oral antifungal therapy may offer only a small benefit [55, 56]. Debridement can provide pain relief and improved patient satisfaction, affording an opportunity to encourage adherence. For patients who opt against pharmacologic treatment, debridement will allow more comfort in shoe gear and reduce potential pressure on the nail bed, especially if diabetic neuropathy is present.

Nail avulsion, the separation of the nail plate from the nail bed, can be achieved non-surgically with daily application of topical 40% urea for 1–2 weeks [57]. Generally, this is followed by application of a topical antifungal once the toenail has been removed, repeating as necessary. Nail avulsion in general is more common in Europe [57]. Nail avulsion achieved via topical urea application can be useful in patients who have a needle/procedure phobia, those who have peripheral vascular disease, or another comorbidity precluding pharmacologic intervention or have a single affected nail. However, removal of the nail itself will not result in clearance of the infection, even when followed by topical antifungal therapy.

For a singularly painful or thickened nail, some patients may opt for a surgical total nail removal. Surgery involves application of local anesthesia to the digit followed by removal of the nail plate in toto. Simple total avulsion of the nail itself is not curative for a mycotic nail, because the procedure does not address the basis of infection which is in the nail bed. A surgical nail avulsion followed by the application of topical antifungals has been described as a treatment plan. Total nail avulsion with the use of a topical azole cream applied twice daily to the exposed nail bed resulted in a high dropout rate in one study. All patients with total dystrophic onychomycosis failed, and only 56% of patients (15/27) were cured with this approach, suggesting that the procedure (nail avulsion plus twice daily azole application) should not be generally suggested for the treatment of onychomycosis [58].

Nail avulsion has been suggested to obtain a better specimen for fungal culture, but should only be used in situations where both systemic and topical antifungal therapies have failed [56]. Contraindications include patients with peripheral vascular disease, autoimmune disorders, collagen vascular disease, diabetes, hemostasis disorders, and acute infection/inflammation of the periungual tissue [59]. Possible keratinization of the nail bed as the nail plate is growing is also a concern.

Laser therapy is a non-surgical, non-pharmacologically based option. Approved devices include Nd:YAG 1064 nm lasers and a diode at 870/930 nm [58]. The US Food and Drug Administration approved laser treatment of certain wavelengths to "temporarily improve the appearance of the nail," making no claims regarding mycological cure owing to device approval being based on substantial equivalence to already existing devices on the market [60]. The mechanism of action is unknown, but proposed to be bulk heating of the nail unit selectively destroying fungal elements [60]. In the onychomycosis laser studies, the definition of "cure" and number of treatments are extremely variable, the fluence (energy applied per surface area) differs from device to device, and the amount of treatments rendered varies from one to several. Consistency within studies on mycological diagnosis varies, and strictness of a pharmaceutical clinical trial lacking. It is difficult to extrapolate settings used on the nail, the length of treatment, and outcomes owing to the differences in just the Nd:YAG laser class. Most likely patients who opt to receive laser as monotherapy will need several treatments over a 12- to 16-month period owing to the lack of recurrence data and possibility for reinfection [60, 61]. It has potential as an adjunct to both oral and topical antifungals, but further research is needed to show efficacy.

## Combination Therapy

New topical antifungals and device-based therapies have expanded therapeutic options in onychomycosis. Combination therapy with multiple drug classes and routes of administration may improve overall efficacy especially in patients proven difficult to treat successfully with more traditional methods.

The rationale for the combination of topical and oral therapy in the treatment of onychomycosis is that systemic antifungals reach the infection via the nail bed, and topical agents are absorbed through the nail surface [62]. In addition, some topical agents may reach the site of infection via the hyponychium. Ideally, combined antifungals should be synergistic in their mode of action and specific activity against the types of fungal infection seen in onychomycosis.

Combination therapy can be used sequentially or in parallel. In patients likely to fail therapy (i.e., those with diabetes or having yellow spikes in the nail (known as dermatophytomas), parallel treatment is invaluable. Sequential treatment (i.e., treating initially with an oral agent and following up with topical treatment) may be helpful in patients who show a poor response to treatment [63].

Combination therapy with oral and lacquer-based topical antifungals has been shown to lead to a marked improvement of mycological and clinical outcomes associated with onychomycosis and may be more cost-effective than using a systemic agent alone [64, 65]. Currently, there is no data with the newer solution-based topical agents (efinaconazole and tavaborole) used in combination with an oral agent to treat onychomycosis, and data is eagerly awaited given the apparent superior efficacy as monotherapy. Data on the combined use of an oral agent and laser therapy also suggest a more rapid and effective clinical outcome in patients with onychomycosis [66].

## Summary

Onychomycosis remains a common, progressive, and difficult disease to manage successfully. Early diagnosis and treatment are important irrespective of risk factors or comorbidities. A multidirectional approach to drug delivery may broaden the utility of topical therapies, such as efinaconazole and tavaborole, in the treatment of onychomycosis, and greater clinical experience will help to guide management practice.

As these are novel agents in treating mycotic nails, it also allows one to go back and revisit the other options already available: systemic, non-surgical, and surgical. With the vast amount of therapeutic possibilities out there (that also have an array of cure rates and complications), it is important for the clinician to choose the best option for the patient's situation and nail disease. Of most importance, confirming the diagnosis of onychomycosis is paramount, especially before starting a systemic medication. Choosing other modalities to treat the infected nail, whether as monotherapy or as a combination regimen, should be tailored to each patient. Overall, the clinician has more options than ever to manage fungal nail disease and ultimately improve quality of life for affected patients.

## References

1. Ghannoum MA, Hajjeh RA, Scher R, et al. A large-scale North American study of fungal isolates from nails: the frequency of onychomycosis, fungal distribution, and antifungal susceptibility patterns. J Am Acad Dermatol. 2000;43:641–8.
2. Thomas J, Jacobson GA, Narkowicz CK, et al. Toenail onychomycosis: an important global disease burden. J Clin Pharm Ther. 2010;35(5):497–519.

3. Borman AM, Campbell CK, Fraser M, et al. Analysis of the dermatophyte species isolated in the British Isles between 1980 and 2005 and review of worldwide dermatophyte trends over the last three decades. Med Mycol. 2007;45:131–41.
4. Saunte DM, Svejgaard EL, Haedersdal M, et al. Laboratory-based survey of dermatophyte infections in Denmark over a 10-year period. Acta Derm Venereol. 2008;88:614–6.
5. Zaias N. Onychomycosis. Dermatol Clin. 1985;3(3):445–60.
6. Westerberg DP, Yoyack MJ. Onychomycosis: current trends in diagnosis and treatment. Am Fam Physician. 2013;88(11):762–70.
7. Gupta AK, Skinner AR, Baran R. Onychomycosis in children: an overview. J Drugs Dermatol. 2003;2:31–4.
8. Hay RJ, Baran R. Onychomycosis: a proposed revision of the clinical classification. J Am Acad Dermatol. 2011;65:1219–27.
9. Faergemann J, Baran R. Epidemiology, clinical presentation and diagnosis of onychomycosis. Br J Dermatol. 2003;149(Suppl 65):1–4.
10. Murphy F, Jiaravuthisan MM, Sasseville D, et al. Psoriasis of the nail: anatomy, pathology, clinical presentation, and review of the literature on therapy. J Am Acad Dermatol. 2007;57(1):1–27.
11. Rich P, Elewski B, Scher RK, et al. Diagnosis, clinical implications, and complications of onychomycosis. Semin Cutan Med Surg. 2013;32(2 Suppl 1):S5–8.
12. Moll JM. Seronegative arthropathies in the foot. Baillieres Clin Rheumatol. 1987;1(2):289–314.
13. Fletcher CL, Hay RJ, Smeeton NC. Onychomycosis: the development of a clinical diagnostic aid for toenail disease. Part I. Establishing discriminating historical and clinical features. Br J Dermatol. 2004;150:701–5.
14. Weinberg JM, Koestenblatt EK, Tutrone WD, et al. Comparison of diagnostic methods in the evaluation of onychomycosis. J Am Acad Dermatol. 2003;49(2):193–7.
15. Reisberger EM, Abels C, Landthaler M, et al. Histopathological diagnosis of onychomycosis by periodic acid-Schiff-stained nail clippings. Br J Dermatol. 2003;148(4):749–54.
16. Borkowski P, Williams M, Holewinski J, et al. Onychomycosis: an analysis of 50 cases and a comparison of diagnostic techniques. J Am Podiatr Med Assoc. 2001;91(7):351–5.
17. Elewski BE. Diagnostic techniques for confirming onychomycosis. J Am Acad Dermatol. 1996;35:56–60.
18. Arca E, Saracli MA, Akar A, et al. Polymerase chain reaction in the diagnosis of onychomycosis. Eur J Dermatol. 2004;14:52–5.
19. Pierard GE, Arrese-Estrada J, Pierard-Franchimont C. Treatment of onychomycosis: traditional approaches. J Am Acad Dermatol. 1993;29:S41–5.
20. Spreadbury C, Holden D, Aufaurre-Brown A, et al. Detection of aspergillus fumigatus by polymerase chain reaction. J Clin Microbiol. 1993;31:615–21.
21. Miyakawa Y, Mabuchi T, Kagaya K, et al. Isolation and characterization of a species-specific DNA fragment for detection of Candida albicans by polymerase chain reaction. J Clin Microbiol. 1992;30:894–900.
22. Baharaeen S, Vishniac HS. 25S ribosomal RNA homologies of basidiomycetous yeasts: taxonomic and phylogenetic implications. Can J Microbiol. 1984;30:613–21.
23. Walberg M, Mørk C, Sandven P, et al. 18S rDNA polymerase chain reaction and sequencing in onychomycosis diagnostics. Acta Derm Venereol. 2006;86:223–6.
24. Ameen M, Lear JT, Madan V, et al. British Association of Dermatologists' guidelines for the management of onychomycosis 2014. Br J Dermatol. 2014;171:937–58.
25. Thatai P, Sapra B. Transungual delivery: deliberations and creeds. Int J Cosmet Sci. 2014;36:398–411.
26. Kobayashi Y, Miyamoto M, Sugibayashi K, et al. Drug permeation through the three layers of the human nail plate. J Pharm Pharmacol. 1999;51:271–8.
27. Gupta AK, Joseph WS. Ciclopirox 8% nail lacquer in the treatment of onychomycosis of the toenails in the United States. J Am Podiatr Med Assoc. 2000;90:495–501.

28. Bohn M, Kraemer K. The dermatopharmacologic profile of ciclopirox 8% nail lacquer. J Am Podiatr Med Assoc. 2000;90(10):491–4.
29. Hamilton JB, Terada H, Mestler GE. Studies of growth throughout the lifespan in Japanese: growth and size of nails and their relationship to age, sex, heredity, and other factors. J Gerontol. 1955;10(4):401–15.
30. Elewski BE, Rich P, Wiltz H, et al. Efficacy and safety of tavaborole topical solution, 5%, a novel boron-based antifungal agent for the treatment of onychomycosis: results from two randomized phase 3 studies. J Am Acad Dermatol. 2015;73(1):62–9.
31. Elewski BE, Rich P, Pollak R, et al. Efinaconazole 10% solution in the treatment of toenail onychomycosis: two phase 3 multicenter, randomized, double-blind studies. J Am Acad Dermatol. 2013;68:600–8.
32. Elewski BE, Pollak RA, Pillai R, et al. Access of efinaconazole topical solution, 10%, to the infection site by spreading through the subungual space. J Drugs Dermatol. 2014;13:1394–8.
33. Gupta AK, Pillai RK. The presence of an air gap between the nail plate and nail bed in onychomycosis patients: treatment implications for topical therapy. J Drugs Dermatol. 2015;14(8):859–63.
34. Singh G, Haneef NS, Uday A. Nail changes and disorders among the elderly. Indian J Dermatol Venereol Leprol. 2005;71(6):386–92.
35. Baran R, Kaoukhov A. Topical antifungal drugs for the treatment of onychomycosis: an overview of current strategies for monotherapy and combination therapy. J Eur Acad Dermatol Venereol. 2005;19(1):21–9.
36. Lecha M, Effendy I, Feuilhade de Chauvin M, et al. Treatment options—development of consensus guidelines. J Eur Acad Dermatol Venereol. 2005;19(Suppl 1):25–33.
37. Jublia (efinaconazole topical solution, 10%) [package insert]. Bridgewater, NJ: Valeant Pharmaceuticals LLC; 2014.
38. Zeichner JA, Stein Gold L, Korotzer A. Penetration of (14C)-Efinaconazole solution does not appear to be influenced by nail polish. J Clin Aesthet Dermatol. 2014;7(9):45–8.
39. Vlahovic T, Merchant T, Chanda S, et al. In vitro nail penetration of tavaborole topical solution, 5% through nail polish on ex vivo human fingernails. J Drugs Dermatol. 2015;14(7):675–8.
40. Del Rosso JQ. Advances in the treatment of superficial fungal infections: focus on onychomycosis and dry tinea pedis. J Am Osteopath Assoc. 1997;97:339–46.
41. Sigurgeirsson B, Billstein S, Rantanen T, et al. L.I.ON. Study: efficacy and tolerability of continuous terbinafine compared to intermittent itraconazole in the treatment of toenail onychomycosis. Br J Dermatol. 1999;141(Supp 56):5–14.
42. Baran R, Tosti A, Hartmane I, et al. An innovative water-soluble biopolymer improves efficacy of ciclopirox nail lacquer in the management of onychomycosis. J Eur Acad Dermatol Venereol. 2009;23:773–81.
43. Baran R, Sigurgeirsson B, de Berker D, et al. A multicenter, randomized, controlled study of the efficacy, safety and cost-effectiveness of a combination therapy with amorolfine nail lacquer and oral terbinafine compared with oral terbinafine alone for the treatment of onychomycosis. Br J Dermatol. 2007;157:149–57.
44. Hay RJ. The future of onychomycosis therapy may involve a combination of approaches. Br J Dermatol. 2001;145:3–8.
45. Rosen T. Evaluation of gender as a clinically relevant outcome variable in the treatment of onychomycosis with efinaconazole topical solution 10%. Cutis. 2015;96(3):197–201.
46. Rodriguez DA. Efinaconazole topical solution, 10% for the treatment of mild and moderate toenail onychomycosis. J Clin Aesthet Dermatol. 2015;8(6):24–9.
47. Markinson B, Caldwell B. Efinaconazole topical solution, 10%: efficacy in onychomycosis patients with co-existing tinea pedis. J Am Podiatr Med Assoc. 2015;105(5):407–11.
48. Rich P. Efinaconazole topical solution, 10%: the benefits of treating onychomycosis early. J Drugs Dermatol. 2015;14(1):58–62.
49. Gupta AK, et al. Cumulative meta-analysis of systemic antifungal agents for the treatment of onychomycosis. Br J Dermatol. 2004;150(3):537–44.

50. Alley MR, Baker SJ, Beutner KR, Plattner J. Recent progress on the topical therapy of onychomycosis. Expert Opin Investig Drugs. 2007;16(2):157–67.
51. Sporanox oral solution [package insert]. Raritan: Ortho Biotech Products, L.P; 2009.
52. Lamisil [package insert]. East Hanover: Novartis Pharmaceuticals Corporation; 2013.
53. Potter LP, Mathias SD, Raut M, et al. The impact of aggressive debridement used as an adjunct therapy with terbinafine on perceptions of patients undergoing treatment for toenail onychomycosis. J Dermatolog Treat. 2007;18:46–52.
54. Malay DS, Yi S, Borowsky P, et al. Efficacy of debridement alone versus debridement combined with topical antifungal nail lacquer for the treatment of pedal onychomycosis: a randomized, controlled trial. J Foot Ankle Surg. 2009;48:294–308.
55. Jennings MB, Pollak R, Harkless LB, et al. Treatment of toenail onychomycosis with oral terbinafine plus aggressive debridement: IRON-CLAD, a large, randomized, open-label, multicenter trial. J Am Podiatr Med Assoc. 2006;96:465–73.
56. Markinson BC, Vlahovic TC, Joseph WS, et al. Diagnosis and management of onychomycosis: perspectives from a joint podiatry-dermatology roundtable. J Am Podiatr Med Assoc. 2015.
57. Gupta AK, Paquet M, Simpson FC. Therapies for the treatment of onychomycosis. Clin Dermatol. 2013;31(5):544–54.
58. Grover C, Bansal S, Nanda S, et al. Combination of surgical avulsion and topical therapy for single nail onychomycosis: a randomized controlled trial. Br J Dermatol. 2007;157(2):364–8.
59. Pandhi D, Verma P. Nail avulsion: indications and methods (surgical nail avulsion). Indian J Dermatol Venereol Leprol. 2012;78:299–308.
60. Ortiz AE, Avram MM, Wanner MA. A review of lasers and light for the treatment of onychomycosis. Lasers Surg Med. 2014;46:117–24.
61. Bristow IR. The effectiveness of lasers in the treatment of onychomycosis: a systematic review. J Foot Ankle Res. 2014;7:34.
62. Evans E. The rationale for combination therapy. Br J Dermatol. 2001;145:9–13.
63. Olafsson JH, Sigurgeirsson B, Baran R. Combination therapy for onychomycosis. Br J Dermatol. 2003;149(Suppl 65):15–8.
64. Avner S, Nir N, Henri T. Combination of oral terbinafine and topical ciclopirox compared to oral terbinafine for the treatment of onychomycosis. J Dermatolog Treat. 2005;16:327–30.
65. Rigopoulos D, Katoulis AC, Ioannides D. A randomized trial of amorolfine 5% solution nail lacquer in association with itraconazole pulse therapy compared with itraconazole alone in the treatment of Candida fingernail onychomycosis. Br J Dermatol. 2003;149:151–6.
66. Xu Y, Miao X, Zhou B, et al. Combined oral terbinafine and long-pulsed 1,064-nm Nd: YAG laser treatment is more effective for onychomycosis than either treatment alone. Dermatol Surg. 2014;40(11):1201–7.

# Chapter 3
# Hammertoe Fixation: Traditional Percutaneous Pin Versus Internal Fixation

**Rachel H. Albright and Adam E. Fleischer**

Hammertoe surgery is one of the most common elective forefoot surgeries performed, yet many foot and ankle surgeons express frustration with long-term outcomes. Despite advancements in surgical technique and improved understanding of the deformity, rates of recurrence are higher than expected and have remained largely unchanged over the years. In addition, excessive postoperative digital edema can sometimes occur and lead to unsatisfactory patient outcomes and difficulty with shoe wear [1, 2]. Other reasons for unsatisfactory results include a less than desired aesthetic appearance of the toe (e.g., unsightly scarring, or over-shortening of toe) and painful pseudoarthrosis or malunion. As such, foot and ankle surgeons now have a multitude of fixation options at their disposal to assist with digital surgery. Most advancements in fixation aim to target one or more of the common complications encountered in digital arthrodesis surgery and offer patented devices/implant systems to help eradicate the problem. This chapter focuses on the various fixation techniques currently available and the evidence behind them.

R. H. Albright
Department of Surgery, Stamford Health, Foot & Ankle, Darien, CT, USA
e-mail: ralbright@stamhealth.org

A. E. Fleischer (✉)
Department of Podiatric Medicine & Radiology, Dr. William M. Scholl College of Podiatric Medicine at Rosalind Franklin University of Medicine & Science, North Chicago, IL, USA
e-mail: adam.fleischer@rosalindfranklin.edu



D. E. Tower (ed.), *Evidence-Based Podiatry*,
https://doi.org/10.1007/978-3-030-50853-1_3

## Hammertoe Correction

### History

As one of the traditional and still most popular fixation techniques, K-wire fixation of the proximal interphalangeal (PIP) joint has been used for both arthroplasty and arthrodesis. K-wire fixation has been described since the 1940s in case series. In the 1980s, more sophisticated designs began to appear in the literature. Taylor, in 1940 [3], published a case series of 12 patients undergoing K-wire fixation for arthrodesis of the PIP joint with "excellent" results. In 1957, Hembree [4] described an arthroplasty of the fifth PIP joint as well as tenotomy and capsulotomy of the metatarsophalangeal joint for painful bilateral heloma molle utilizing an incision over the metatarsal-phalangeal (MTP) joint that extends distally. Proper alignment of the toe could not be obtained with arthroplasty alone; therefore a 0.045 intramedullary pin was used to fixate the toe. The pin was left intact for 8 days. At that time, the patient returned to work with a shoe modification and was discharged from care on postoperative day 25. Hembree's colleagues at the time noted pin fixation is rarely needed for fifth toe deformities [4]. Moving forward, the late 1980s through the 1990s showed an increase in publications and quality regarding surgical correction for hammertoes. In 1987, Coughlin's textbook chapter [1] described fixation of the PIP joint in the flexible hammertoe and provided insight into deformities involving subluxation at the MTP joint, which, up to this point, was described only briefly. He described several clinical situations including severity of deformity, with treatment recommendations for each. For example, for MTP joint subluxation, he found retrograding a K-wire into the metatarsal head provided stability after a tenotomy and capsulotomy was performed. Removal of the pin occurred 3 weeks after surgery, and taping the toe to allow ground contact with ambulation was recommended for 6 weeks. For more severe MTP joint subluxation, a partial metatarsal head resection was recommended. In addition, he discussed transverse plane deviation of the toe and MTP joint where he found success with soft tissue releases of deforming structures. For the most severe transverse plane issues, he mentions a flexor to extensor tendon transfer with K-wire fixation. Coughlin's text has been largely accepted, and still today, many are using these recommendations for deformities falling along all levels of severity. Much of the literature in the early 1990s consisted of outcomes research describing cohorts of patients undergoing similar procedures described by Coughlin [1, 2], along with variants of the procedures to improve common intraoperative challenges.

In 1995 Lehman and Smith [5] examined a retrospective case series of 76 consecutive patients (100 feet) undergoing PIP joint arthrodesis with 1-year follow-up. A peg and socket technique was used to facilitate K-wire fixation. Using patient surveys, the authors were able to identify areas of patient dissatisfaction. Forty-four percent of patients reported they were satisfied without reservation, while the remaining cohort were either dissatisfied or were satisfied with reservations. Patients who were over the age of 65 were less likely to report a satisfactory outcome. Curiously, evidence of postoperative malalignment on physical exam was not a clear source of dissatisfaction. For example, elevation of the tip of the toe was noted in 14 feet, however, only 4 of these patients were dissatisfied, and none of the dissatisfied patients expressed concern of the elevation on the questionnaire. Transverse plane malalignment was noted at the fusion site in 11 feet, with only one of these patients being dissatisfied on questionnaire. Flexion at the distal interphalangeal (DIP) joint (44%) and angulation at the PIP joint (14.4%) were common postoperative findings, but did not seem to contribute to patient perception of success (7/33 patients with flexion deformity were dissatisfied). This article offered one of the first instances suggesting patient's perception of success may differ from the surgeon's perception of success (that is, where the surgeon's perception of success is typically based upon postoperative alignment and pain levels).

In 2000, Coughlin and colleagues [2] conducted a case series of 61 patients undergoing hammertoe correction via arthroplasty with K-wire fixation with additional procedures as needed for other deformities present. He described a transverse plane incision over the PIP joint to reduce the scar appearance, and used a percutaneous K-wire technique for fixation. His results were overall positive with 84% of patients rating the surgery satisfactory; however, a 10% complication rate enlightened surgeons to a range of complications and patient dissatisfaction that could occur. Complications ranged from calluses to malrotation of the toe, hyperextension at the DIP joint, inability to wear over-the-counter shoe gear, transverse plane malalignment, need for second surgery, toe amputation, mallet toe, and recurrence. As surgeons began to further investigate possible causes of patient dissatisfaction, more fixation techniques became available to offer eradication of the issues.

## *Technique, K-Wire*

The technique for arthroplasty and arthrodesis of the PIP joint has remained largely consistent. The patient is positioned supine with monitored anesthesia care (MAC) being the anesthetic of choice. General anesthesia may be indicated for a patient requiring intervention with a bilateral combination procedure or additional forefoot surgery. Typically a local anesthesia block is administered and ankle tourniquet is utilized. Two incision types are commonly used: a longitudinal incision overlying the PIP joint extending approximately 0.5 cm proximal and distal from the joint line and two semi-elliptical incisions oriented transversely over the PIP joint. The transverse approach is believed to offer more aesthetic scarring while still allowing the surgeon adequate visualization (see Fig. 3.1). There is no evidence currently to suggest one incision type has significant correlation with patient-reported outcome measures (PROMs) postoperatively. The longitudinal incision is considered the traditional approach and allows for proximal extension to incorporate additional soft tissue procedures as necessary, while the transverse type would require additional incisions to accommodate proximal work. The incision is deepened sharply until the extensor tendon is identified. The tendon is transversely cut and carefully freed proximally and distally from surrounding tissues to allow re-approximation at the end of the procedure. Full exposure of the head of the proximal phalanx is achieved with release of both medial and lateral collateral ligaments. An oscillating sagittal saw is typically used to remove the head of the proximal phalanx at the surgical neck. This can also be achieved using a bone rongeur. A bone burr can be used to smooth roughened edges. If an arthrodesis is being performed, the

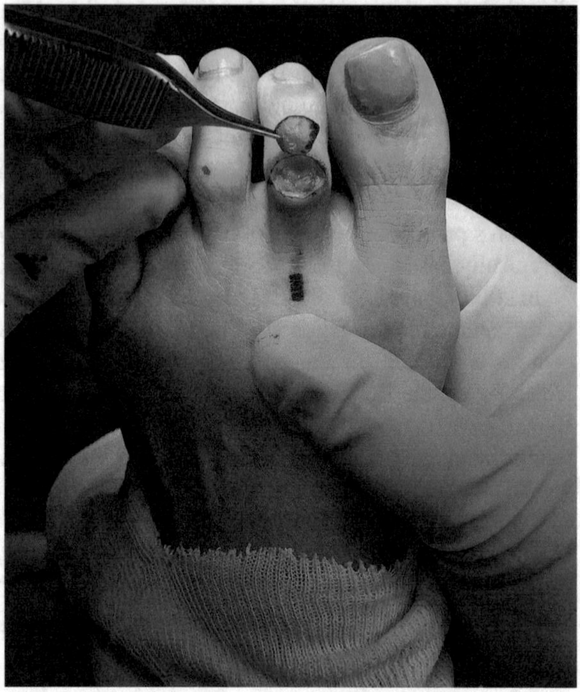

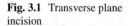

**Fig. 3.1** Transverse plane incision

base of the middle phalanx can be resected with an oscillating saw, a bone rongeur, or the articular surface can be denuded with a bone burr. Some surgeons choose to facilitate arthrodesis with a "chevron" or "peg-in-hole" type method of joint preparation. For the chevron technique, a small bone rongeur is typically utilized to denude both the head of the proximal phalanx and the base of the middle phalanx. The proximal phalanx will display a chevron-shape with dorsal and plantar surfaces resected to produce an apex distally (see Fig. 3.2). The middle phalanx medullary bone will then be evacuated to produce a complementary shape for proper fit of the proximal phalanx head (see Fig. 3.3). For arthroplasty, the middle phalanx is left intact and the head of the proximal phalanx is resected. A 0.045 K-wire is driven through the middle and distal phalanges, exiting the distal aspect of the digit and continued until the wire is not impeding reduction of the PIP joint. Using the index finger and thumb of the surgeon's non-dominant hand, the toe should be held in rectus position relative to the other toes. Using the dominant hand, the K-wire may be retrograded back through the proximal phalanx. Driving the K-wire across the MTP joint is based on surgeon preference, and was described by Coughlin previously to increase joint stability [1]. For arthroplasty, it is not necessary for the proximal and middle phalanges to be in close proximity, and the "chevron" technique is not indicated. For arthrodesis on the other hand, maximal contact between osseous structures is preferred to obtain either an osseous or fibrous union (see section "Current Concepts" for more information on "Fibrous Union Versus Osseous Union"). The surgeon should be careful to fixate the toe in a rectus position in both the transverse and sagittal planes with no signs of deviation in relation to the non-operative toes. This can be checked with forefoot loading and visualizing the toe from both dorsoplantar and lateral views. Intraoperative fluoroscopy can be used to ensure proper positioning of the K-wire, which is sometimes difficult to decipher from clinical exam alone. It may be

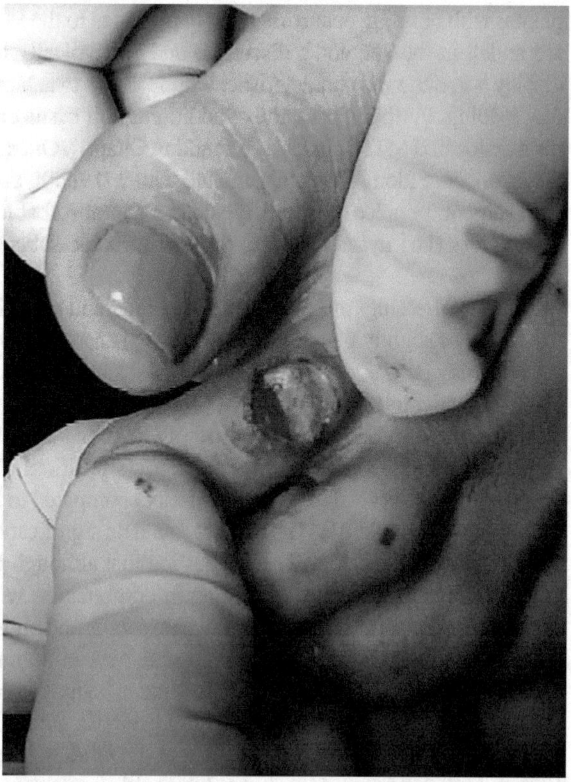

**Fig. 3.2** Preparation of the proximal phalanx using Chevron technique. A distal apex can be noted here, with the superior and inferior portions of the joint removed with a bone rongeur

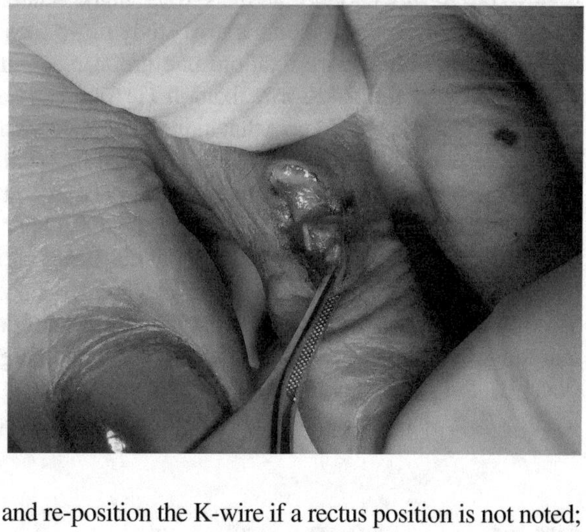

**Fig. 3.3** Close approximation of the osseous surfaces can be achieved with the Chevron-type technique, depicted here

necessary to re-align the toe and re-position the K-wire if a rectus position is not noted; however, the surgeon should be aware that frequent repositioning of the K-wire may predispose the toe to vascular compromise. Excessive re-drilling of the wire should be avoided. Two K-wires may be used in a crossing fashion. Both wires should be drilled through the middle and distal phalanges first before attempting to reduce the joint. The first wire may be oriented lateral proximal dorsal to medial distal plantar and the second K-wire oriented in complementary fashion medial proximal dorsal to lateral distal plantar with crossing occurring slightly proximal to the PIP joint. Soft tissue procedures are added at the surgeon's discretion and are typically implemented when the toe(s) display a trackbound characteristic, with inability to achieve a rectus position with forefoot loading. Further discussion of additional soft tissue procedures that may be utilized for a dislocated MTP joint can be found in Chap. 4. Once adequate fixation is achieved, the extensor tendon is re-approximated with 3-0 vicryl, and the skin is re-approximated with surgeon's choice of suture, typically a non-absorbable suture for simple or horizontal mattress (i.e., nylon, prolene) or an absorbable subcuticular suture (i.e., monocryl, vicryl).

Surgical dressings are considered important and typically involve splinting the toe(s) in a rectus or slightly plantarflexed position to ensure toe purchase upon weight bearing. Patients may be weight bearing in a surgical shoe. Holinka et al. [6] conducted a study evaluating two intervention groups, one receiving PIP joint arthroplasty with K-wire fixation and one with arthroplasty without fixation but with a careful postoperative bandage which strapped the toe in a plantigrade position. The authors found the K-wire group had 93% survival (e.g., no recurrence) compared to the strapping group with 88% survival ($p$-value <0.001). The authors found no significant differences in AOFAS scores or VAS scores between groups, suggesting that although K-wire has superior results in relation to recurrence rates, strapping in combination with arthroplasty does seem to play a role in relation to postoperative pain scores and physical function. This article has helped solidify the notion that strapping can have important implications post-hammertoe surgery, and the confidence that fixation is better than no fixation.

The length of time a K-wire should remain intact has varied in the literature, based mostly on surgeon's preference and confidence in stability. The typical time a K-wire remains intact is 4–6 weeks – with a percentage of surgeons choosing to remove the K-wire earlier than the 4-week mark. Klammer, in 2012 [7], performed a two-group, prospective comparative study of 46 toes undergoing arthroplasty of the PIP joint with K-wire fixation: one group receiving 3-week duration and the other 6-week duration of K-wire fixation. He found no statistical differences between groups on PROMs but did note that higher complication rates occurred in the 3-week duration group. Despite fear of K-wire-related infections with a longer duration of intact hardware, the authors found no difference in complications between groups. The authors concluded 6 weeks was preferred. Other studies have noted higher infection rates up to 18% when hardware has been left intact for 6 weeks [8] compared to rates ranging from 0% to 4.7% when left intact for 4 weeks [2, 7, 9–11]. This debate continues, but our current highest level of data does not support notions that longer duration of intact hardware contribute to higher pin tract infection rates (level II). Surgeons may therefore use other criteria to determine duration of K-wire fixation (i.e., stability or severity of deformity, patient compliance).

## *Effectiveness of K-Wires* (Table 3.1)

There have been several studies examining the effectiveness of K-wires from a case series and retrospective cohort perspective.

**Table 3.1** Effectiveness of K-wires for hammertoe correction

| Author (year) | Study design/ description | Sample size | Summary | Level of evidence |
|---|---|---|---|---|
| Baig et al. (1996) [12] | Retrospective case series of arthrodesis with K-wire fixation | 19 (42 toes) | 31% developed DIP joint deformity which was a cause of dissatisfaction. Overall patient satisfaction ranged from 78% to 88% | IV |
| Coughlin et al. (2000) [2] | Retrospective case series of arthroplasty with K-wire fixation | 63 (118 toes) | Chief complaint was relieved in 78% of patients. Reported a 10% complication rate. Overall, K-wire fixation is reliable | IV |
| Kramer et al. (2015) [10] | Retrospective cohort of arthroplasty with K-wire fixation | 876 (1,115 procedures) | Overall K-wire is reliable with low complication rates (94 pin migrations (3.5%), 9 pin tract infections (0.3%), and 2 pin breakages (0.1%). 150 recurrent deformities (5.6%) and 94 toes (3.5%) required revision hammertoe surgery. Malalignment in 55 toes (2.1%). Vascular compromise occurred in 16 toes (0.6%), with 10 (0.4%) requiring amputation. 94 toes (3.5%) required revision surgery because of symptomatic recurrence of deformity | III |
| Holinka et al. (2013) [6] | Retrospective cohort of arthroplasty with K-wire versus no fixation with strapping | 54 (62 procedures) | Significantly lower recurrence of deformity in K-wire group | III |
| Klammer et al. (2012) [7] | Prospective cohort of arthroplasty with K-wire fixation with wire remaining for 3 weeks or 6 weeks | 52 toes | The 6-week K-wire group showed a lower rate of recurrence with no increase in infection compared to the 3-week group | II |
| Lehman et al. (1995) [5] | Retrospective case series of arthrodesis with K-wire | 76 (100 toes) | Reported a patient satisfaction rate of 85%. DIP joint contracture developed in 44% | IV |
| Mueller et al. (2018) [13] | Retrospective cohort of arthroplasty with two K-wires (stratified by age) | 58 patients | Outcomes within both age groups were similar with comparable satisfaction and complication rates | III |

(continued)

**Table 3.1** (continued)

| Author (year) | Study design/ description | Sample size | Summary | Level of evidence |
|---|---|---|---|---|
| Zingas et al. (1995) [14] | Retrospective cohort of any lesser toe procedure using K-wire | 824 patients | K-wires of smaller size (0.045 compared to 0.062) were more likely to break. Spanning the wire across the MTP joint increases risk of breakage | III |
| Schrier et al. (2016) [15] | Randomized controlled trial of arthrodesis versus arthroplasty with K-wire | 26 (39 toes) in arthroplasty group; 29 (50 toes) in arthrodesis group | No significant differences between groups for rigid PIP joint deformity. Both groups with good results | II |
| Boffeli et al. (2016) [16] | Retrospective case series of arthrodesis with two K-wires | 60 (91 procedures) | Complication rate was 3.33%. One patient underwent revision. No postoperative infections were noted | IV |
| Creighton et al. (1995) [17] | Case series of arthrodesis with buried K-wire | 30 (46 procedures) | K-wire provides rigid digital fixation without high rates of infection; however K-wire extrusion occurred in 33% | IV |

In one of the largest cohort studies to-date on any fixation technique, Kramer et al. in 2015 [10] reinvigorated the interest in K-wires when he was able to "debunk" many of the concerns K-wires carried, such as pin tract infections, migration, and breakage. He found a 0.3% pin tract infection rate in one of the largest cohorts to-date (2,698 toes) and a 0.1% wire failure rate – a stark difference in rates reported among small cohorts and case series which described rates of pin tract infection up to 18%. He was able to identify predictors of hammertoe recurrence (i.e., transverse plane deformity, previous toe surgery, hardware complications) and concluded that infection due to K-wires themselves is rare, and is not a justified reason to abstain from utilization. The authors note that, overall, K-wires are an effective technique.

Coughlin identified issues with new hammertoe formation in adjacent toes, along with new interdigital corns and distal flexion deformities following hammertoe correction with K-wire fixation [2]. Rotational deformities were also noted. These imperfections lead to 15% (19/118) of the study population reporting "dissatisfied," or "satisfied with reservations." Despite these complications, Coughlin agreed that K-wires provided good results with low incidence of severe complications.

Other studies with much smaller sample sizes have also provided insight into specific postoperative complications after K-wire fixation. Baig et al. [12] reviewed 42 toes undergoing arthrodesis with K-wire fixation and noted 31% developed a DIP joint deformity postoperatively. Despite a third of the population experiencing this complication, most reported satisfaction with their results (satisfaction rate of 78–88%). Lehman et al. [5] also reported a high rate of DIP joint deformity (44%) in his sample of 100 toes undergoing arthrodesis with K-wire fixation. Lehman's satisfaction rate was 85% overall. Zingas et al. [14] performed a large review of all hammertoe surgeries in their institution ($n$ = 824) who had either a 0.045 or a 0.062 K-wire to examine failure rates of K-wires (e.g., K-wire breakage). The second toe had the greatest incidence of K-wire breakage (5.6%) with a total breakage rate of 3.3% in the entire population.

The highest level of evidence on K-wire fixation is level II (prospective cohort or lesser quality RCT).

## *K-Wire Variants*

Buried K-wires (i.e., the absence of protrusion of the wire from the distal aspect of the toe) have been discussed in the literature as a permanent implant for hammertoe fixation. This fixation technique mimics that of intramedullary implants, where the wire is retained indefinitely and arthrodesis of the joint is the only option. Creighton et al. [17] published their case series of 46 arthrodesis procedures with buried K-wire. The authors noted rigid fixation but experienced wire extrusion in 33% of patients. Scholl et al. [18] reported on a retrospective comparative study between patients undergoing fixation with implant (shape memory, $n$ = 58) versus buried K-wires ($n$ = 28). No statistically significant differences were noted between groups regarding revision rates or complications. Literature showing superiority of this technique over others is currently lacking.

# Commercial Intramedullary Implants

Since 2000, another surge in publications emerged on hammertoe surgery, due in part to commercial implants entering the market. Although implants are an attractive alternative to K-wires, they do not lend themselves to arthroplasty of the PIP joint. Commercial implants, therefore, by nature, have less flexibility than K-wires in determining procedure type. Patients who are candidates for arthrodesis (e.g., traditionally toes with a non-reducible, rigid deformity) are appropriate for implant use. However, if an arthroplasty is the preferred procedure (e.g., traditionally reducible, flexible deformities), implants are typically inappropriate for achieving this goal. Within this text, when implants are described, it is assumed that arthrodesis has been performed.

## *Technique, Commercial Implant*

It is first important to recognize differences among current commercial implants on the market. There are currently over 20 implantable devices available in the USA and European Union, less than 50% of which have received recognition in the literature. Guelfi et al. [19] performed one of the only literature reviews in 2015, depicting different types of commercial implants on the market. Since then, more implant choices have emerged but can still fall into the four categories described by the authors: (1) one-piece solid or cannulated, (2) shape memory, (3) bone allograft, and (4) two-piece.

Patient positioning and preparation is similar in technique to K-wire fixation, where the patient is placed supine and local anesthesia is preferred unless additional forefoot reconstruction or bilateral procedures are required. Dissection technique is identical to the above technique for K-wires; however, arthrodesis is exclusively performed with the use of commercial implants. The surgeon, in theory, should prepare both the proximal phalanx and middle phalanx joint surfaces, which is typically undertaken with an oscillating sagittal saw, or a bone rongeur. However, each implant type does recommend slightly different joint preparation techniques, which will be generically explained here but, however, should be explored preoperatively using the respective companies' technique guide. Further details into the four types of currently available commercial implants and their techniques are outlined below.

The surgical techniques for each implant type described below are in reference to a generic version of each type and are not inclusive of all steps, instrumentations, or variants of the technique. Surgeons should consult the technique guides provided by implant manufacturers to familiarize themselves with the nuances and instruments needed for the specific implant type.

## *One-Piece Implants*

The one-piece implant may resemble that of a headless screw with threads on each end to facilitate compression, where the implant is utilized as a traditional headless screw. In other systems, the distal piece, although resembling a threaded piece, is not utilized for dual compression in the same manner as a traditional headless screw (i.e., where the distal threads are not engaged using a driver). One-piece implants may recommend typical resection of both the head of the proximal phalanx and base of the middle phalanx or recommend minimal resection of the head of the proximal phalanx, and no middle phalanx preparation, dependent upon company recommendations. Implants recommending no middle phalanx resection typically incorporate fenestration of the middle phalanx and use of a broach, or may allow for cartilage preparation later in the procedure. Some one-piece implants are packaged with a set of single-use sterile instruments needed to insert the implant, eliminating the need for sterile processing. For companies offering a larger range of implant options, there is often color-coded instrumentation to avoid confusion. The sterile set will vary depending on the implant used, but a typical set may contain planars and impactors, solid drills, drill handles, forceps, cannulated drills, separate handles according to size and angulation of implant, and sizing guides. These implants are available in multiple sizes, both in length and width to accommodate bone quality and size. Some one-piece implants will additionally offer a degree of angulation ranging from 0 degrees (completely horizontal) to 10 degrees plantarflexed.

Angulation is chosen based on the degree of elevation noted within the clinical deformity upon forefoot loading. Some surgeons will choose to fuse the elevated toe at 0 degrees and correct the elevation with soft tissue procedures, whereas others prefer to fuse the toe in a corrected position. In general, for cannulated systems, dissection is undertaken as above (see section "Technique, K-Wire"), and the head of the proximal phalanx is resected, minimally, with a sagittal saw. A guide wire is placed within the middle phalanx first, in the same manner as if utilizing K-wire fixation technique, where the wire exits the distal aspect of the toe, and ideally extends down the longitudinal shaft of both the middle and distal phalanges. If planars are available within the set, these are used to prepare the middle phalanx joint surface using the guide wire. A pilot hole using the guide wire within the middle phalanx is created in the proximal phalanx. This is the first opportunity for the surgeon to ensure the PIP joint is properly reduced. The middle and proximal phalanges are then pre-drilled using instrumentation provided within the sterile set. The implant is then inserted into the middle phalanx and press-fitted into the proximal phalanx using the pre-drilled hole. The ability to use cannulated instrumentation to further compress the joint will vary by company, but is typically available. At this point, the surgeon may be given the option to advance the guide wire across the MTP joint for proximal stability, in which case the guide wire will remain in place for up to 6 weeks postoperatively, and removed in the outpatient setting. The implant remains in place, without the need for removal unless a complication is encountered. In a solid (non-cannulated) system, the surgeon will "free-hand" the pre-drilled holes within the proximal and middle phalanges using a guide wire, aiming for the central canal. Planars are not typically used for the middle phalanx preparation, and fenestration with the same K-wire as well as hammering of a broach is instead undertaken in the middle phalanx, or the middle phalanx will be resected initially using a sagittal saw in the same manner as arthrodesis with K-wire fixation. The implant is then inserted into the proximal phalanx first, and the middle phalanx is press-fitted onto the distal portion of the implant. A common technique variation with one-piece solid implants is noted with the pre-drilling portion, where the proximal phalanx is pre-drilled and the middle *and* distal phalanges are drilled, with the driver exiting the distal aspect of the toe. The handle is removed, but the driver is left within the joint to engage the screw (e.g., for one-piece implants which incorporate traditional headless screw technique) and facilitate compression. The implant is screwed into the proximal phalanx with the distal threaded portion left unengaged. The handle is then placed on the distal end of the driver that exits the toe, and with the middle and distal phalanges held firmly in place with one hand, the surgeon will use the driver to engage the head of the screw within the joint, into the middle phalanx. The driver is used to pull the distal threads into engagement with the middle phalanx (typically in a counter-clockwise fashion; however, this should be confirmed using the company's technique guide). Once the middle phalanx is engaged by the distal threads, the driver is used to compress the middle and proximal phalanges (typically in a clockwise fashion). This is facilitated by the dual-threaded design which, once properly engaged within each end of the joint, will compress the joint surface. As one can imagine, the distal aspect of the toe must be held firmly during this technique, to prevent distal rotational deformity. The driver is then removed. We have outlined a generic surgical technique for one-piece implants for both cannulated and solid types. It is important for the surgeon to understand the companies' individual recommendations, as further variations within the surgical technique may be present.

## *Effectiveness of One-Piece Implants* (Table 3.2)

Basile and colleagues [21] reported on patients who underwent fixation with one-piece implants ($n$ = 117 toes). Overall, the authors noted improvements in VAS and AOFAS scores compared to preoperative scores, providing some

**Table 3.2** Effectiveness of various commercial implant types for hammertoe correction

| Author (year) | Study design/ description | Sample size | Summary | Level of evidence |
|---|---|---|---|---|
| Kominsky et al. (2013) [20] | Case series of bone allograft implant (arthrodesis) | 32 | All patients reported satisfaction with results; no complications noted | IV |
| Basile et al. (2015) [21] | Prospective cohort of one-piece implant arthrodesis (no comparison group) | 57 (117 toes) | Improvements were noted in VAS and AOFAS scores | IV |
| Averous et al. (2015) [22] | Case series of one-piece implant (radiolucent) | 142 (180 procedures) | No complications reported; patient satisfaction rate of 94%. No recurrence at 1 year | IV |
| Guelfi et al. (2015) [19] | Systematic review of all implant options (qualitative analysis only) | 9 articles included | Implants seem to have good results with no significant differences between implant groups | IV |
| Khan et al. (2015) [23] | Prospective cohort of shape memory implant for arthrodesis of PIP joint (no comparison group) | 82 patients | Foot and ankle disability index at 6 months postoperatively showed trends toward satisfaction (no statistical analysis) | IV |
| Catena et al. (2014) [24] | Case series of shape memory implant | 29 patients (53 toes) | AOFAS scores and VAS pain scores improved at final follow-up | IV |
| Witt et al. (2012) [25] | Case series of one-piece implant | 7 toes | No postoperative complications at 1 year with radiographic alignment maintained | IV |
| Sandhu et al. (2013) [26] | Case series of shape memory implant | 65 implants; 35 patients | Complication rates of 6.1% with no revisions needed | IV |
| Harmer et al. (2017) [27] | Case series of one-piece implant | 38 patients | 94.7% felt their condition was better or much better. Two patients felt worse. At 3 years postoperative, 92.8% felt their condition was better | IV |

evidence of effectiveness of the one-piece technique. Richman et al. [28] published a retrospective cohort of one-piece implant ($n = 54$) versus K-wire ($n = 95$) for arthrodesis of the PIP joint. The implant group seemed to perform better overall with fewer complications ($p = 0.027$) and only one episode of recurrence ($p = 0.095$). Obrador et al. [29] performed an observational intervention study ($n = 96$) looking at three fixation techniques: one-piece implants, shape memory implants, and K-wire fixation for arthrodesis of the PIP joint. Results were similar for all three groups with trends toward better patient satisfaction in both implant groups, although statistical significance was not achieved. Averous et al. [22] published a case series of patients undergoing fixation with one-piece implants ($n = 180$ procedures) and noted a patient satisfaction rate of 94%. No complications were noted within the series, and no recurrence of deformity was noted at 1-year follow-up. The highest level of evidence on one-piece implants is level III (retrospective cohort).

## *Shape Memory*

The shape memory implants are one-piece memometal nitinol implants that typically have a claw-like appearance on both ends to facilitate compression and quality bone contact, while controlling rotation. Shape memory implants conform to the shape of the medullary canal and are activated into compression by body temperature. These implants are typically stored cooled at approximately 0 degrees Celsius for a minimum of 2 hours preoperatively. Once in contact with body temperature, the implant expands to conform to the anatomy. This takes approximately 2–3 minutes once implanted. Care should be taken to not have the implant opened on the back table before it is needed, as exposure to room air will also encourage the implant to expand, although this will happen at a slower rate than if exposed to body temperature. Once activated, these implants may be difficult to remove or alter. If using a shape memory implant, the surgeon should be aware there is a limited time period available for the device to be implanted before it can no longer be altered. Shape memory implants come in a variety of sizes as well as a 10-degree plantarflexed position similar to one-piece implants. Instrumentation is not typically one-time use, requiring hospital sterilization preoperatively. The traditional set will include a sizing guide and color code, implant holding forceps, positioning rod, proximal and distal drill bits, surfacing reamer, and broaches of varying sizes. A standard longitudinal or transverse incision is made, and dissection is carried out as described in previous paragraphs. Resection of the head of the proximal phalanx should be limited to 2–3 mm. The proximal phalanx is then pre-drilled, aiming for the central canal to a depth specified by manufacturer's guidelines (typically corresponding to laser lines on the drill bit). The middle phalanx is pre-drilled using a different drill bit in a similar manner. The cartilage on the base of the middle phalanx is then denuded using the provided surfacing reamer in the instrumentation set, or using a bone rongeur at the surgeon's discretion. A separate T-handle broach is used for the proximal and middle phalanges to prepare the surfaces for implantation. These broaches are typically color coordinated and labeled to correspond with the size of the implant chosen before the start of the procedure, based on clinical and radiographic examination. It is very important not to turn or toggle the broach within the canal. At this time, the surgeon has an opportunity to ensure the toe will be reduced in the proper position, by lining up the joint and clinically inspecting the toe in relation to the adjacent digits. The foot should be loaded at this time to simulate weight bearing position. The implant can then be removed from cold storage and will have been packaged in accordance with its proper insertion. Using the provided forceps in the instrumentation set, the implant is removed, and the "longer" end, or that with a more oblong shape, is inserted into the proximal phalanx. The forceps are left in place and not removed from the implant. If the implant is difficult to insert, a mallet may be used to gently coax the implant into the predrilled hole. For bone that feels soft, a positioning rod can be used to prevent the proximal end of the implant from slipping deeper into the proximal phalanx while the middle phalanx is being manually compressed. The rod is placed into the provided space on the implant, keeping the forceps in place. The middle phalanx is then manually compressed onto the implant and proximal phalanx. The forceps should remain engaged until the middle phalanx is at least partially reduced onto the implant. The forceps can then be removed, and the middle phalanx can be compressed further onto the implant. The rod may then be removed and the compression completed. It is recommended to hold the rectus position for approximately 1 minute to ensure the implant has adequate time for expansion into the canal. To speed up the process, warm saline can be used in the operative site. Many shape memory implants boast dynamic compression, however, most product guides do not endorse immediate weight bearing despite this benefit. A surgical shoe is recommended postoperatively for protected weight bearing.

## *Effectiveness of Shape Memory Implants* (Tables 3.2 and 3.3)

Rothermel et al. [30] conducted a comparative cadaveric study of arthrodesis with K-wire versus shape memory implants to evaluate strength of fixation type when placed under mechanical stress ($n = 6$ per group). The authors found that K-wires provided a stronger construct compared to shape memory implants. Angirasa et al. [31] conducted a comparative study of arthrodesis using K-wires ($n = 15$) versus shape memory implants ($n = 13$). The authors concluded that the implant group had higher patient satisfaction, although no statistical analysis was performed to truly evaluate important differences. The highest level of evidence on using shape memory implants is level III (retrospective cohort).

**Table 3.3** Comparison of K-wire versus various commercial implants for hammertoe correction

| Author (year) | Study design/ description | Sample size | Summary | Level of evidence |
|---|---|---|---|---|
| Rothermel et al. (2018) [30] | Comparison K-wire and shape memory implant; cadaveric study (arthrodesis) | 6 in each group; 12 pairs | K-wires provided stronger constructs compared to shape memory implants | |
| Angirasa et al. (2012) [31] | Comparative cohort of arthrodesis with K-wire versus shape memory implant | 28 (15 with K-wire, 13 with implant) | Implants outperformed K-wires in terms of satisfaction (no statistical analysis performed) | III |
| Richman et al. (2017) [28] | Retrospective cohort of arthrodesis with K-wire versus one-piece implant | 60 (95 toes) with K-wire; 39 (54 toes) with implant | Implant group resulted in fewer complications, only one recurrence and no re-operations compared to K-wire group | III |
| Scholl et al. (2013) [18] | Retrospective cohort of arthrodesis with buried K-wire versus shape memory implant | 86 toes (58 with implant, 28 buried K-wire) | No statistically significant differences between groups regarding complications and revision rates | III |
| Obrador et al. (2018) [29] | Retrospective cohort of arthrodesis with two types of implant (shape memory and one-piece) versus K-wire | 96 | Results were comparable within all three groups with slightly better patient satisfaction in the implant groups (not statistically significant) | III |
| Albright et al. (2018) [38] | Cost-effectiveness analysis of K-wire versus commercial implants (all types) for arthrodesis | 5,612 patients (pooled studies; 4,320 with K-wire; 1,292 with implant) | K-wires were more cost-effective when compared to implants. If implant prices decreased to $300, they would be a more competitive option | II |
| Sung et al. (2014) [39] | Retrospective comparative study of arthrodesis with K-wire, arthroplasty with no fixation or one-piece flexible implant | 114 patients | VAS pain scores improved for all three groups; complication rates were between 35% and 56% | III |

(continued)

**Table 3.3** (continued)

| Author (year) | Study design/ description | Sample size | Summary | Level of evidence |
|---|---|---|---|---|
| Jay et al. (2016) [9] | Randomized controlled trial of K-wire versus two-piece implant | 46 toes allocated to K-wire; 45 toes to implant | The implant group experienced better union rates and better quality of life scores in the early postoperative period (i.e., first 6 months) | II |
| Yassin et al. (2017) [40] | Prospective cohort of open arthrodesis with K-wire versus percutaneous osteotomy of phalanx with Coban dressing | 675 toes (454 open K-wire; 221 percutaneous) | Both procedures led to good results; percutaneous group experienced less infection and recurrence | III (noncontemporaneous cohorts) |

## *Bone Allograft*

Bone allograft implants are one-piece implants to facilitate arthrodesis of the PIP joint with graft incorporation, eliminating the need for metallic hardware. Straight and angulated types are offered in several sizes to meet the requirements of an individual's anatomy. These grafts are typically ridged to prevent rotational forces and pull-out. Some feature a tapered design to facilitate ease of insertion into the proximal phalanx. Variation in graft origin exists between companies. It is therefore the surgeon's responsibility to ensure the ideal graft type is used for the patient. Both sterilized and aseptic grafts are available, which speak to the biologic property potential. Sterilized grafts will typically have fewer biological properties available, functioning like bone matrix and typically machine engineered. Aseptic grafts may advertise some osteoinductivity available to facilitate arthrodesis and may originate from cortical bone. The grafts are stored at room temperature and most do not require reconstitution before implantation.

Surgical technique is similar to that of one-piece metallic implants where manual compression is used for joint reduction once the implant is in place. Single-use instrumentation is offered where preoperative sterilization is not required. Instrumentation will typically include sizing guides, drill bits, reamers, and handling forceps. Once the PIP joint is exposed, minimal resection of the proximal phalanx is performed with a sagittal saw. Middle phalanx cartilage can be removed with a bone rongeur or sagittal saw. If a saw is used, care should be taken to remove only the articular surface. The appropriate depth reamer for the proximal phalanx is selected and oriented toward the central canal at 90 degrees to the resected surface. The same technique should be used for the middle phalanx, using the appropriately sized reamer. The allograft may then be removed from the packaging. Handling forceps are typically provided in the sterile set and used to insert the proximal end of the bone graft (longer end) into the proximal phalanx. Holding the graft at the site of transition (i.e., if using a graft with angulation, the site of transition will be at the vertex), slow and steady pressure is used to insert the graft until a "click" is noted and the forceps touch the proximal phalanx. The forceps are left in place and the middle phalanx is manually compressed until at least partial reduction is achieved over the implant. The forceps may then be removed, and continued compression applied until the joint surfaces are in close proximity. A cannulated approach is also offered by select companies to aid in ensuring proper reduction of the deformity and for the pre-drilling portion of the technique. This option allows the surgeon to visualize the wire placement through the distal end of the toe and also allows the use of fluoroscopy for deformity reduction confirmation. The bone allograft, however, is solid; therefore the K-wire must be removed before implantation of the allograft.

The current literature reports satisfactory results with bone allograft implants with respect to fusion rates and postoperative complications; however, it should be noted that only case series have been published, which feature no control group or statistical analysis of findings (level IV). One may argue that fusion rates are not a clinically important outcome to measure (see sections "Current Concepts" and "Fibrous Union Versus Osseous Union"). There is no current evidence to prove these implanted devices offer superior outcomes to other devices on the market today.

## *Implant Variant: Bioabsorbable Implant*

Bioabsorbable implants follow similar ideals to that of bone allograft implants, relying on incorporation of the implant into the surrounding bone. One such implant is made of 82% poly-L-lactic acid and 18% polyglycolic acid and has been tested in a biomechanical study for feasibility of use [32]. Patton published a case series of patients undergoing PIP joint fixation with a bioabsorbable implant. The authors did not find evidence of foreign body reaction or infection within their series [33]. This implant was composed of similar materials to that of PDS suture. Konkel [34] published a case series using a similar implant type. The authors noted this implant is best indicated in a patient with a stable MTP joint, good skin condition, and an intramedullary canal of at least 2 mm. Other implants of similar material have been utilized in other parts of the body for fixation of osteotomies, including bunionectomies [35, 36]. The highest level of evidence existing for hammertoe fixation with this technique is level IV (case series).

## *Two-Piece Implant*

Two-piece implants feature a dual threaded design with separate proximal phalanx and middle phalanx pieces which lock together at the joint line. These implants typically offer some adjustment in situ and can be found in multiple sizes with 10 degrees of plantarflexion available. Although more complicated to employ in relation to other types, two-piece implants offer the advantage of easier removal postoperatively where the implant can be disassembled at the joint line. Typical instrumentation kits are single-use and contain a driver handle, drill bit, reamers for both the proximal and middle phalanges, and bone holder forceps. Some companies will contain color-coded sets to decipher the proximal and distal portions of the implant. Implants are stored at room temperature.

Once the PIP joint is exposed, the head of the proximal phalanx is resected with a sagittal saw. This is done at the surgical neck, and less care is needed to preserve bone compared to other implant types. The bone holder forceps may be used for stability at this step. If a plantarflexed position is desired, then a 10-degree cut can be used at the proximal surface for joint preparation. If the implant itself has an angulated position, these 10-degree cuts should also be used to ensure proper bone contact. The surgeon should reference the manufacturer's technique guide to confirm variations specific to implant type. In lieu of 10-degree bone cuts, for implants where the angulation is within the implant itself, the surgeon may opt to use a reaming method to prepare the joint surfaces. In the reaming method, pilot holes are made in both the proximal and middle phalanges using provided instrumentation, aiming for the central canal. The reamer pin is inserted into the pilot hole, and the cartilage is denuded on both the proximal and distal ends of the PIP joint with the reamer. A bone rongeur is then used to smooth surfaces as needed. If the sagittal saw technique is used, pilot holes are made in the proximal and middle phalanges in the same manner, aiming for the central canal. Some systems will feature a "dead stop," where the drill will stop automatically when it has made contact with the bone surface. For softer bone, a smaller drill bit is recommended. For the middle phalanx, the smallest drill bit should be used, and the pilot hole should be stopped short of the natural "dead stop," where care is taken to not engage the drill to the cortical wall. Some may prefer to engage the drill only a few millimeters below the surface to avoid overdrilling of the middle phalanx. For implantation of the device, some drivers will feature a gender-specific side, where one end of the drill is "male" (corresponding to the proximal phalanx) and the other end is "female" (middle phalanx). For two-sided drivers such as this, the handle can be attached to either side, so the surgeon should take care to ensure the proper end is being utilized at the appropriate time. The proximal piece of the implant is loaded onto the driver and hand driven into the proximal phalanx until the driver end is flush with the bone surface. The proximal implant can be countersunk if needed (although this seems rarely necessary). The proximal implant should "bite" the bone appropriately, which can be tested with two-finger resistance, and should be flush with the bone surface. If the proximal implant is spinning with two-finger resistance, a larger implant should be substituted. The same driver can be used to remove the proximal piece, but instrumentation to grasp the implant if the driver does not engage is also provided within the set. Fluoroscopy can be used if the grasper is not easily engaging with the implant. For a truly loose piece, a hemostat may be used to gently twist the implant out. Pulling the implant forcefully out should be avoided and will compromise a tight fit of a larger size. The distal piece of the implant is then loaded onto the appropriate driver and inserted into the middle phalanx until the threads are fully engaged. Sitting proud and connected to the middle phalanx portion, the lockable portion of the implant is then placed within the proximal implant portion. Manual compression is used, and the middle phalanx portion is press-fitted into the proximal portion. Some implants have several locking levels. Any level is appropriate with the goal of good bone-to-bone contact. Implants with this feature will typically have plantarflexion built within the construct of the implant itself, and cannot be adjusted during the positioning of the implant. A variation of this involves both the proximal and middle phalangeal pieces sitting flush with the bone surface, and a separate, third piece is used to facilitate the locking of the two ends. This piece is placed within the proximal phalanx portion, and plantarflexion can be applied at this point. The middle phalanx is then press-fitted into the proximal portion. Some two-piece implants offer an advantage where if inadequate positioning is noted (e.g., the implant is too shallow or too deep within the bone), the implant can be "unlocked" and re-adjusted.

## *Effectiveness of Two-Piece Implants* (*Table 3.2*)

Literature on two-piece implants is one of the scarcest in comparison to other implant types. Despite the small number of publications on specifically this type of implant, the articles that do exist display higher-quality study designs (level II). A randomized controlled trial allocated patients to K-wire fixation or two-piece implant for hammertoe correction [9]. Patient satisfaction and quality of life was assessed with the foot function index and Bristol foot score. A better radiographic union rate was noted within the implant group. Although not statistically significant, a greater average mean score was noted for the implant group for patient outcome measures in the immediate postoperative period. This article does report a financial conflict.

## *Implant Removal*

Implants are not routinely removed. In the event of a non-union or postoperative complication, implant removal may be necessary. Dissection can be carried down to the joint surface, and small osteotomes may be used to gently remove overlying bone to expose the implant within the PIP joint. Two-piece implants feature a central locking area within the joint that can be unlocked in the event of a complication. One such device requires twisting of the implant to a 45-degree angle, which may be limited by the soft tissue structures and overlying bone proliferation. Nonetheless, once the device is unlocked and the joint distracted, the driver used to insert the implant can be used to twist each piece out. This is the preferred method if possible. If the driver fails to engage the implant, additional instrumentation is typically offered which will lock into the proximal piece (which will be flush with the bone surface) and require axial pulling of the implant. Regardless of the method used, the same implant cannot be used again. If the device does not feature an "unlocking" advantage, the implant can be exposed at the joint level in the same manner. The proximal phalanx can then be elevated (e.g., pushed upward) to allow for grasping of the implant itself (assuming a non-union is present and joint approximation is poor). Curettes or small bone rongeurs may be used to remove excess bone and expose the implant further to facilitate removal. Toggling or axial pulling of the implant may be necessary and can often be a frustrating process. The surgeon should remember to take care with implant removal and to preserve as much bone surface as possible to allow the patient another technique of reduction. Implant removal can be difficult. Referencing the original procedure can assist the surgeon in removing the implant in a reverse manner.

## *Postoperative Care*

Surgical dressings can be implemented in a similar fashion to the K-wire technique (see section "Technique, K-Wire"). Patients are typically weight bearing as tolerated in a surgical shoe for 6 weeks. It is at the surgeon's discretion to decide when arthrodesis has been achieved and when transition into supportive shoe gear is indicated.

## *Complications*

Complications following digital surgery include recurrence of deformity, chronic edema, vascular compromise, infection, pain, hardware failure, and floating or misaligned toe [1, 2, 7, 10]. Most complications will occur within the immediate postoperative period, but deformity recurrence may occur several years after success is believed to have been achieved. Longevity of good outcomes in hammertoe surgery continues to be a problem that increases with severity of initial deformity. Kramer and colleagues [10] identified risk factors for hammertoe recurrence within their cohort study in 2015, stating that toes with transverse plane deviation pre-operatively were 2.25 times more likely to result in recurrence than toes that did not ($p$-value = 0.0003; 95% CI 1.45, 3.48). Additional risk factors identified included procedures which were considered a revision ($p$-value = 0.0031) and MTP capsulotomy ($p$-value <0.0001) which was reserved for patients with more "severe" deformity. Albright and colleagues [37] found similar results, where transverse plane deviation of the toe was a risk factor for recurrence (HR 1.03 $p$-value<0.001; 95% CI 1.02, 1.04). Additional risk factors for recurrence were second toes, which were 2.23 times more likely to recur than third or fourth toes ($p = 0.0033$; 95% CI 1.31, 3.81). Second toes began to recur most significantly after 2.7 years postoperatively, suggesting long-term results of hammertoe procedures are suboptimal, with most recurring well after patient discharge. This suggests that future hammertoe studies should aim to have a follow-up of at least 3–4 years, in order to fully capture recurrence rates.

## Current Concepts

### *K-Wire Versus Implants* (*Table 3.3*)

Within the foot and ankle community, controversy exists regarding which fixation technique is superior. This debate is largely fueled by cost, the belief of better outcomes with implants, and the belief of higher postoperative infections with K-wires, increasing the probability of a rare, yet costly inpatient admission. This argument has led surgeons to feel that despite the higher upfront cost of implants, they are worthwhile to avoid a possible expensive complication associated with K-wires. This same ideal also suggests implants may have better effectiveness overall to justify a larger upfront cost. With this debate in mind, several authors have attempted to tackle this subject.

Scholl and colleagues [18] published a head-to-head retrospective comparison between a commercial implant (Smart Toe) and buried K-wire for PIP joint arthrodesis. No statistical significance was noted in regard to non-union and revision rates. However, the authors utilized a buried K-wire technique eliminating the percutaneous nature of the wire, and thus reducing fears of pin tract infection. Although some would argue the lack of the traditional K-wire technique voids this article of being considered an accurate head-to-head comparison of the two fixation types, one could also say it compares stability and strength outcomes, in which K-wires were found to be no different than implants. Richman [28] performed a similar head-to-head comparison using a one-piece implant compared to traditional, percutaneous K-wires. He found significantly more complications (total) within the K-wire group, but no difference in revision rates. There was also no difference in infection rate between groups when evaluated independently. The authors ultimately concluded the implant is an adequate alternative to K-wires. Obrador et al. [29] in 2018 demonstrated another head-to-head comparison using two implant types (shape memory and bone allograft) versus K-wire (total $n = 96$). The authors assessed patient-reported pain, physical function and satisfaction, complications, and union rate. There were no differences in pain or postoperative complications, although "satisfaction" was higher in the implant group when compared to K-wires. At the same time, no difference was found in the "very satisfied," "unsatisfied," or "very unsatisfied" groups, leading to skepticism if this finding has clinical significance. Overall, they concluded K-wires do not pose enough disadvantages to consider implants the new standard of care. Another small, retrospective comparison was published by Angirasa et al. [31], evaluating a shape memory implant versus K-wire ($n = 28$). The authors found no statistically significant differences between groups regarding pain scores or patient satisfaction; however, they concluded the implant group trended toward superiority in patient satisfaction categories. High-level research is scarce involving head-to-head comparisons, with most articles being retrospective comparisons between groups. Confounding and bias are concerns in the retrospective design and can threaten study validity if not adequately addressed. One of the only prospective, randomized controlled trials to date has been from Jay et al. [9] who randomized patients into a two-piece implant group and K-wire group for PIP joint arthrodesis. He found no statistically significant differences between the groups with respect to revision and complication rates but did note higher satisfaction scores on PROMs within the implant group. Rothermel and colleagues [30] published a cadaveric comparison of two shape memory implants versus K-wires to test strength and stability, using mechanical stress testing. The K-wires were able to withstand a significantly greater amount of force before failure compared to both implants (91N versus 63.3N for K-wire and implant #1, respectively ($p$-value<0.01), and 102.3N versus 53.3N for K-wire and implant #2, respectively ($p$-value = 0.0038)). It should be noted the study was undertaken at time zero after surgery, which may not accurately reflect ongoing stability of the implants. In 2018, Albright et al. [38] conducted an economic analysis to test the idea that implants may give patients better outcomes, justifying their cost. The authors ultimately concluded commercial implants were slightly more effective than K-wires, but not effective enough to justify their high upfront cost. Costly inpatient admissions for K-wire complications are rare, and did not appear to be a valid concern for the technique's disuse. The authors concluded that K-wires are the more cost-effective technique and will continue to be so until the price of implants decreases to $300 (versus current pricing ranging from $500 to $1,500). Although the literature has increased on the subject, more studies are needed to provide a definitive answer to this question; however, one could argue the consistency in the literature can support the inference that K-wires are equally as effective as implants. Given the lower price tag of K-wires, the authors believe this technique is most justified and worthwhile, except for very specific patient populations who have low tolerance for protruding wires.

## *Fibrous Union Versus Osseous Union*

Although an osseous union is a prerequisite for optimal outcomes within other joints of the foot and ankle, this has not held true for the small joints within the toe. The published literature suggests an osseous union is not required for pain-free patient outcomes. In fact, Coughlin et al. [2] found no statistically significant differences in patient satisfaction between those achieving a fibrous union or an osseous union ($p$-value = 0.910) and noted it was difficult to differentiate union type on physical exam alone. Scholl et al. [18] found similar results in his comparative intervention study of commercial implant versus K-wire for arthrodesis of the PIP joint. The authors noted a 68.8% osseous union rate within the implant group radiographically. However, despite this low union rate, the authors found most patients with a fibrous union were asymptomatic, resulting in only 8.6% of their study population actually needing revision surgery. Despite the lack of evidence to show that an osseous union is necessary, this continues to be the primary outcome measure in a majority of available articles. We would not argue that osseous union is desirable; however, based on current evidence, this radiographic outcome does not seem to correlate well with patient's perception of success and, therefore, lacks much clinical importance. It should therefore, in our opinion, likely be abandoned as a primary outcome measure in future research and should serve as a secondary or tertiary outcome only, unless further research can strongly suggest otherwise. Commercial implant literature has used osseous union as a primary outcome measure to help demonstrate superiority, yet this most likely lacks any true value. Modern viewpoints should move toward achieving union of any kind (fibrous or osseous) within the PIP joint to achieve satisfactory patient outcomes.

There are several options available for fixation in hammertoe surgery. It is the surgeon's responsibility to be aware of the costs, efficacy, risks, and benefits of each device. Surgeons and patients can then decide together which is the best option for them based on their postoperative goals.

Footnote: The images used within this chapter, Hammertoe Fixation: Traditional Percutaneous Pin versus Internal Fixation, are courtesy of Dr. Charles Reilly, DPM of Advocate Illinois Masonic Medical Center in Chicago, IL.

## References

1. Coughlin MJ. Lesser toe deformities. Orthopedics. 1987;10(1):63–75.
2. Coughlin MJ, Dorris J, Polk E. Operative repair of the fixed hammertoe deformity. Foot Ankle Int. 2000;21(2):94–104.
3. Taylor R. An operative procedure for the treatment of Hammer-Toe and Claw-Toe. J Bone Joint Surg. 1940;22:608–9.
4. Hembree JW. Reduction of a hammertoe by use of an intramedullary pin. J Natl Assoc Chirop. 1957;47(10):517–8.
5. Lehman DE, Smith RW. Treatment of symptomatic hammertoe with a proximal interphalangeal joint arthrodesis. Foot Ankle Int. 1995;16(9):535–41.
6. Holinka J, Schuh R, Hofstaetter JG, Wanivenhaus AH. Temporary Kirschner wire transfixation versus strapping dressing after second MTP joint realignment surgery: a comparative study with ten-year follow-up. Foot Ankle Int. 2013;34(7):984–9.
7. Klammer G, Baumann G, Moor BK, Farshad M, Espinosa N. Early complications and recurrence rates after Kirschner wire transfixion in lesser toe surgery: a prospective randomized study. Foot Ankle Int. 2012;33(2):105–12.

8. Reece AT, Stone MH, Young AB. Toe fusion using Kirschner wire. A study of the postoperative infection rate and related problems. J R Coll Surg Edinb. 1987;32(3):158–9.
9. Jay RM, Malay DS, Landsman AS, Jennato N, Huish J, Younger M. Dual-component intramedullary implant versus Kirschner wire for proximal interphalangeal joint fusion: a randomized controlled clinical trial. J Foot Ankle Surg. 2016;55(4):697–708.
10. Kramer WC, Parman M, Marks RM. Hammertoe correction with k-wire fixation. Foot Ankle Int. 2015;36(5):494–502.
11. Lamm BM, Ribeiro CE, Vlahovic TC, Fiorilli A, Bauer GR, Hillstrom HJ. Lesser proximal interphalangeal joint arthrodesis: a retrospective analysis of the peg-in-hole and end-to-end procedures. J Am Podiatr Med Assoc. 2001;91(7):331–6.
12. Baig AU, Geary NPJ. Fusion rate and patient satisfaction in proximal interphalangeal joint fusion of the minor toes using Kirschner wire fixation. Foot. 1996;6(3):120–1.
13. Mueller CM, Boden SA, Boden AL, et al. Complication rates and short-term outcomes after operative hammertoe correction in older patients. Foot Ankle Int. 2018;39(6):681–8.
14. Zingas C, Katcherian DA, Wu KK. Kirschner wire breakage after surgery of the lesser toes. Foot Ankle Int. 1995;16(8):504–9.
15. Schrier JC, Keijsers NL, Matricali GA, Louwerens JW, Verheyen CC. Lesser toe PIP joint resection versus PIP joint fusion: a randomized clinical trial. Foot Ankle Int. 2016;37(6):569–75.
16. Boffeli TJ, Thompson JC, Tabatt JA. Two-pin fixation of proximal interphalangeal joint fusion for hammertoe correction. J Foot Ankle Surg. 2016;55(3):480–7.
17. Creighton RE, Blustein SM. Buried Kirschner wire fixation in digital fusion. J Foot Ankle Surg. 1995;34(6):567–70; discussion 595
18. Scholl A, McCarty J, Scholl D, Mar A. Smart toe(R) implant versus buried Kirschner wire for proximal interphalangeal joint arthrodesis: a comparative study. J Foot Ankle Surg. 2013;52(5):580–3.
19. Guelfi M, Pantalone A, Cambiaso Daniel J, Vanni D, Guelfi MG, Salini V. Arthrodesis of proximal inter-phalangeal joint for hammertoe: intramedullary device options. J Orthop Traumatol. 2015;16(4):269–73.
20. Kominsky SJ, Bermudez R, Bannerjee A. Using a bone allograft to fixate proximal interphalangeal joint arthrodesis. Foot Ankle Spec. 2013;6(2):132–6.
21. Basile A, Albo F, Via AG. Intramedullary fixation system for the treatment of hammertoe deformity. J Foot Ankle Surg. 2015;54(5):910–6.
22. Averous C, Leider F, Rocher H, et al. Interphalangeal arthrodesis of the toe with a new radiolucent intramedullary implant (Toegrip). Foot Ankle Spec. 2015;8(6):520–4.
23. Khan F, Kimura S, Ahmad T, D'Souza D, D'Souza L. Use of Smart Toe((c)) implant for small toe arthrodesis: a smart concept? Foot Ankle Surg. 2015;21(2):108–12.
24. Catena F, Doty JF, Jastifer J, Coughlin MJ, Stevens F. Prospective study of hammertoe correction with an intramedullary implant. Foot Ankle Int. 2014;35(4):319–25.
25. Witt BL, Hyer CF. Treatment of hammertoe deformity using a one-piece intramedullary device: a case series. J Foot Ankle Surg. 2012;51(4):450–6.
26. Sandhu JS, DeCarbo WT, Hofbauer MH. Digital arthrodesis with a one-piece memory nitinol intramedullary fixation device: a retrospective review. Foot Ankle Spec. 2013;6(5):364–6.
27. Harmer JL, Wilkinson A, Maher AJ. A midterm review of lesser toe arthrodesis with an intramedullary implant. Foot Ankle Spec. 2017;10(5):458–64.
28. Richman SH, Siqueira MB, McCullough KA, Berkowitz MJ. Correction of hammertoe deformity with novel intramedullary PIP fusion device versus K-wire fixation. Foot Ankle Int. 2017;38(2):174–80.
29. Obrador C, Losa-Iglesias M, Becerro-de-Bengoa-Vallejo R, Kabbash CA. Comparative study of intramedullary hammertoe fixation. Foot Ankle Int. 2018;39(4):415–25.
30. Rothermel SD, Aydogan U, Roush EP, Lewis GS. Proximal interphalangeal arthrodesis of lesser toes utilizing k-wires versus expanding implants: comparative biomechanical cadaveric study. Foot Ankle Int. 2019;40(2):231–6.

31. Angirasa AK, Barrett MJ, Silvester D. SmartToe(R) implant compared with Kirschner wire fixation for hammer digit corrective surgery: a review of 28 patients. J Foot Ankle Surg. 2012;51(6):711–3.
32. Pietrzak WS, Lessek TP, Perns SV. A bioabsorbable fixation implant for use in proximal interphalangeal joint (hammer toe) arthrodesis: biomechanical testing in a synthetic bone substrate. J Foot Ankle Surg. 2006;45(5):288–94.
33. Patton GW, Shaffer MW, Kostakos DP. Absorbable pin: a new method of fixation for digital arthrodesis. J Foot Surg. 1990;29(2):122–7.
34. Konkel KF, Menger AG, Retzlaff SA. Hammer Toe correction using an absorbable intramedullary pin. Foot Ankle Int. 2007;28(8):916–20.
35. Taylor GC. Absorbable Fixation Devices. PI Update Chapters: The Podiatry Institute; 1990. http://www.podiatryinstitute.com/pdfs/Update_1990/1990_20.pdf.
36. Mariash S, Taylor GC. Absorbable Fixation in Podiatric Surgery. PI Update Chapters: The Podiatry Institute; 1992. http://www.podiatryinstitute.com/pdfs/Update_1992/1992_24.pdf.
37. Albright RH, Hassan M, Randich J, O'Keefe R, Klein EE, Weil L Jr, Weil L Sr, Fleischer AE. Risk factors for suboptimal outcomes in hammertoe surgery. Foot Ankle Int. 2020;41(5):562–71.
38. Albright RH, Waverly BJ, Klein E, Weil L Jr, Weil LS Sr, Fleischer AE. Percutaneous Kirschner wire versus commercial implant for Hammertoe repair: a cost-effectiveness analysis. J Foot Ankle Surg. 2018;57(2):332–8.
39. Sung W, Weil L Jr, Weil LS Sr. Retrospective comparative study of operative repair of hammertoe deformity. Foot Ankle Spec. 2014;7(3):185–92.
40. Yassin M, Garti A, Heller E, Robinson D. Hammertoe correction with K-wire fixation compared with percutaneous correction. Foot Ankle Spec. 2017;10(5):421–7.

# Chapter 4
# 2nd Metatarsophalangeal Joint Pathology: Pre-dislocation Syndrome

**Erin E. Klein and Lowell Weil Jr**

## Relevant Anatomy of the 2nd Metatarsophalangeal Joint

The lesser metatarsophalangeal (MTP) joint (Fig. 4.1) is composed of the metatarsal head, the base of the proximal phalanx, the joint stabilizing structures/capsule, and the extensor and flexor tendons. The lesser MTP joint has many intricacies that, once understood, can aid the physician in identifying and understanding pathology in this region.

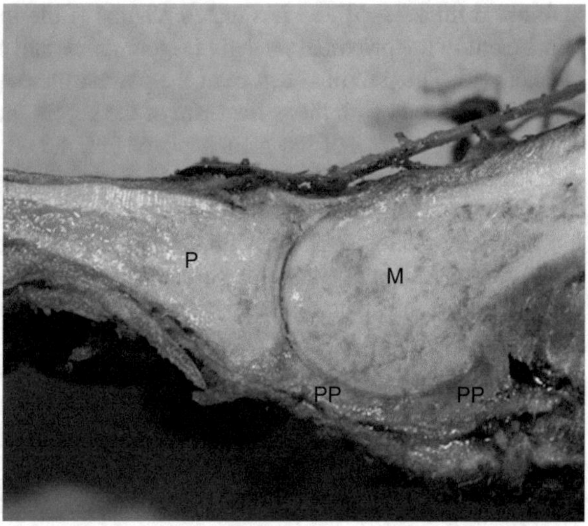


**Fig. 4.1** Sagittal section of the 2nd MTP joint region. P base of the proximal phalanx, M metatarsal head, PP plantar plate

E. E. Klein (✉) · L. Weil Jr
Weil Foot and Ankle Institute, Mount Prospect, IL, USA
e-mail: eek@weil4feet.com



D. E. Tower (ed.), *Evidence-Based Podiatry*,
https://doi.org/10.1007/978-3-030-50853-1_4

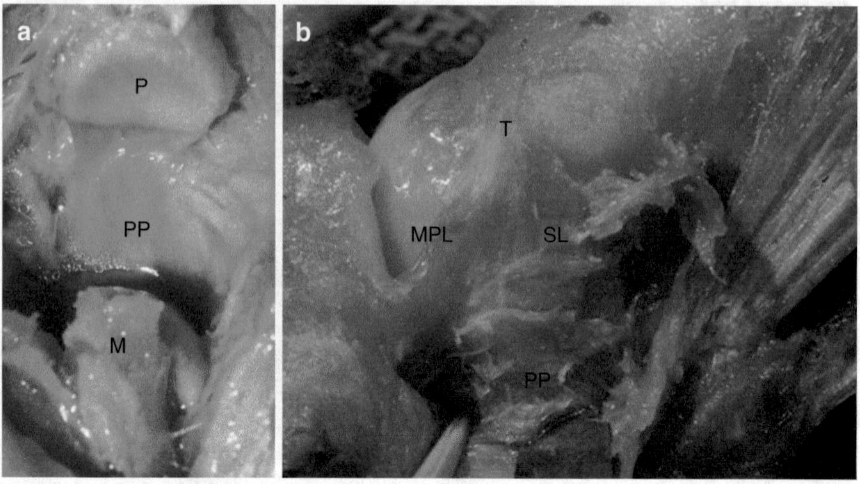


**Fig. 4.2** (**a**) Dorsal aspect of the plantar plate. P base of the proximal phalanx, PP plantar plate, M metatarsal head. (**b**) Collateral ligament complex. T tubercle, MPL metatarsophalangeal ligament, SL suspensory ligament, PP plantar plate

## *The Plantar Plate*

The plantar plate of the 2nd MTP joint is approximately 20 mm long, 9 mm wide, and 2 mm thick [1–5] and is situated plantar to the metatarsal head. Distally, the attachment to the proximal phalanx is stout, thick and can have one or two bundles of fibers [2]. The proximal aspect of the plantar plate is tissue that is thinner, more mobile and blends with the periosteum of the second metatarsal [2].

The dorsal surface of the plantar plate (Fig. 4.2) has an articular like structure composed primarily of type 1 collagen [1–3] (which resembles fibrocartilage). The fibers on the dorsal surface of the plantar plate are orientated in a longitudinal fashion, which would be consistent with its overall anatomic course. The plantar third of the plantar plate has fibers that are organized in a transverse fashion to facilitate the attachments of the plantar plate to the deep transverse metatarsal ligament (DTML) [1–3, 6].

The medial and lateral aspects of the plantar plate are continuous with two structures: the DTML and the collateral joint ligaments. The DTML runs medial to lateral across the foot and provides a strong ligamentous structure that prevents undue splaying of the forefoot [7] and is a critical component of the stability of the lesser MTP joint [6, 8, 9]. Cadaveric dissection has identified that sectioning of the DTML may decrease the force needed to sublux or dislocate the lesser MTP joint [6, 8].

The lesser metatarsals have a tubercle on the dorsomedial and dorsolateral aspects of the metatarsal head, just proximal to the articular cartilage (Fig. 4.2). The lesser MTP joint has two collateral ligaments, one on each side of the metatarsal head (medially and laterally). The collateral ligaments attach to the tubercles on either side of the metatarsal head and extend to the plantar medial and plantar lateral aspects of the proximal phalangeal base, respectively. The metatarsophalangeal ligament attaches to the anterior superior portion of the tubercle located proximal to the expansion of the articular cartilage on the metatarsal head. The metatarsophalangeal ligament courses anteriorly and inferiorly to attach to the plantar medial or plantar lateral portion of the base of the proximal phalanx [10]. The metatarsoglenoid ligament (suspensory ligament) attaches to the inferior posterior portion of the metatarsal head tubercle [10] and widens as it courses inferiorly to attach to the plantar plate [10]. Cadaveric dissection has identified that the collateral ligaments are important in the stability of the lesser MTP joint [8]. Ruptured collateral ligaments have been identified in cadaveric specimens with crossover toes [11, 12]. Sectioning of (1) only the plantar plate; (2) only the collateral ligaments; and, (3) both the plantar plate and collateral ligaments decreased the amount of force needed to dislocate the 2nd MTP joint by 30%, 46%, and 80%, respectively [8].

The plantar plate has an important relationship with the plantar fascia. Multiple authors [7, 13, 14] have identified that the plantar fascia divides into superficial and deep layers at the level of the necks of the metatarsals. There is also division that occurs that splits the plantar fascia into five sections – and each section travels toward its corresponding toe. Closer to the metatarsal head, each section divides into two slips. The slips of the plantar fascia then encompass the flexor tendon [10, 13]. The combination of the plantar fascia, the plantar plate and the flexor tendon (Fig. 4.3), provides flexion at the lesser MTP joint as the flexor tendon has no direct attachment to the metatarsal head or the proximal phalanx in this region [10].

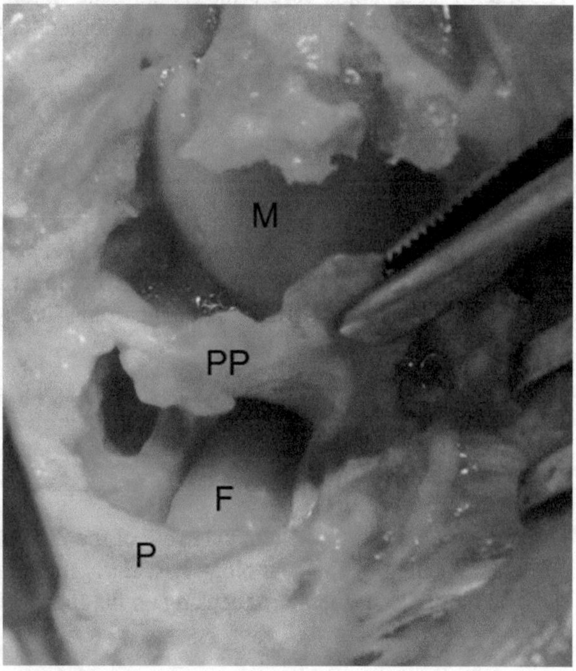


**Fig. 4.3** Relationship between the plantar fascia, plantar plate, and flexor tendon complex. M metatarsal head, PP plantar plate, F flexor tendon, P base of the proximal phalanx

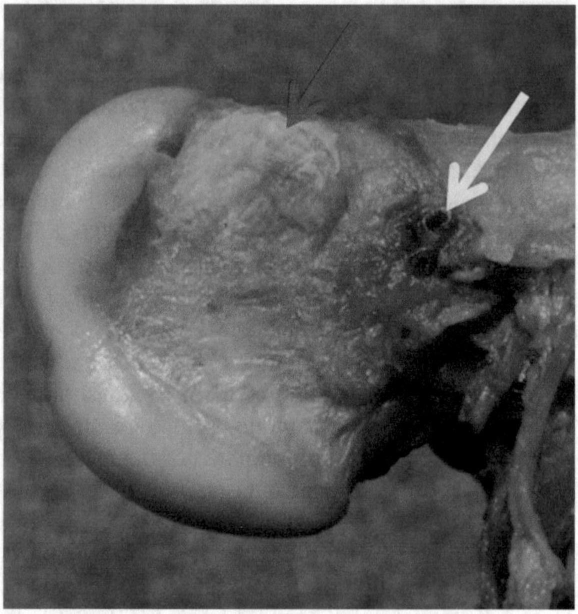

**Fig. 4.4** Vascular supply. This is a cadaveric picture where the metatarsal head was dissected. The pink arrow identifies the attachment of the collateral ligaments. The yellow arrow is the nutrient artery to the metatarsal head/neck

## *Vascular Supply*

The main blood supply to the metatarsal head enters the neck of the metatarsal slightly proximal to the tubercle and the attachment of the collateral ligaments [15] (Fig. 4.4).

## *Interdigital Nerve*

The interdigital nerve courses in a small space between the lesser MTP joint capsules (Fig. 4.5). If there is capsular distension or alteration in anatomy, the nerve can become compressed. This may result in neuroma-like symptoms in the absence of a true neuroma formation.

## Patient History

The literature related to the clinical exam of the 2nd MTP joint has evolved just as our understanding of this pathology has. Early literature focused on the crossover toe with more recent literature focusing on the foot with less obvious deformity.

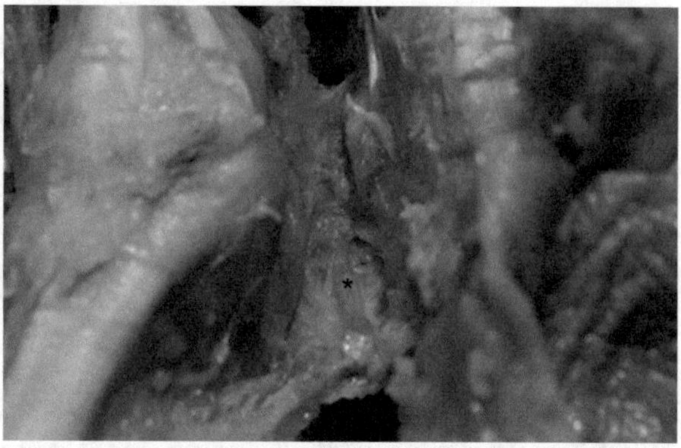


**Fig. 4.5** Interdigital nerve. This is a cadaveric picture of the interdigital nerve interposed between the 2nd and 3rd metatarsal heads. It is easy to see that edema of nearby structures could compress the nerve

Patient history should be obtained, and, although this can vary from patient to patient, a few factors remain a common theme in the current literature. Pain can be acute in onset but tends not to necessarily be related to sports and/or trauma [16]. Pain tends to have a gradual onset over time [17]. The vast majority of patients who present with this problem are women between 45 and 60 years of age [16, 18]. The previous use of higher heeled shoes is common but not always present [16]. Patients may have had a previous first ray surgery without complete restoration of motion at the 1st MTP joint [17], which may limit the patient's ability to fully load the 1st MTP joint, leading to lateralization of pressure while walking. Approximately 25% of patients who have had a previous cortisone injection in the region of the 2nd MTP joint may later experience plantar plate pathology [17].

## Physical Exam

On physical exam, the following parameters have been discussed in the literature: pain, edema, drawer sign, neuritic symptoms, plantar grip, toe touching the ground, separation of toes, and crossover toes.

### *Pain*

Pain could be present at the 2nd metatarsal head, associated sulcus, and/or base of the proximal phalanx [16, 17]. Pain has been demonstrated to increase as the injury progresses from a grade 0 to a grade III injury and then drastically reduces with grade IV injuries [16]. Classification of plantar plate injuries will be covered later in the chapter. Pain has been reported to have a high odds ratio (OR = 6.125) for plantar plate pathology [17].

## *Edema*

There is generally edema plantar to the metatarsal head [17], but this may not be present, particularly in grade IV injuries [16] or in feet with dislocations and cross-over toes [17].

## *Drawer Test*

The drawer test, sometimes referred to as the Lachman test, is a vertical stress test [19]. When the test is performed, the non-dominant hand should hold the forefoot stable with the ankle at 90 degrees. The dominant hand should firmly grasp the proximal phalanx and displace the proximal phalanx vertically on the metatarsal head (Fig. 4.6). Thompson and Hamilton [19] proposed a classification system for the positivity of the drawer test. In their classification system, the positivity of the drawer test is graded from 0 (stable joint) to 4 (dislocated joint) (Fig. 4.7).

The drawer test has been identified as both sensitive (80.6%) and specific (99.8%) [17] for plantar plate pathology. As the grade of the plantar plate injury increases from grade 0 to grade IV, the degree of subluxation/dislocation may increase as well [16]. When a positive drawer test is correctly interpreted and combined with the position of the third toe on radiographs, this may correctly identify a high-grade tear of the plantar plate [20].

## *Neuritic Symptoms*

There have been several authors [17, 21] reporting on the concept of neuritic symptoms that have not resolved with traditional treatments. Instances of lack of improvement may be related to plantar plate instability, localized capsular edema, and irritation of the digital nerve.

## *Plantar Grip*

Plantar grip is a test of strength of the plantarflexion mechanism at the MTP joint [22, 23]. The patient is asked to stand, and a narrow strip of paper is placed under the toe to be tested. The patient is asked to grip/hold the paper strip to the ground, so the examiner cannot pull the paper away. If the patient is able to keep the paper strip under the toe, it is considered a positive or normal exam. If the patient is only partially able to resist this force, the strength is considered diminished. If the patient has no ability to resist the force and the paper is pulled away, the test is considered

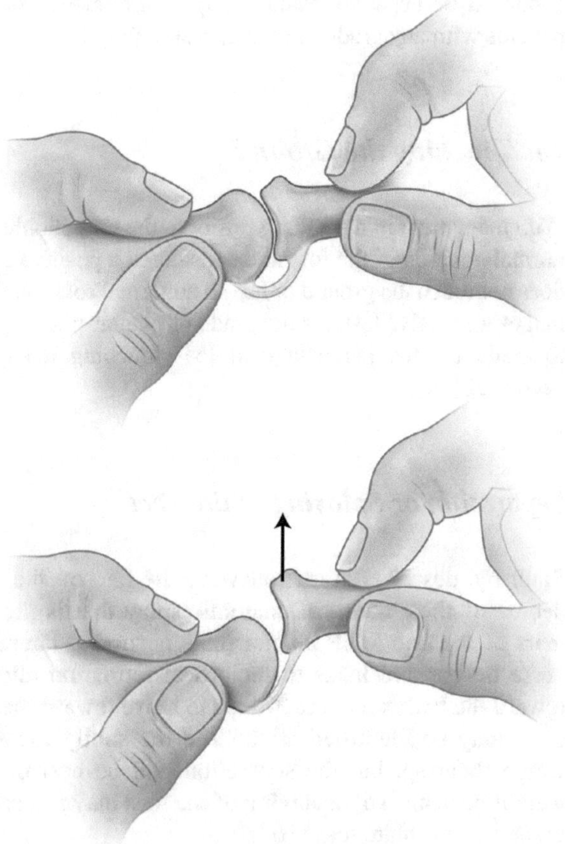

**Fig. 4.6** Drawer test. This is a vertical stress test on the lesser MTP joint [19]

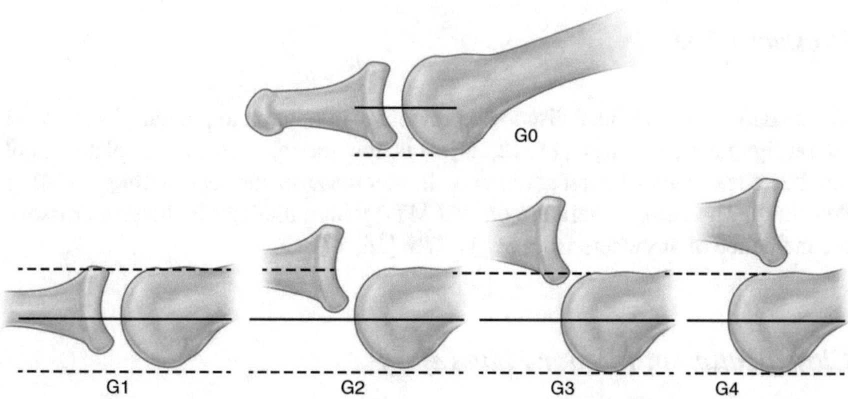


**Fig. 4.7** Thompson and Hamilton classification for the positivity of the drawer test. G0-stable joint, G1-slightly unstable (<50% subluxable), G2-moderately unstable (>50% subluxable), G3-grossly unstable (dislocatable joint), G4-dislocated joint [19]

abnormal or negative. Plantar grip is diminished or abnormal/negative in most patients with any grade of plantar plate injury [16].

## *Toe Touching the Ground*

With the patient in a standing position, the toes should touch the ground; this is the normal position of the foot and considered a positive test. When the patient's toe(s) does not touch the ground or has an abnormal rotation to it, this is considered abnormal or a negative test. As the grade of plantar plate injury progresses from grade 0 to grade IV, the percentage of toes touching the ground in a normal fashion decreases [16].

## *Separation or Splaying of the Toes*

Stainsby described the transverse tie-bar of the forefoot (Fig. 4.8) which decreases the amount of anatomic splay that is present [7]. With many of the tears of the 2nd MTP plantar plate occurring laterally, this disrupts the transverse tie-bar and leads to reciprocal retraction allowing the 2nd toe to move toward the hallux and the 3rd toe to move toward the 4th toe [20]. This phenomenon may be identified as the 2nd toe subtly touching the hallux when non-weight bearing, but the separation will be best observed when the patient is weight bearing [16]. Splaying of the toes may indicate the presence of a higher-grade plantar plate tear [16, 20].

## *Crossover Toes*

The crossover toe has been discussed previously in relation to plantar plate and collateral ligament pathology [11, 12, 24]. It is now thought that plantar plate pathology has a spectrum of presentations with the crossover toe representing end-stage deformity. The current literature on 2nd MTP joint pathology includes a crossover toe incidence of anywhere from 8% to 77% [16, 17].

## *Classification of Plantar Plate Injury*

Plantar plate injuries can be classified via (1) a clinical staging system and (2) an anatomic grading system. The two classifications were presented in a study of 68 patients (100 metatarsophalangeal joints) conducted by Nery et al., in 2015 [16].

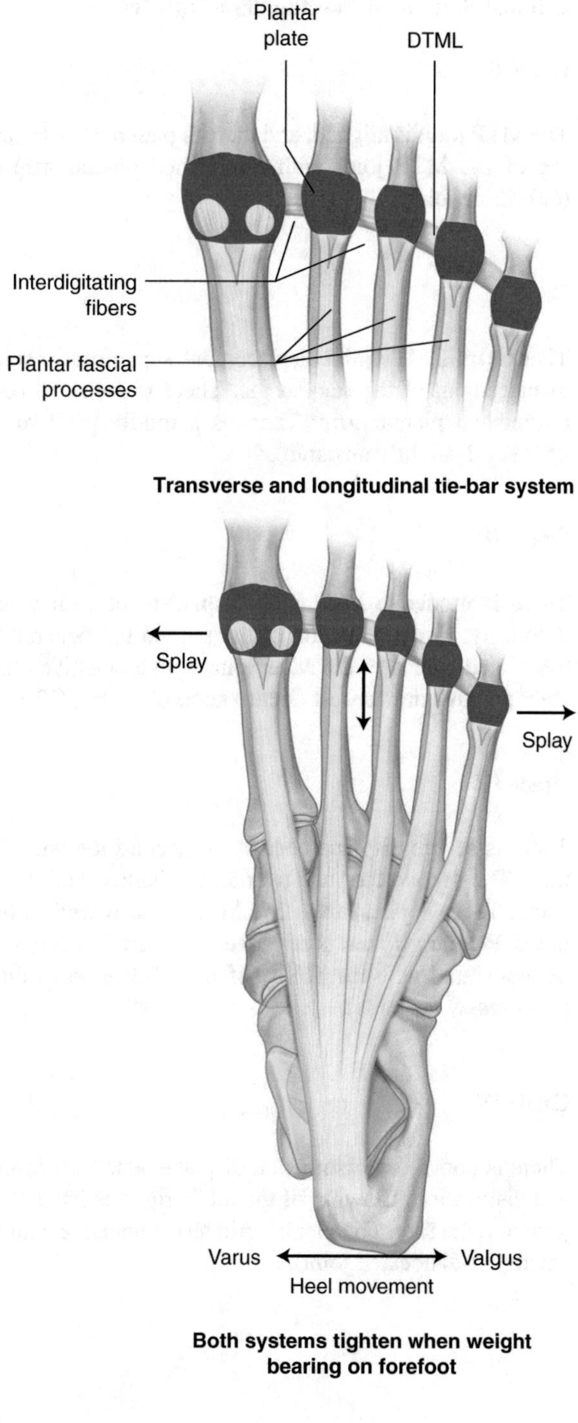


**Fig. 4.8** Transverse tie-bar of the foot [7]

## Clinical Staging of Plantar Plate Injuries

### Grade 0

The MTP joint is aligned, and there is pain but no deformity. There may be thickening of the MTP joint with diminished plantar grip and a negative drawer test (G0-stable joint).

### Grade I

There is mild MTP joint displacement, separation or splaying of the toes, and medial displacement of the second toe. There is pain and edema in the MTP joint with diminished plantar grip. There is a mildly positive drawer test (subluxation of <50%; G1-slightly unstable).

### Grade II

There is moderate MTP joint displacement with medial, lateral, or dorsomedial deformity. Hyperextension of the second toe occurs. There is joint pain with less associated edema in the MTP joint with a negative plantar grip. There is a moderately positive drawer test (subluxation of >50%; G2-moderately unstable).

### Grade III

There is severe displacement of the second toe with dorsal or dorsomedial deformity. The second toe may overlap the hallux, and flexible clawing of the toe may occur. There is pain in the 2nd MTP joint as well as the foot with minimal edema noted. Plantar grip test is negative, and there is a very positive drawer test. This may be associated with the ability of the MTP joint to dislocate with the drawer test (G3-grossly unstable).

### Grade IV

There is dorsal or dorsomedial displacement with severe 2nd MTP joint deformity and dislocation. Clawing of the toe is rigid or fixed. There is pain in the 2nd MTP joint and the foot. The plantar grip test is negative, and the MTP joint may be dislocated (G4-dislocated joint).

**Anatomic Grading of Plantar Plate Injuries** [12, 16] (Fig. 4.9)

Grade 0

Attenuation and/or capsular dislocation of the plantar plate

Grade 1

Distal transverse lesion (adjacent to the insertion) at the proximal phalanx (lesion is <50% of the width of the plantar plate); medial/lateral/central area and/or intra-substance lesion (<50%)

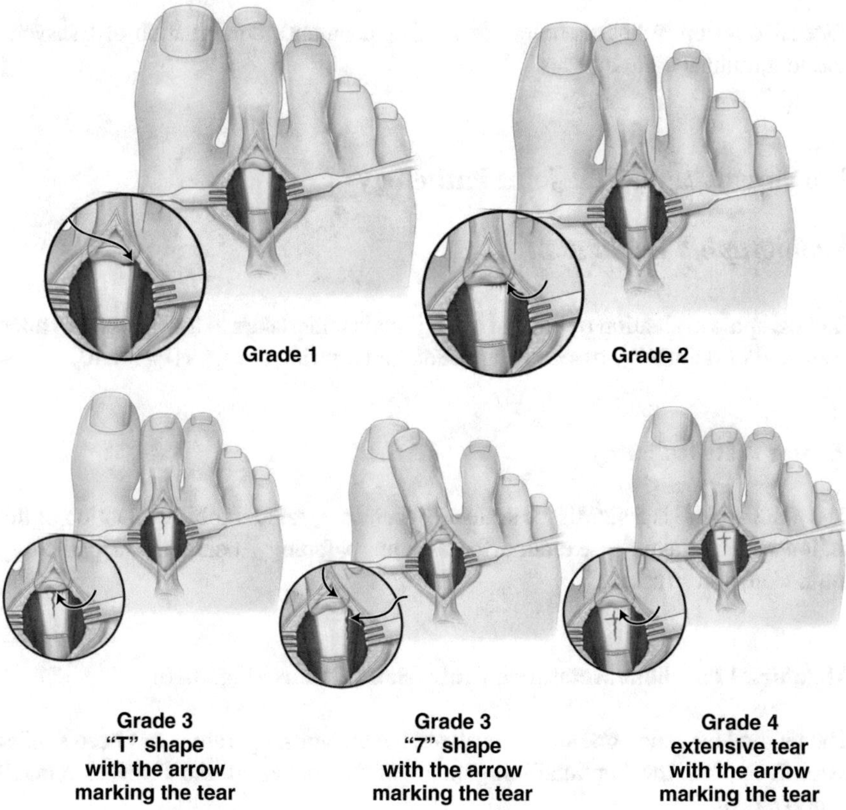


**Fig. 4.9** Anatomic grading system with distal metatarsal head removed [12, 16]

Grade 2

Distal transverse lesion (>50%); medial/lateral/central area and/or intra-substance lesion (>50%)

Grade 3

Transverse lesion and/or extensive longitudinal lesion (may involve collateral ligament structures)

Grade 4

Extensive lesion in "buttonhole" shape (displacement); combination of transverse and longitudinal plate injuries

## Imaging of 2nd MTP Joint Pathology

### *Radiographic Evaluation*

Radiographic evaluation of the 2nd MTP joint is undertaken to assess osseous alteration and/or deformity, osseous alignment, and arthritic changes (Fig. 4.10).

#### Plantar Plate Pathology

The plantar plate is a soft tissue structure; therefore, radiographic evaluation of this region is undertaken to examine for osseous pathology, contaminant pathology, alignment, and structure.

#### **Metatarsal Parabola/Metatarsal Protrusion Distance** (Fig. 4.10)

The method by which one should evaluate the metatarsal parabola has been studied extensively, but the "optimal" alignment of the bones of the forefoot remains controversial.

Hardy and Clapham [25] described a method to evaluate the metatarsal parabola. An arc compares the first metatarsal length to the second metatarsal length with ±2 mm being established as a parameter of normalcy [26].

Reese and Scoffield [27] described a method of measuring the 2nd metatarsal protrusion distance. In this measurement, a line connects the articular surface of the

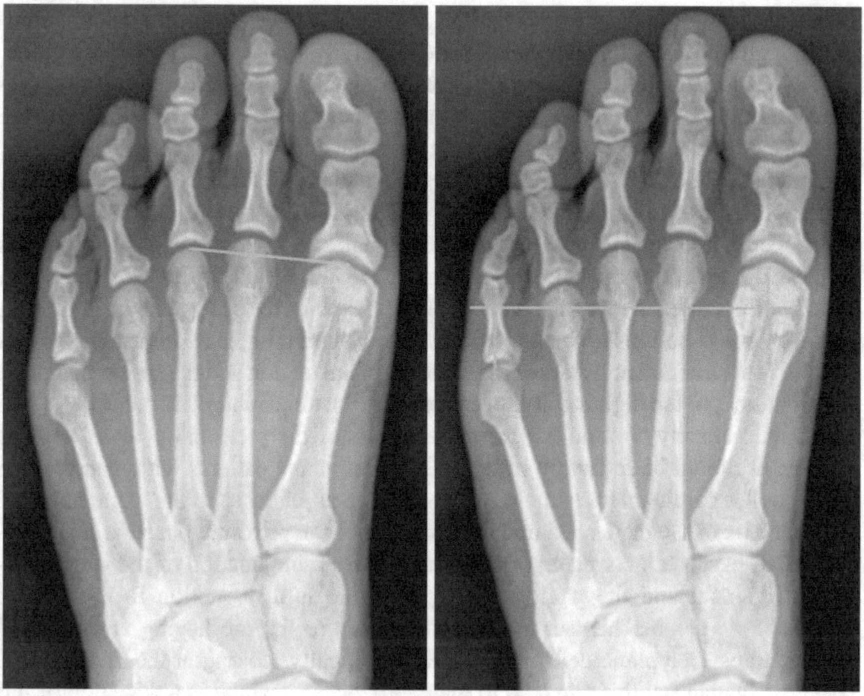

**Fig. 4.10** Radiographic evaluation. Left: Second metatarsal protrusion distance [24, 28]. This is created by a line that connects the distal most portion of the first and third metatarsals. The portion of the second metatarsal distal to the line is measured in millimeters. Right: The measurement of the parabola as described by Maestro [28]

1st metatarsal articular cartilage to the articular cartilage of the 3rd metatarsal allowing measurement of the protrusion of the 2nd metatarsal. This method was later popularized by Coughlin [24].

The most studied method of measuring the metatarsal parabola was reported by Maestro et al. [28]. This method of measurement starts with a line drawn parallel to the medial cortex of the 2nd metatarsal. A second line is created that is perpendicular to the first line and bisects the fibular sesamoid. Each metatarsal is then assessed for length relative to the line that bisects the fibular sesamoid. This method has been found to be reliable and reproducible [29]. Maestro was initially interested in defining the "most harmonious" morphotype of the forefoot [28] and attempted to establish "normal" values for each of the metatarsal lengths. In his initial study of 40 feet, where 48% of patients had identical foot morphology, Maestro established that the "most harmonious" position of the 2nd metatarsal was 1–2 mm longer than the 1st metatarsal. The 2nd metatarsal was 3.4 mm longer than the 3rd metatarsal, and the axis perpendicular to the sagittal foot axis should pass through the center of the 4th metatarsal head [28]. Maestro also noted that the relationships in the forefoot are extremely complex, and small deviations or alterations (i.e., even as small as 2 mm) are enough to cause pain and plantar callosities [28].

With examining the metatarsal parabola, particularly when comparing the symptomatic foot to the contralateral/asymptomatic foot, there may be asymmetry in the 2nd metatarsal length between sides with an elongated 2nd metatarsal found on the symptomatic side [30] when measured by the method set forth by Reese [27].

Early studies of plantar plate pathology identified an association between elongated second metatarsals and risk of plantar plate tears. Subsequent literature has suggested a potential causative relationship [31, 32]. Much of this work has been heavily criticized; however, the authors of these studies have suggested that the soft tissue/osseous relationship in the forefoot is very similar to the relationship between a flatter foot structure and tears of the posterior tibial tendon and the spring ligament.

Alignment of the digit has also been associated with plantar plate pathology [31]. In the theoretically "normal" foot, the long axis of the proximal phalanx and the metatarsal should be relatively straight. However, many patients with plantar plate and/or collateral ligament pathology demonstrate an increase in the angle between the long axis of the metatarsal and the long axis of the proximal phalanx. It is theorized that, because most plantar plate tears occur at the junction of the lateral collateral ligament and the plantar plate [33], there is a disruption in the plantar transverse tie-bar mechanism [7, 20]. This leads to the toe having an increased angular transverse plane deformity. When specifically looking at the 2nd and 3rd proximal phalanges, this can lead to increased "splay," which is a deviation of the 2nd proximal phalanx toward the hallux and a deviation of the 3rd proximal phalanx toward the 4th toe.

## *Ultrasound*

Multiple studies have investigated the use of ultrasound to identify plantar plate pathology.

### Normal and Abnormal Appearance

Gregg [34] was one of the first to investigate the use of ultrasound to identify plantar plate pathology on cadaveric specimens. The normal plantar plate was described as a slightly echoic, homogenous, curved structure (Fig. 4.11). Torn plantar plates appear as a hypoechoic or heterogeneous focus replacing the normally homogenously echoic insertion [34, 35] (Fig. 4.12). Isoechoic change has been described, and, if this occurs, the plantar plate will be only slightly altered in echogenicity, but the direction of the fibers will be disorganized [34, 35].

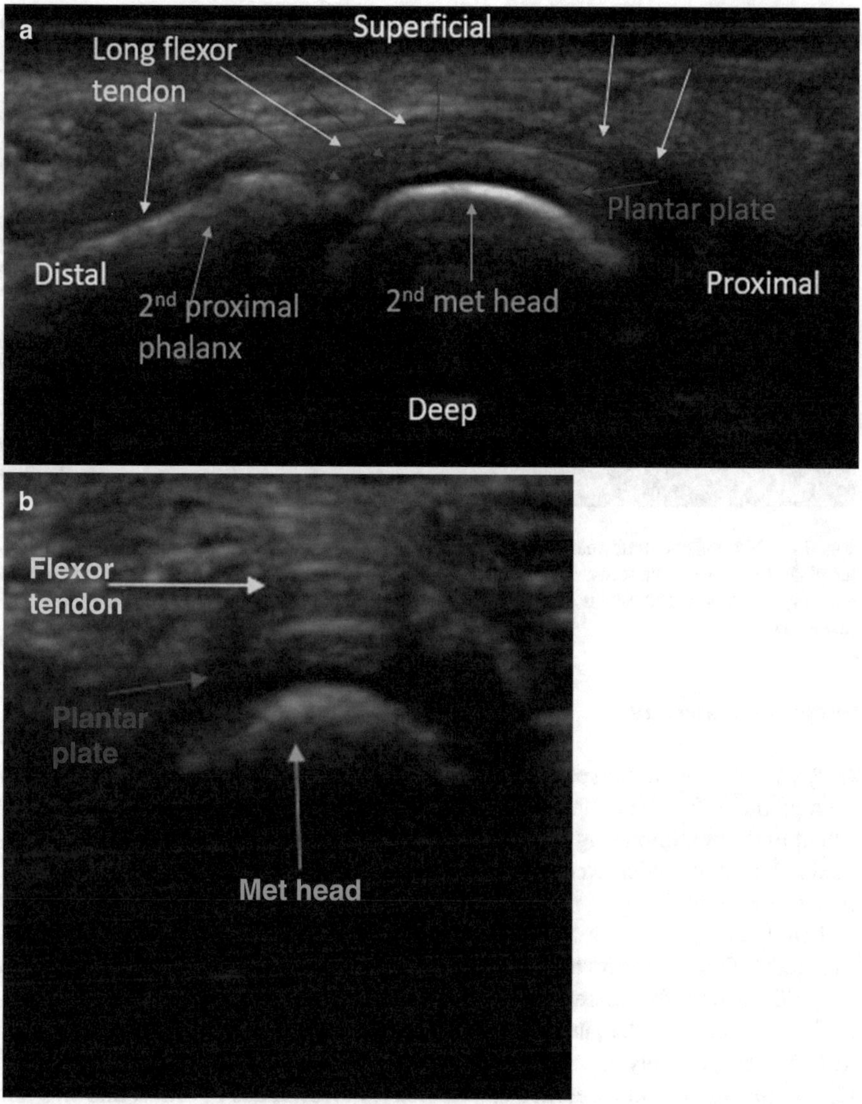


**Fig. 4.11** Normal appearance of plantar plate on ultrasound. Image (**a**) The longitudinal images are created by placing the probe over the plantar 2nd MTP joint in line with the long axis of the 2nd metatarsal. Image (**b**) is created by turning the probe 90 degrees (or perpendicular) from the long axis [18]

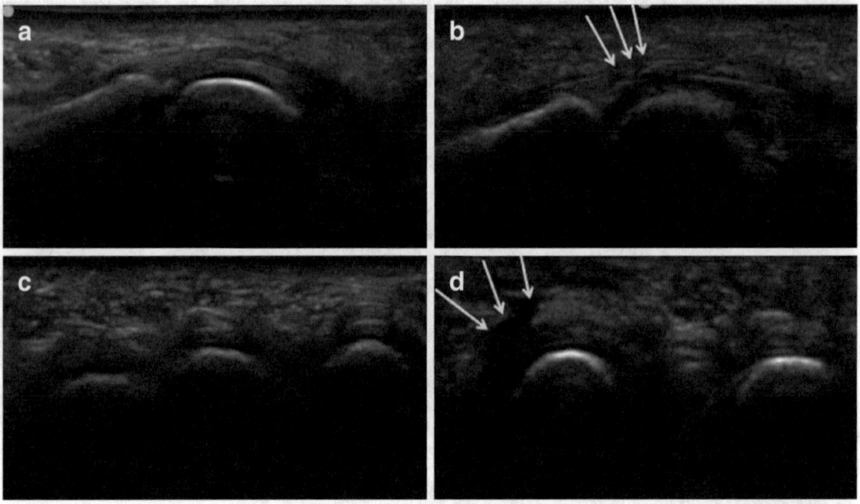


**Fig. 4.12** Normal and abnormal appearance of plantar plate on ultrasound. Pathology of the plantar plate. (**a**) Normal anatomy. (**b**) The pathology is identified by the yellow arrows. (**c**) Normal anatomy. (**d**) The pathology is identified by the large defect in the tissue identified by the yellow arrows

## Supportive Literature

Gregg's subsequent prospective study [36] compared 40 symptomatic and 40 asymptomatic feet (160 plantar plates in each group). This study focused on ultrasound findings while using MRI as the gold standard for reference. Operative correction was only undertaken in 10 subjects. The authors concluded that ultrasound may be the better imaging modality for detection of plantar plate tears.

Utilizing Gregg's work as a starting point, Klein [18] et al. performed a prospective study of 50 consecutive patients where intraoperative inspection was utilized as the gold standard for reference compared to ultrasound. The sensitivity, specificity, positive predictive value, and negative predictive values were 91.1%, 25%, 91.1%, and 25%, respectively. Utilization of longitudinal ultrasound images was adequate for identification of the presence of pathology; however, use of ultrasound was not as adequate for identifying where the pathology was located.

Subsequent authors have identified that both static and dynamic ultrasound exams can be utilized to identify plantar plate tears with relatively high accuracy. In a prospective, diagnostic study of 45 2nd MTP joints in 36 patients, Feuerstein [37] et al. directly compared the diagnostic accuracy of static ultrasound exams of the lesser MTP joint with the dynamic examination of the same region. Both types of ultrasound examination had value in identifying plantar plate pathology; however, the dynamic exam was more sensitive with a higher negative predictive value noted. The authors urge that static ultrasound examinations be interpreted with caution in the forefoot.

Ultrasound is generally considered to be a low-cost, easy to perform examination. However, the technician performing the exam needs to be familiar with the anatomy and the possible pathology of the region in order to be able to accurately capture useful images of the region.

## *Magnetic Resonance Imaging*

Magnetic resonance imaging (MRI) has been studied in relation to identifying plantar plate pathology.

### Normal and Abnormal Appearance

On MRI, the plantar plate is a thin, smooth, curvilinear, low signal structure abutting the plantar aspect of the metatarsal head [34]. The plantar plate can be seen attaching to the base of the proximal phalanx and, if the image has high enough resolution, can be seen blending with the joint capsule and periosteum proximally [34] (Fig. 4.13).

Findings of a plantar plate tear include discontinuity of the plantar plate with an area of increased signal in the region of the suspected tear [34]. There may be associated intra-articular edema or effusion.

### Supportive Literature

Sung [38] et al. performed one of the first studies of imaging of the plantar plate utilizing intraoperative inspection as the gold standard of reference. Forty-one patients (45 feet) were prospectively enrolled in a study aimed at determining if a plantar plate-specific MRI protocol could identify plantar plate pathology preoperatively. Accuracy, sensitivity, specificity, positive, and negative predictive values were stated as 96%, 95%, 100%, 100%, and 67%, respectively.

It should be noted that contrast was *not* utilized in this study as the radiologist on the study felt that contrast would obscure the plantar plate. MR arthrography has been described for identification of plantar plate pathology [39] and has been used in older studies. One study suggests that up to 29% of lesions require gadolinium contrast to be seen [40]. Interestingly, as technology has evolved, the use of arthrography has not been as present in the literature.

MRI utilizes a standardized protocol which creates a more predictable image. MRI can also assess all of the structures in the region of the 2nd MTP (as well as the rest of the forefoot). MRI can generally identify collateral ligament tears, osteochondral defects, bone marrow edema, stress fractures, and neuromas (among other pathology). Although more costly and time consuming to perform, the MRI may provide a more complete picture of what is occurring in the forefoot.

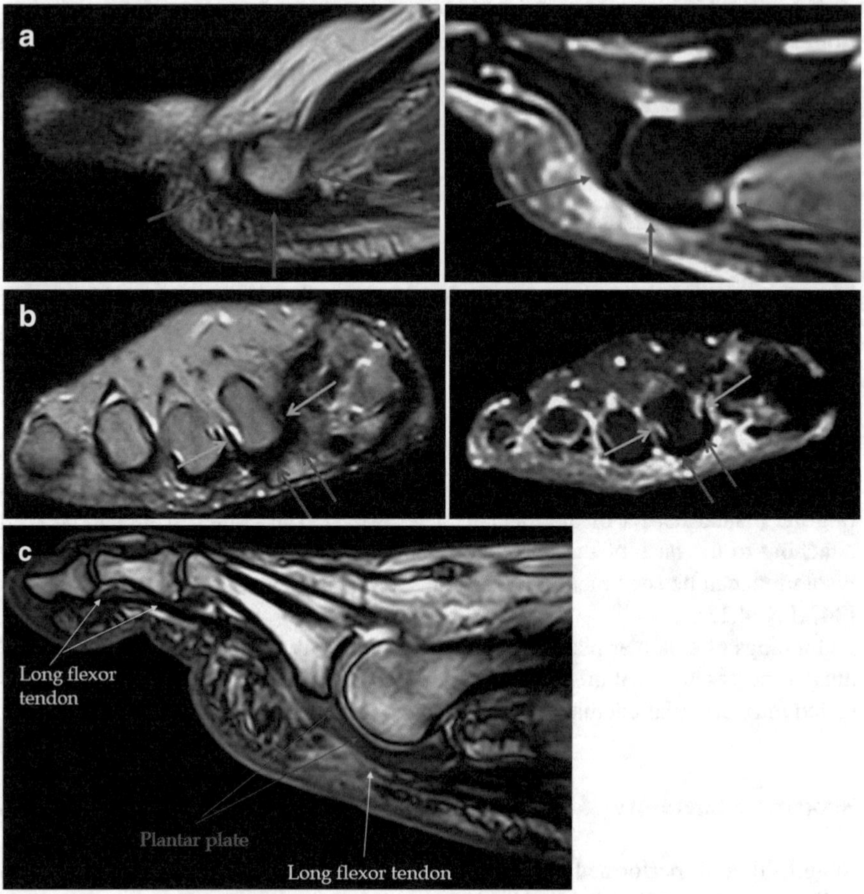


**Fig. 4.13** MRI images of an intact plantar plate. (**a**) Sagittal view: The purple arrows highlight the plantar plate. (**b**) Short axis images. The pink arrows highlight the plantar plate. The green arrows identify the collateral ligament complexes. (**c**) 3D SHARC reconstruction sagittal plane images [38]

## *What Is the Comparison Between Ultrasound and MRI?*

Ultrasound and MRI have both been rather extensively studied in relation to the plantar plate and pathology in this region.

Klein [41] et al. performed a direct comparison of MRI and US with intraoperative inspection being utilized as the gold standard of reference. Prospective examination of 42 consecutive patients (51 feet) identified that US was the more sensitive exam, while MRI was the more specific exam. Additionally, MRI was better able to detect additional pathology (i.e., collateral ligament tears), while US was unable to do this as the exam was targeted at only the plantar plate.

A more recent case series [42] directly compared high-resolution dynamic ultrasonography to MRI utilizing intraoperative examination as the gold standard of reference. The sensitivity, specificity, positive predictive value, negative predictive value, and overall accuracy were 60%, 100%, 100%, 33%, and 66%, respectively, for MRI. High-resolution dynamic ultrasound had values of 100%, 100%, 100%, 100%, and 100%, respectively. The differences between these values were not found to be statistically significant, and the authors concluded that both modalities were acceptable for imaging plantar plate tears.

A meta-analysis of 246 plantar plates compared MRI to ultrasound [43]. Meta-analyses are limited in value based on the techniques utilized to obtain information. As such, this meta-analysis included only papers that included arthroscopy or surgical inspection as the gold standard of reference. This meta-analysis also compared the sensitivity, specificity, positive likelihood ratio and negative likelihood ratio of MRI, and ultrasound for plantar plate tears. These values were 95%, 54%, 2.08, and 0.08 for MRI, respectively, and 93%, 33%, 1.20, and 0.35, respectively, for ultrasound. The authors concluded that MRI has better accuracy for detection of plantar plate tears. However, the authors of this study also note that the results should be interpreted cautiously as there was some heterogenicity of the data (rather than homogeny), and the protocol for examination and interpreting radiologists were different for each included study [43].

### *Computed Tomography*

As the plantar plate is a soft tissue structure, use of MRI and US are more common. The ability of the CT scan to identify soft tissue pathology is limited. At this time, there is a single case study [44] in the literature where a plantar plate injury was detected by a CT scan.

## Surgical Techniques: Plantar Plate

### *Suture Button*

This technique includes use of a suture button to reconstruct the plantar plate after failed digital surgery [45]. The authors opine that, because of decreased VAS scores and improvement in the Bristol Foot Score, this is a useful technique for reconstruction of the MTP joint after failed digital surgery.

## *Dorsal Approach*

In his initial study, Weil et al. [46] suggested that the plantar plate could be repaired through a Weil osteotomy approach. These authors created a Weil metatarsal osteotomy [47] through a dorsal approach. The capital fragment of the osteotomy was then retrograded and *temporarily* fixated. This allows a view of the plantar plate that was exceptional and not previously discussed in the literature. A suture passer was utilized to pass suture directly through the plantar plate. The configuration of the suture was determined based on the pathology that was present. The ends of that suture were then passed through osseous tunnels in the base of the proximal phalanx. The capital fragment of the metatarsal was repositioned and fixated. In their initial case series of 15 feet in 13 patients with an average of 22.5 months of follow-up, patients reported a decrease in VAS score from 7.3 to 1.7. AOFAS scores were 85.7/100 postoperatively. The authors concluded that this procedure was viable and reproducible to decrease pain and restore function to the 2nd MTP joint.

An author on this original study has subsequently published a technique tip that suggests that one can use an interference screw with a knotless, synthetic, high strength tape in the region of the compromised structures utilizing the same dorsal approach [47]. This author opines that this technique would be a suitable alternative to a flexor tendon transfer.

## *Plantar Approach*

McAlister and Hyer [48] describe a direct plantar approach for plantar plate repair. The authors opine that there is pathology present on the plantar surface of the plantar plate. This approach allows for direct visualization of the plantar portion of the plantar plate and direct repair from this approach. The authors mention that contaminant procedures can be performed from other approaches (i.e., dorsal approach for a hammer toe repair or a Weil metatarsal osteotomy) if needed to correct the pathology that is present. The authors address that the prominent plantar scar does not occur frequently and that patients recover well from this procedure.

## *Combined Dorsal-Plantar Approach*

Donegan and Caminear [49] describe a combined dorsal and plantar approach with direct plantar plate repair. The authors opine that this approach allows for direct repair of the plantar plate with imbrication of the flexor digitorum longus sheath creating a “robust” repair. Long-term follow-up and patient reported outcome measures were not presented.

### *Coblation with Weil Metatarsal Osteotomy*

Nery et al. [50] presented a case series of 19 patients with 35 slightly unstable 2nd MTP joints. These patients were treated with radiofrequency coblation and a Weil metatarsal osteotomy. Pain was decreased, AFOAS score increased, and stability was restored. The authors concluded that this technique is a viable treatment option for patients with grade 0 or 1 lesions with some instability.

### *Arthroscopic Techniques*

Lui [51, 52] reported on an arthroscopic, minimally invasive correction for cross-over toe. This technique is indicated for symptomatic crossover toe that is unresponsive to non-operative care. This technique sutures the plantar plate to the extensor tendon to correct the deformity. The author cautions that this technique is contraindicated in patients with degeneration of the metatarsophalangeal joint, dislocation of the metatarsophalangeal joint, the presence of neuroma, or if the crossover toe is caused by deformity of the metatarsal head or base of the proximal phalanx.

### *Flexor Tendon Transfer*

This procedure has been discussed by multiple authors for the management of chronic, severe, combined sagittal, and/or transverse plane dislocation of the lesser MTP joint. Bouch [53] et al. published a case series of 18 patients (20 feet) who underwent a flexor digitorum longus tendon transfer. The postoperative AOFAS score was 87.7/100, and all patients were satisfied with the procedure.

## Postoperative Considerations

Every surgical procedure has the potential for complications. A review of complications related to the Weil metatarsal osteotomy was undertaken. In 1,131 Weil metatarsal osteotomies, floating toes were reported in 233 (36%). Recurrence of the initial deformity/pain was reported in 15% of the cases. Transfer metatarsalgia was reported in 7% of cases. Delayed, non-union, and malunion were reported (collectively) in 3% of cases [54].

Very few papers discuss management of complications and prevention of sequelae of surgical procedures that address plantar plate repair. Some authors opine that surgeons must be cognizant of possible complications, prepare the patient for possible poor outcomes, and actively engage in techniques that would proactively prevent possible complications [55].

The "floating toe" may be the most widely discussed complication after 2nd MTP joint surgery with an incidence of 20% to 68% [56–59]. This can be a painless positional problem or it can be painful. The theory of the etiology of the floating toe has been related to excessive shortening, as many articles with high rates of floating toe shorten the metatarsal more than the 2–3 mm suggested in the original article on Weil's metatarsal osteotomy [61]. Other authors, however, believe that the floating toe occurs because of a lack of plantarflexion and/or loss of plantarflexory power, particularly with weight bearing [60–62]. Shortening the metatarsal with a Weil osteotomy (without a plantar plate repair) may decrease or "dampen" the flexor mechanism, ultimately leading to a floating toe [60].

There are both intraoperative techniques and postoperative considerations that can help prevent toes from floating after a Weil metatarsal osteotomy. From an intraoperative standpoint, shortening the metatarsal only 2–3 mm as originally described will assure that the metatarsal is not overly shortened. If more than 2–3 mm of shortening is desired due to the initial metatarsal length, taking a small parallel section of metatarsal might be required.

Postoperatively, bracing the toe in plantarflexion may help the dorsal tissues heal in an elongated position and decrease tension on the plantar tissues while healing. Postoperative bracing and assertive physical rehabilitation play active roles in preventing floating toes [55]. Other authors opine that performing a flexor digitorum brevis transfer at the PIPJ may also treat this problem [63].

## Long-Term Outcome-Based Studies

To date, only two studies with intermediate to longer-term follow-up have been published on the outcomes of surgical correction of the plantar plate.

Flint et al. [64] performed a prospective analysis of 138 plantar plate repairs in 97 feet utilizing the dorsal approach technique [47]. Patients were followed for 12 months with data being collected pre- and postoperatively. Eighty percent of patients were "good" or "excellent" 12 months postoperatively. Visual analog pain scale scores decreased from 5.4 to 1.5. AOFAS scores increased from 49 to 81 points. Forty-two percent of patients passed the paper pull out test at baseline, while 54% passed at final follow-up. The authors of this study concluded that the plantar plate could be repaired through the dorsal approach with reliable outcomes and improved patient function.

Klein et al. [65] followed 53 consecutive patients for an average of 2 years postoperatively. All patients underwent a dorsal approach to plantar plate repair [46] by one of the two senior authors. Visual analog scale for pain scores decreased from an average of 6.5 preoperatively to 1.5 postoperatively. FAOS scores improved significantly in 4 of 5 subscales at final follow-up.

## References

1. Deland JT, et al. Anatomy of the plantar plate and its attachments in the lesser metatarsal phalangeal joint. Foot Ankle Int. 1995;16:480–6.
2. Johnston RB 3rd, Smith J, Daniels T. The plantar plate of the lesser toes: an anatomical study in human cadavers. Foot Ankle Int. 1994;15:276–82.
3. Umans HR, Elsinger E. The plantar plate of the lesser metatarsophalangeal joints: potential for injury and role of MR imaging. Magn Reson Imaging Clin North Am. 2001;9:659–69.
4. Cruveilhier J, Pattison GS, Madden WH. The anatomy of the human body. The 1st American, from the last Paris ed. New York: Harper & Brothers; 1844. p. xv, 907.
5. Johnston RB 3rd, Soth J, Daniels T. The plantar plate of the lesser toes: an anatomical study in human cadavers. Foot Ankle Int. 1994;15(5):276–82.
6. Wang B, et al. Deep transverse metatarsal ligament and static stability of lesser metatarsophalangeal joints: a cadaveric study. Foot Ankle Int. 2015;36(5):573–8.
7. Stainsby GD. Pathological anatomy and dynamic effect of the displaced plantar plate and the importance of the integrity of the plantar plate-deep transverse metatarsal ligament tie-bar. Ann R Coll Surg Engl. 1997;79:58–68.
8. Bhatia D, et al. Anatomical restraints to dislocation of the second metatarsophalangeal joint and assessment of a repair technique. J Bone Joint Surg. 1994;79A(9):1371–5.
9. Chalayon O, et al. Role of plantar plate and surgical reconstruction techniques on static stability of lesser metatarsophalangeal joints: a biomechanical study. Foot Ankle Int. 2013;34(10):1436–42.
10. Sarrafian SK, Topouzian LK. Anatomy and physiology of the extensor apparatus of the toes. J Bone Joint Surg Am. 1969;51(4):669–79.
11. Deland JT, Sung IH. The medical crossover toe: a cadaveric dissection. Foot Ankle Int. 2000;21(5):375–8.
12. Coughlin MJ, et al. Metatarsophalangeal joint pathology in crossover second toe deformity: a cadaveric study. Foot Ankle Int. 2012;33(2):133–40.
13. Bojsen-Moller F, Falgstad KE. Plantar aponeurosis and internal architecture of the ball of the foot. J Anat. 1976;121:599–611.
14. Poirier P. Traite d'Anatomie Humaine, Vol. 2. Paris: L Battaille et Cie; 1892.
15. Peterson WJ. The arterial supply of the lesser metatarsal heads: a vascular injection study in human cadavers. Foot Ankle Int. 2002;23(6):491–5.
16. Nery C, et al. How to classify plantar plate injuries: parameteres from history and physical examination. Rev Bras Ortop. 2015;50(6):720–8.
17. Klein EE, et al. Clinical exam of plantar plate abnormality: a diagnostic perspective. Foot Ankle Int. 2012;34(6):800–4.
18. Klein EE, et al. Musculoskeletal ultrasound for preoperative imaging of the plantar plate. Foot Ankle Spec. 2013;6(3):196–200.
19. Thompson FM, Hamilton WG. Problems of the second metatarsophalangeal joint. Orthopedics. 1987;10:83–9.
20. Klein EE, et al. Positive drawer test combined with radiographic deviation of the third metatarsophalangeal joint suggests high grade tear of the second metatarsophalangeal joint plantar plate. Foot Ankle Spec. 2014;7(6):466–70.
21. Doty JF, Coughlin MJ. Metatarsophalangeal joint instability of the lesser toes. J Foot Ankle Surg. 2014;53(4):440–5.
22. Haddad SL, et al. Results of a flexor to extensor and extensor brevis tendon transfer for correction of the crossover second toe deformity. Foot Ankle Int. 1999;20:781–8.
23. Mendicino RW, et al. Pre dislocation syndrome: a review and retrospective analysis of eight patients. J Foot Ankle Surg. 2001;40:214–24.
24. Coughlin MJ. Second metatarsophalangeal joint instability in the athlete. Foot Ankle. 1993;14:309–91.

25. Hardy RH, Clapham JC. Observations on hallux valgus: based on a control series. J Bone Joint Surg Br. 1951;33-B:376–91.
26. Heden RI, Sorto LA Jr. The buckle point and the metatarsal protrusion's relationship to hallux valgus. J Am Podiatry Assoc. 1981;71:200–8.
27. Reese HW, Scoffield M. Metatarsal shortening osteotomy with shortening osteotomy guide. J Am Podiatry Assoc. 1987;77:304–7.
28. Maestro M, et al. Forefoot morphotype study and planning method for forefoot osteotomy. Foot Ankle Clin. 2003;8:695–710.
29. Deleu PA, et al. Reliability of the Maestro radiographic measuring tool. Foot Ankle Int. 2010;31(10):884–91.
30. Klein EE, et al. The underlying osseous deformity in plantar plate tears: a radiographic analysis. Foot Ankle Spec. 2013;6(2):108–18.
31. Fleischer AE, et al. Association of abnormal metatarsal parabola with second metatarsophalangeal joint plantar plate pathology. Foot Ankle Int. 2017;38(3):289–97.
32. Fleischer AE, et al. Association between second metatarsal length and forefoot loading under the second metatarsophalangeal joint. Foot Ankle Int. 2018;39(5):560–7.
33. Kier R, et al. MR arthrography of the second and third metatarsophalangeal joints for the detection of tears of the plantar plate and joint capsule. AJR. 2010;194:1079–81.
34. Gregg J, et al. Sonography of plantar plates in cadavers: correlations with MRI and histology. AJR. 2006;186:948–55.
35. Stone M, et al. Accuracy of sonography in plantar plate tears in cadavers. J Ultrasound Med. 2017;36(7):1355–61.
36. Gregg J, et al. Sonographic and MRI evaluation of the plantar plate: a prospective study. Eur Radiol. 2006;16:2661–9.
37. Feuerstein CA, et al. Static versus dynamic musculoskeletal ultrasound for detection of plantar plate pathology. Foot Ankle Spec. 2014;7(4):259–65.
38. Sung W, et al. Diagnosis of plantar plate injury by magnetic resonsance imaging with reference to intraoperative findings. J Foot Ankle Surg. 2012;51:570–4.
39. Yao L, Cracchiolo A, Farahani K. Plantar plate of the foot: findings on a controversial arthrography and MR imaging. AJR. 1994;163:641–4.
40. Dinoa V, et al. Evaluation of lesser metatarsophalangeal joint plantar plate tears with contrast enhanced and fat suppressed MRI. Skelet Radiol. 2016;45(5):635–44.
41. Klein EE, et al. Magnetic resonance imaging versus musculoskeletal ultrasound for identification and localization of plantar plate tears. Foot Ankle Spec. 2012;5(6):359–65.
42. Donegan RJ, et al. Comparing magnetic resonance imaging and high-resolution ultrasonography for diagnosis of plantar plate pathology: a case series. J Foot Ankle Surg. 2017;56(2):371–4.
43. Duan X, et al. Role of magnetic resonance imaging versus ultrasound for detection of plantar plate tear. J Orthop Surg Res. 2017;12(1):14.
44. Stevens CJ, et al. Plantar plate tear diagnosis using dual-energy computed tomography colagen material decomposition application. J Comput Assist Tomogr. 2013;37(3):478–80.
45. Judge MS, Hild G. A suture button technique for stabilization of the plantar plate and lesser metatarsophalangeal joint. J Foot Ankle Surg. 2018;57(4):645–53.
46. Weil L Jr, et al. Anatomic plantar plate repair using the weil metatarsal osteotomy approach. Foot Ankle Spec. 2011;4(3):145–50.
47. Sung W. Technique using interference fixation repair for plantar plate ligament disruption of lesser metatarsophalangeal joints. J Foot Ankle Surg. 2015;54(3):508–12.
48. McAlister JE, Hyer CF. The direct plantar plate repair technique. Foot Ankle Spec. 2013;6(6):446–51.
49. Donegan RJ, Caminear D. Anatomic repair of plantar plate with flexor tendon shealth reinforcement: case series. Foot Ankle Spec. 2016;9(5):438–43.
50. Nery C, et al. Plantar plate radiofrequency and Weil osteotomy for subtle metatarsophalangeal joint instability. J Orthop Surg Res. 2015;10:180.

51. Lui TH. Correction of crossover toe deformity by arthroscopically assisted plantar plate tenodesis. Arthosc Tech. 2016;5(6):e1273–9.
52. Lui T. Correction of crossover deformity of the second toe by combined plantar plate tenodesis and extensor digitorum brevis transfer: a minimally invasive approach. Arch Orthop Trauma Surg. 2011;131:1247–52.
53. Bouch RT, Heit EJ. Combined plantar plate and hammer toe repair with flexor digitorum longus tendon transfer for chronic, severe sagittal plant instability of the lesser metatarsophalangeal joints: preliminary observations. J Foot Ankle Surg. 2008;47(2):125–37.
54. Highlander P, VonHerbulis E, Gonzalez A, Joshua B, Buchman J. Complications of the Weil metatarsal osteotomy. Foot Ankle Spec. 2011;4(3):165–70.
55. Sorensen MD, Weil L Jr. Lesser metatarsal osteotomy. Clin Podiatr Med Surg. 2015;32(3):275–90.
56. Migues A, et al. Floating toe deformity as a complication of the Weil ostoetomy. Foot Ankle Int. 2004;25:609–13.
57. O'Kane C, Kilmartin TE. The surgical management of central metatarsalgia. Foot Ankle Int. 2002;23:415–9.
58. Trnka HJ, et al. Comparison of the results of the Weil and Helal osteotomies for the treatment of metatarsalgia secondary to dislocation of the lesser metatarsophalangeal joints. Foot Ankle Int. 1999;20:72–9.
59. Hoffsaetter SG, et al. The Weil osteotomy: a seven year follow up. J Bone Joint Surg Br. 2005;87:1507–11.
60. Perez HR, Reber LK, Christensen JC. The role of passive plantar flexion in floating toes following Weil osteotomy. J Foot Ankle Surg. 2008;47(6):520–6.
61. McGlamry ED. Floating toe syndrome. J Am Podiatr Assoc. 1982;72:561–8.
62. Hicks JH. The mechanics of the foot: II. The plantar aponeurosis and the arch. J Anat. 1954;88:25–30.
63. Lee LC, Charlton TP, Thordarson DB. Flexor digitorum brevis transfer for floating toe prevention after Weil osteotomy: a cadaveric study. Foot Ankle Int. 2013:34(12);1724–8.
64. Flint WW, Macias DM, Jastifer JR, Doty JF, Hirose CB, Coughlin MJ. Plantar plate repair for lesser metatarsophalangeal joint instability. Foot Ankle Int. 2017:38(3):234–42.
65. Klein EE, et al. Intermediate term outcomes of the dorsal approach plantar plate repair. in press.

# Chapter 5
# Lapidus Bunionectomy

**Daniel J. Hatch**

## History

The Lapidus bunionectomy has evolved over the years and has become increasingly popular with foot and ankle surgeons for a variety of reasons. Albrecht first described this procedure in 1911 [1]. Truslow coined the term metatarsus primus varus in 1925 [2], which was in reference to the adduction deformity of the first metatarsal in the transverse plane and not varus as we understand it today in the frontal plane. In 1934, Lapidus stated "the only mechanically sound osteotomy for metatarsus primus varus should be at the metatarsocuneiform joint which is at the apex of the angulation between the first metatarsal and cuneiform joint" [3]. A true Lapidus procedure involves arthrodesis of the first tarsometatarsal joint and the bases of the first and second metatarsals. Modifications are commonly performed by only either fusing the first tarsometatarsal joint (TMTJ) or employing screw stabilization or arthrodesis between the first and second rays if instability is observed in either the sagittal or transverse planes.

D. J. Hatch (✉)
Clinical Instructor: Scholl College of Podiatric Medicine, North Chicago, IL, USA

Director of Surgery: North Colorado Podiatric Surgical Residency, Greeley, CO, USA

Private Practice: Foot and Ankle Center of the Rockies, Denver, CO, USA
e-mail: dhatch@facrockies.com



D. E. Tower (ed.), *Evidence-Based Podiatry*,
https://doi.org/10.1007/978-3-030-50853-1_5

## Indications

### *Historical*

Classic indications for the Lapidus bunionectomy have been based on severity-oriented algorithms and include hypermobility in the transverse and sagittal planes; increased deformity of the intermetatarsal (IM) angle; presence of osteoarthritis of the first TMTJ; and, significant elevation of the first ray. Condon et al. in 2002 described a severity-based algorithm for hallux valgus repair in which a severe deformity was classified as an IM angle of 16 degrees or greater [4]. This also was supported by Coughlin and Jones in 2007 [5]. Traditionally, it has been in this class of severe deformity that the Lapidus procedure would be performed. Additionally, hypermobility of the first ray has been a criterion for the Lapidus procedure. While still a precise clinical enigma, many descriptions of first ray hypermobility have been attempted. Due to the difficulty in defining hypermobility, many now prefer to call this condition first ray insufficiency or instability. Many authors believe that hypermobility of the first ray unlocks the forefoot predisposing it to hallux abducto valgus (HAV) deformity [3, 6, 7]. D'Amico wrote an excellent review of first ray mechanics in 2016 [8]. In his article he stated "hypermobility of the first ray…occurs primarily at the medial cuneiform-navicular articulation caused by subtalar and midtarsal joint pronation as a result of inherently induced phylogenetic and ontogenic induced imperfections." In 2017, Kimura et al. stated that hypermobility occurs along the entire first ray [9].

The majority of articles discuss hypermobility in the sagittal plane. It was discussed in 1977 by Root et al. as motion in excess of equal amounts of dorsal and plantar displacement of the first ray compared to the second ray [10]. Roukis and Landsman described a dynamic Hicks test in their review of the literature in 2003 [11]. In this case, the windlass mechanism would be engaged while evaluating the degree of sagittal plane deviation of the first ray. The power of the windlass mechanism was detailed by Rush et al. in 2000 [12]. They found significant loss of the windlass mechanism when hallux valgus deformity was present. Additionally, realignment of the first ray and sesamoids provides successful engagement of the windlass mechanism. Shibuya et al. found in their systematic review that there was 3.62 mm displacement of the first ray in the sagittal plane in the hallux valgus group [13]. Radiographic signs of sagittal plane instability include second ray overload with stress fractures and plantar gapping of the first TMTJ (Fig. 5.1).

Transverse instability or "splay" as an indication for the Lapidus bunionectomy is less pronounced in the literature. Weber et al. described a "splay test" that represented transverse plane instability especially in a Romash 1 foot type [14]. This was later reinforced by Fleming et al. who found that in patients with hallux valgus, 73.8% had transverse plane instability [15].

Hypermobility not only influences the HAV deformity, but it increases the chance of recurrence and overload to the second ray as pointed out by Feilmeier et al. [16].

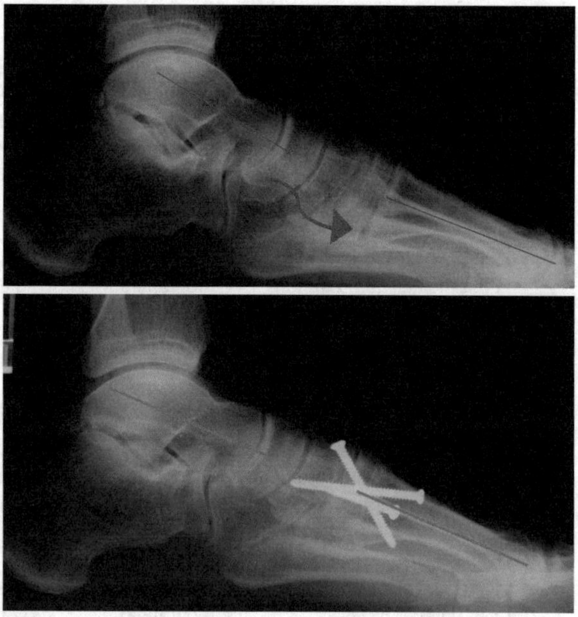

**Fig. 5.1** Lateral view of foot illustrating plantar gapping at the first tarsometatarsal joint and subsequent repair. (Photo courtesy of Meagan Jennings, DPM, FACFAS)

## *Current Indications*

Current indications for the Lapidus bunionectomy are based on the historical perspective along with an improved understanding of three-dimensional analysis of the first ray. The anatomic-based approach has been discussed by Hatch et al. in 2018 [17] (Table 5.1) and involves an understanding of the frontal plane component of the first ray as elucidated in current literature. An improved understanding of the three-dimensional aspects of the first ray has evolved since Mizuno first described hypertorsion of the first metatarsal in 1956 [18]. Scranton and Rutkowski, in their 1980 study, found patients with HAV had 14.5 degrees of valgus rotation of the first ray versus 3.1 degrees in those without HAV [19]. Eustace, in 1994, described a valgus rotation of the first metatarsal with bunion deformity [20]. Talbot and Saltzman found that pronation of the first metatarsal changed the apparent position of the sesamoids on the AP radiographic view [21]. Okuda et al. described a lateral rounding of the first metatarsal in the HAV group indicating rotation in the frontal plane [22]. This rotation was also substantiated by Yamaguchi et al. in 2015 [23]. Mortier, in 2012, found the first ray to be pronated in the HAV group by an average of 12.7 degrees [24]. Dayton et al. pointed out that our evaluations of the bunion deformity may be flawed and also found significant valgus rotation of the first ray in HAV patients [25]. With improved imaging provided by three-dimensional computerized tomography (CT), it has become clear that a majority of patients with hallux valgus possess a valgus rotation of the first ray. This rotation may be intrinsic as described by Ota et al. [26] or extrinsic as elucidated by many recent authors. Unless the valgus rotation is addressed surgically, recurrences can be expected due to

**Table 5.1** Classification of triplane HAV deformity by Hatch et al. 2018

| Triplane Hallux Valgus Classification and Treatment Algorithm | | | |
|---|---|---|---|
| Class | Anatomic findings | MTP joint status | Treatment recommendation |
| 1 | Increased HVA and IMA<br>No first metatarsal pronation evident on AP and sesamoid axial radiograph<br>Sesamoids may be subluxed | No clinical or radiographic evidence of DJD | Metatarsal osteotomy or TMT correction. Sesamoid release to help realign complex |
| 2A | Increased HVA and IMA<br>First metatarsal pronation evident on AP and sesamoid axial radiograph<br>No sesamoid subluxation on axial | No clinical or radiographic evidence of DJD | Triplane correction including first metatarsal inversion<br>+/- Lateral capsulotomy |
| 2B | Increased HVA and IMA<br>First metatarsal pronation evident on AP and sesamoid axial radiograph<br>With sesamoid subluxation on axial | No clinical or radiographic evidence of DJD | Triplane correction including first metatarsal inversion<br>Conservative lateral capsular release prior to correction |
| 3 | Increased HVA and IMA<br>>20 degrees MTA | No clinical or radiographic evidence of DJD | Metatarsal 2 and 3 transverse plane correction<br>Metatarsal osteotomy or TMT correction per class 1 and 2 recommendations |
| 4 | Increased HVA and IMA<br>+/- First metatarsal pronation | Clinical and or radiographic evidence of DJD | First MTP arthrodesis preferred; joint arthroplasty |

Definitions: *MTP* Metatarsophalangeal, *HVA* Hallux valgus angle, *IMA* Intermetatarsal angle, *AP* Anterioposterior, *DJD* Degerative joint disease, *MTA* Metatarsus adductus, *TMT* Tarsometatarsal

malalignment of the sesamoid complex [27]. The center of rotation and angulation (CORA) is defined by Paley as either mechanical or anatomic [28]. The first TMTJ location is the most easily accessed site surgically to address the triplane component of HAV and also represents the anatomic CORA of the deformity between the medial cuneiform and the first metatarsal [25, 29, 30]. The mechanical axis of the first ray has been discussed by LaPorta et al. in 2016 [31]. They described the mechanical axis being very proximal in the rearfoot. Indeed, the majority of motion within the first ray is at the navicular-medial cuneiform joint [8].

## Radiographic Evaluation

Preoperative planning is essential for adequate bunion correction. The weight bearing (WB) AP projection is used to evaluate the IM and the hallux valgus angles (HVA). These angles are the only ones that have been validated over various studies.

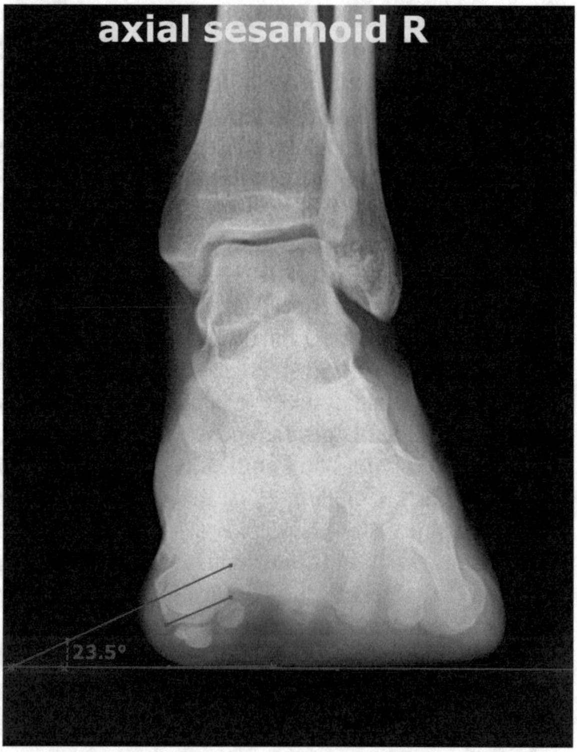


**Fig. 5.2** Axial view showing the amount of metatarsal rotation in frontal plane

The distal metatarsal articular angle (DMAA), also known as the proximal articular set angle (PASA), has proven to be less reliable [5, 32, 33]. The WB lateral projection is utilized to assess Meary's angle and the Seiberg index. If elevation of the first ray is observed, then it should be addressed at the time of surgery. There is a renewed importance of the WB axial sesamoid view since Kim et al. demonstrated frontal plane rotation of the first metatarsal via 3-D CT analysis [34]. The axial view will evaluate the amount of eversion of the metatarsal when it exists and the degree, if any, of sesamoid subluxation (Fig. 5.2). When sesamoid subluxation occurs, a first metatarsophalangeal joint (MTPJ) lateral release should be performed to properly align the sesamoid complex upon realignment of the metatarsal.

## Anatomy and Surgical Biomechanics

It has long been thought that the obliquity of the medial cuneiform was a primary etiological factor in hallux valgus. Truslow, in 1925, coined the term "metatarsus primus varus" with his understanding of the deviation of the first metatarsal-cuneiform joint in the transverse plane even though we understand varus to be a component of the frontal plane [2]. DJ Morton described metatarsus atavicus in

1927 [6]. Lapidus described the "atavistic" foot in 1934 as an etiological factor in hallux valgus [3]. However, more recent studies show that the obliquity of this joint does not correlate with HAV deformity [35–38]. Vyas specifically found that the morphology of the medial cuneiform was not involved in HAV deformity [35].

Doty et al. gave an excellent description of the first metatarsal-cuneiform joint [36], and their cadaveric study revealed an average depth of 28.3 mm and width of 13.1 mm. The joint is typically continuous (59%) vs bi-lobed (38%) [36]. The lateral inclination angle, formed by the TMTJ and the WB surface observed on the lateral view, averages 26.5 degrees [36]. The first ray is inherently unstable. As such, there are static and dynamic stabilizers of the first ray that should be appreciated. Static stabilizers are the articulations of the first TMTJ, intercuneiform joint, and the medial cuneiform and second metatarsal base [10, 39, 40]. Additionally, the plantar first metatarsal-medial cuneiform ligament is a static force [41]. Dynamic stabilizers include the plantar aponeurosis and the peroneus longus. The effects of the plantar aponeurosis on stabilization of the first ray have been described by Rush et al. [12]. Later, Coughlin et al. also noted this effect [42]. The peroneus longus locks the first ray in eversion [43–45]. This action is inhibited by significant ankle equinus and pronation of the subtalar and midtarsal joints [8, 46]. Bierman et al. discussed the effects of the Lapidus on peroneal longus function [47] and found increased efficiency of the longus in stabilizing the first ray after the Lapidus procedure. The peroneus longus also everts the medial cuneiform and elevates the talus. Lastly, as previously stated, the windlass mechanism is now more functionally employed [12, 46].

## Surgical Considerations

There are many variations of this surgical technique ranging from the traditional Lapidus to more contemporary approaches. The common denominator is the fusion of the first TMTJ. Adjacent ray fusion is employed when transverse or sagittal plane instability is observed or noted [14, 15]. The adjacent ray fusion may incorporate the medial cuneiform to second metatarsal base or intercuneiform joints (Fig. 5.3). Incisional exposure is based on surgeon preference and may be a long dorsal incision or a smaller dorsal incision at the base of the first TMTJ and an additional medial incision if needed over the first MTPJ.

Literature has supported the importance of proper sesamoid alignment postoperatively to prevent recurrence of the HAV deformity [27]. Further analysis of the sesamoid- metatarsal complex has evolved through current 3-D CT and has demonstrated that the deformity is indeed a triplanar condition that must be addressed surgically. Hatch et al. have developed a new classification scheme that is based upon this 3-D anatomy [48]. In Hatch et al.'s classification system, the sesamoids may be rotated with the metatarsal and or displaced. When displaced, especially in long-standing conditions, the sesamoid complex must be released in order to be properly realigned (Fig. 5.4). When the sesamoids

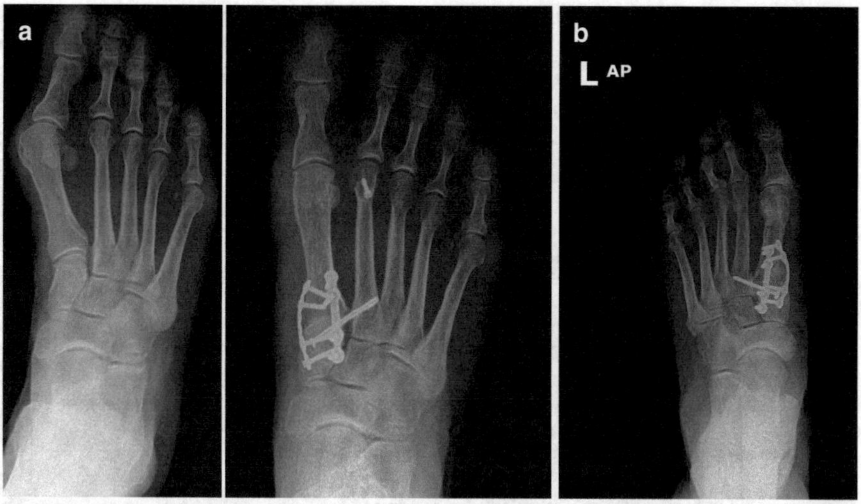


**Fig. 5.3** When there is noticeable gapping at the medial cuneiform – 2nd metatarsal base or intercuneiform joint along with clinical transverse plane instability, a fusion is performed between the 1st and 2nd rays. (**a**) This example shows the AP preop and postop. (**b**) This is a postoperative example

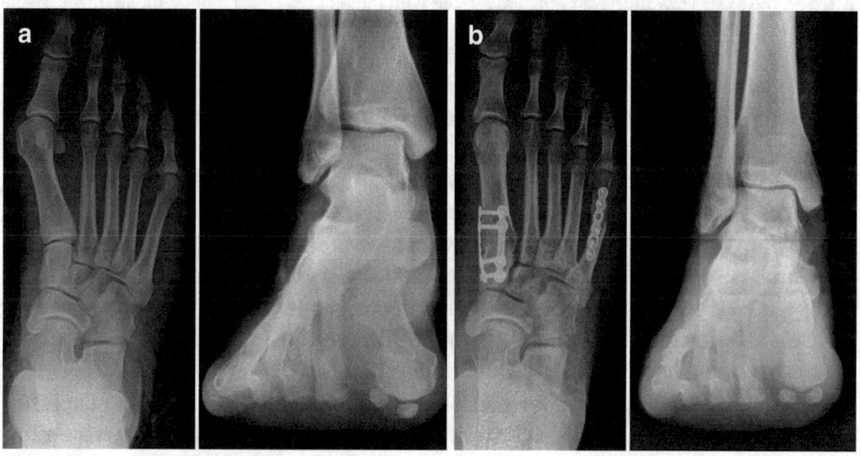


**Fig. 5.4** (**a**) Preoperative AP and axial views demonstrate sesamoid subluxation. (**b**) Postoperative AP and axial alignments are three dimensionally anatomic

are deviated in the AP projection but aligned in the axial, it is a sign of net first ray rotation that must be addressed at the time of surgery (Fig. 5.5).

Fixation constructs have evolved over time with the quest for earlier postoperative WB. Traditionally, a 2–3 screw construct has been employed. Hansen realized that precompressing a joint with axial loading created shear at the site [49]. Since

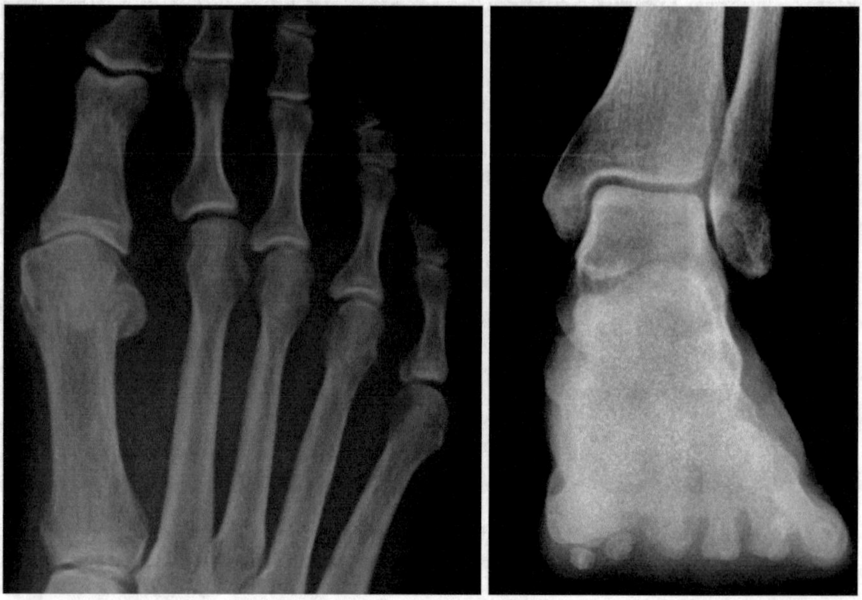

**Fig. 5.5** Radiographs demonstrating apparent sesamoid subluxation on AP view, but when analyzed on the axial view the sesamoids are rotated with the metatarsal segment with an intact cristae and are not subluxed

the foot is loaded tangentially to the long axis of the bone, shear forces are created with weight bearing, and joint compression is generated with standard rigid internal fixation. The bone graft allows micromotion and secondary bone healing which has shown to be quicker and stronger by Perren's studies [50]. Hence, Hansen developed a shear-strain-relieved bone graft to mitigate the shear effect, which has also been supported by Mani et al. in 2015 [51]. Traditionally, postoperative protocols included 6 weeks of non-weight bearing (NWB) followed by 6 weeks of protected WB in a CAM boot. Although, King et al. with screw constructs, reported early partial WB at 12 days and full WB at 4 weeks [52]. Patient acceptance of lengthy NWB or partial WB parameters was low, and hence surgeons began to strive for newer and stronger surgical constructs that would allow earlier WB. Several recent studies have advocated early WB with conventional screw constructs [52, 53]. Plate and screw combinations have evolved and allowed for earlier WB [54]. Newer biplanar constructs, advocated by Peren in 2002, take into account the concept of "biologic healing" [50]. Micromotion at the arthrodesis site allows for callus formation yielding a faster and stronger arthrodesis. A large level III study was performed by Prissel et al. (2016) and compared early versus delayed WB; they found no difference in union rates [55]. Some of the newer fixation constructs may allow for early WB (from immediate to early [2 weeks]) (Fig. 5.6).

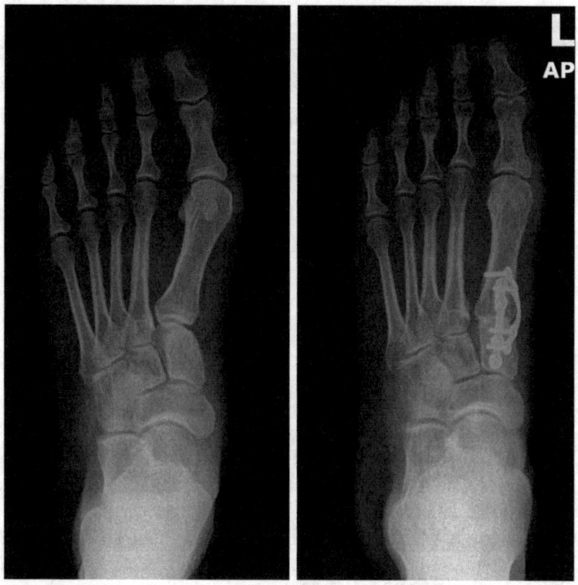


**Fig. 5.6** Example of "biologic" fixation without rigid internal fixation for the HAV deformity. Shown is AP preop and AP postop

## Complications

Complications of the Lapidus bunionectomy are similar to other types of bunion procedures and include shortening or elevation of the first metatarsal; nonunion of the fusion site(s); and recurrence of deformity. Shortening of the first metatarsal is minimized by using cutting jig guides or curettage technique during joint resection/preparation. Elevation of the first metatarsal is avoided by proper technique and checking with lateral image fluoroscopy during the surgical procedure. Reports of nonunion for the Lapidus bunionectomy have ranged from 3.3% to 12% [56]. Barp et al. reported nonunion rates of 6.7% in 147 procedures [57]. Even more encouraging was a Mani et al. study in 2015 reporting a 2.7% nonunion rate if meticulous joint preparation, internal fixation, and a shear-strain bone graft were utilized [51]. Recurrence of the deformity is due to lack of sesamoid alignment [27, 58] and under-correction of the IM angle [59]. Achieving a collinear alignment of the first ray will optimize the direct pull of the tendons inserting onto the hallux. With a dorsal incision, there may be compromise or irritation to the medial dorsal cutaneous nerve.

## Summary

The Lapidus bunionectomy is a dependable procedure that helps minimize the chance of recurrence while providing a surgically amenable site to address the triplane deformity of the first ray. The first TMTJ site is considered the anatomic

CORA of the deformity. However, this does not discount that more proximal motions are pathologic for the condition, especially motion at the intercuneiform and navicular-cuneiform joints. When excessive motion occurs at the intercuneiform and navicular-cuneiform joints, stabilization may be achieved by intercuneiform or medial cuneiform-second metatarsal base arthrodesis. The triplane deformity of the first ray may be easily addressed at the first TMTJ, and as a result of arthrodesis of the first TMTJ, the effects of peroneus longus and the windlass mechanism are enhanced to stabilize the first ray.

## References


1. Albrecht GH. The pathology and treatment of hallux valgus. Russ Vrach. 1911;10:14.
2. Truslow W. Metatarsus primus varus or hallux valgus. JBJS. 1925;7:98–108.
3. Lapidus P. Operative correction of the metatarsal varus primus in hallux valgus. Surg Gynecol Obsetet. 1934;58:183–91.
4. Condon F, Kaliszer M, Conhyea D, O'Donnell T, Shaju A, Masterson E. The first intermetatarsal angle in hallux valgus: an analysis of measurement reliability and the error involved. Foot Ankle Int. 2002;23:717–21.
5. Coughlin MJ, Jones CP. Hallux valgus: demographics, etiology, and radiographic assessment. Foot Ankle Int. 2007;28:759–77.
6. Morton DJ. Metatarsus Atavicus. JBJS. 1927;9:531–4.
7. Hansen ST Jr. Introduction: the first metatarsal: it's importance in the human foot. Clin Podiatr Med Surg. 2009;26:351–4.
8. D'Amico JC. Understanding the first ray. Podiatry Management. 2016;9:109–20.
9. Kimura T, Kubota M, Taguchi T, Suzuki N, Hattori A, Marumo K. Evaluation of first-ray mobility in patients with hallux valgus using weight-bearing CT and a 3-D analysis system: a comparison with normal feet. J Bone Joint Surg Am. 2017;99:247–55.
10. Root ML, Orien WP, Weed JH. Normal and abnormal function of the foot. Clin Biomech. 1977;Vol 2.
11. Roukis TS, Landsman AS. Hypermobility of the first ray: a critical review of the literature. J Foot Ankle Surg. 2003;42:377–90.
12. Rush SM, Christiansen JC, Johnson CH. Biomechanics of the first ray. Part II: metatarsus primus varus as a cause of hypermobility. A three dimensional kinematic analysis in a cadaver model. J Foot Ankle Surg. 2000;39:68–77.
13. Shibuya N, Roukis T, Jupiter DC. Mobility of the first ray in patients with or without hallux valgus deformity: systematic review and meta-analysis. J Foot Ankle Surg. 2017;56:1070–5.
14. Weber AK, Hatch DJ, Jensen JL. Use of the first ray splay test to assess transverse plane instability before first metatarsocuneiform fusion. J Foot Ankle Surg. 2006;45:278–82.
15. Fleming JJ, Kwaadu KY, Brinkley JC, Ozuzu Y. Intraoperative evaluation of medial intercuneiform instability after lapidus arthrodesis: intercuneiform hook test. J Foot Ankle Surg. 2015;54:464–72.
16. Feilmeier M, Dayton P, Wienke JC Jr. Reduction of intermetatarsal angle after first metatarsophalangeal joint arthrodesis in patients with hallux valgus. J Foot Ankle Surg. 2014;53:29–31.
17. Hatch DJ, Santrock RD, Smith B, Dayton P, Weil L. Triplane hallux abducto valgus classification. J Foot Ankle Surg. 2018;57(5):972–81.
18. Mizuno S, Sima Y, Yamazaki K. Detorsion osteotomy of the first metatarsal bone in hallux valgus. J Jpn Orthop Assoc. 1956;30:813–9.
19. Scranton PE Jr, Rutkowski R. Anatomic variations in the first ray: part I. Anatomic aspects related to bunion surgery. Clin Orthop Relat Res. 1980;151:244–55.

20. Eustace S, Byrne JO, Beausang O, Codd M, Stack J, Stephens MM. Hallux valgus, first metatarsal pronation and collapse of the medial longitudinal arch--a radiological correlation. Skelet Radiol. 1994;23:191–4.
21. Talbot KD, Saltzman CL. Assessing sesamoid subluxation: how good is the AP radiograph? Foot Ankle Int. 1998;19:547–54.
22. Okuda R, Kinoshita M, Yasuda T, Jotoku T, Kitano N, Shima H. The shape of the lateral edge of the first metatarsal as a risk factor for recurrence of hallux valgus. JBJS. 2007;89:2161–72.
23. Yamaguchi S, Sasho T, Endo J, Yamamoto Y, Akagi R, Sato Y, Takahashi K. Shape of the lateral edge of the first metatarsal head changes depending on the rotation and inclination of the first metatarsal: a study using digitally reconstructed radiographs. J Orthop Sci. 2015;20:868–74.
24. Mortier J-P, Bernard J-L, Maestro M. Axial rotation of the first metatarsal head in a normal population and hallux valgus patients. Orthop Traumatol Surg Res. 2012;98:677–83.
25. Dayton P, Kauwe M, Feilmeier M. Is our current paradigm for evaluation and management of the bunion deformity flawed? A discussion of procedure philosophy relative to anatomy. J Foot Ankle Surg. 2015;54:102–11.
26. Ota T, Nagura T, Kokubo T, Kitashiro M, Ogihara N, Takeshima K, Seki H, Suda Y, Matsumoto M, Nakamura M. Etiological factors in hallux valgus, a three-dimensional analysis of the first metatarsal. J Foot Ankle Res. 2017;10:43.
27. Shibuya N, Kyprios EM, Panchani P, Martin LR, Thorud J, Jupiter DC. Factors associated with early loss of hallux valgus correction. J Foot Ankle Surg. 2018;57:236–40.
28. Paley D. Principles of deformity correction. Berlin, Heidelberg: Springer Berlin Heidelberg; 2002.
29. Tanaka Y, Takakura Y, Kumai T, Samoto N, Tamai S. Radiographic analysis of hallux valgus. JBJS. 1995;77A:205–13.
30. Paley D, Foot N, Correction D. Principles of foot deformity correction: ilizarov technique. In: Gould JS, editor. Operative foot surgery. Phildelphia: WB Saunders; 1994. p. 476–514.
31. LaPorta GA, Nasser EM, Mulhern JL, Malay DS. The mechanical axis of the first ray: a radiographic assessment in Hallux abducto valgus evaluation. J Foot Ankle Surg. 2016;55:28–34.
32. Coughlin MJ, Freund E. The reliability of angular measurements in hallux valgus deformities. Foot Ankle Int. 2001;22:369–79.
33. Lee KM, Chung CY, Park MS, Lee SH, Cho JH, Choi IH. Reliability and validity of radiographic measurements in hindfoot varus and valgus. J Bone Joint Surg Am. 2010;92:2319–27.
34. Kim Y, Kim JS, Young KW, Naraghi R, Cho HK, Lee SY. A new measure of tibial sesamoid position in hallux valgus in relation to the coronal rotation of the first metatarsal in CT scans. Foot Ankle Int. 2015;36:944–52.
35. Vyas S, Conduah A, Vyas N, Otsuka NY. The role of the first metarsocuneiform joint in juvenile hallux valgus. J Pediatr Orthop B. 2010;19:399–402.
36. Doty JF, Coughlin MJ, Hirose C, et al. First metatarsocuneiform joint mobility: radiographic, anatomic, and clinical characteristics of the articular surface. Foot Ankle Int. 2014;35:504–11.
37. Hatch DJ, Smith A, Fowler T. Radiographic relevance of the distal medial cuneiform angle in hallux valgus assessment. J Foot Ankle Surg. 2016;55:85–9.
38. Houghton GR, Dickson JR. Hallux valgus in the younger patient. JBJS. 1979;61:176–7.
39. Hicks JH. The mechanics of the foot. J Anat. 1954;88:25–30.1.
40. Dykyj D, Ateshian GA, Trepal MJ, MacDonald LR. Articular geometry of the medial TMTJ comparison of metatarsus primus adductus and metatarsus primus rectus. J Foot Ankle Surg. 2001;40:357–65.
41. Mizel MS. The role of the plantar first metatarsal first cuneiform ligament in weightbearing on the first metatarsal. Foot Ankle. 1993;14:82–4.
42. Coughlin MJ, Jones CP, Viladot R, Golanó P, Glanó P, Grebing BR, Kennedy MJ, Shurnas PS, Alvarez F. Hallux valgus and first ray mobility: a cadaveric study. Foot Ankle Int. 2004;25:537–44.
43. Johnson CH, Christensen JC. Biomechanics of the first ray part I. The effects of peroneus longus function: a three-dimensional kinematic study on a cadaver model. J Foot Ankle Surg. 1999;38:313–21.

44. Dullaert K, Hagen J, Klos K, Gueorguiev B, Lenz M, Richards RG, Simons P. The influence of the Peroneus Longus muscle on the foot under axial loading: a CT evaluated dynamic cadaveric model study. Clin Biomech. 2016;34:7–11.
45. Klemola T, Leppilahti J, Laine V, Pentikäinen I, Ojala R, Ohtonen P, Savola O. Effect of first tarsometatarsal joint derotational arthrodesis on first ray dynamic stability compared to distal chevron osteotomy. Foot Ankle Int. 2017:38:1–8.
46. Faber F, Mulder P, Verhaarr J. Role of first ray hypermobility in the outcome of the Hohmann and the Lapidus procedure. JBJS. 2004;86A:486–95.
47. Bierman RA, Christensen JC, Johnson CH. Biomechanics of the first ray. Part III. Consequences of lapidus arthrodesis on peroneus longus function: a three-dimensional kinematic analysis in a cadaver model. J Foot Ankle Surg. 2001;40:125–31.
48. Dayton PD, editor. Radiographic assessment. In: Evidence-based bunion surgery. Springer International: New York; 2018. p. 61–72.
49. Hansen ST. Functional reconstruction of the foot and ankle. Philadelphia: Lippincott Williams & Wilkins; 2000.
50. Perren SM. Evolution of the internal fixation of long bone fractures. J Bone Joint Surg (Br). 2002;84:1093–110.
51. Mani SB, Lloyd EW, MacMahon A, Roberts MM, Levine DS, Ellis SJ. Modified lapidus procedure with joint compression, meticulous surface preparation, and shear-strain-relieved bone graft yields low nonunion rate. HSS J. 2015;11:243–8.
52. King CM, Richey J, Patel S, Collman DR. Modified lapidus arthrodesis with crossed screw fixation: early weightbearing in 136 patients. J Foot Ankle Surg. 2015;54:69–75.
53. Basile P, Cook EA, Cook JJ. Immediate weight bearing following modified lapidus arthrodesis. J Foot Ankle Surg. 2010;49:459–64.
54. Cottom JM, Vora AM. Fixation of lapidus arthrodesis with a plantar interfragmentary screw and medial locking plate: a report of 88 cases. J Foot Ankle Surg. 2013;52:465–9.
55. Prissel MA, Hyer CF, Grambart ST, et al. A multicenter, retrospective study of early weightbearing for modified lapidus arthrodesis. J Foot Ankle Surg. 2016;55:226–9.
56. Patel S, Ford LA, Etcheverry J, Rush SM, Hamilton GA. Modified lapidus arthrodesis: rate of nonunion in 227 cases. J Foot Ankle Surg. 2004;43(1):37–42.
57. Barp EA, Erickson JG, Smith HL, Armeida K, Millonig K. Evaluation of fixation techniques for the metatarsocuneiform arthrodesis. J Foot Ankle Surg. 2017;56(3):468–73.
58. Park CH, Lee W-C. Recurrence of hallux valgus can be predicted from immediate postoperative non-weight-bearing radiographs. J Bone Joint Surg Am. 2017;99:1190–7.
59. Raikin SM, Miller AG, Daniel J. Recurrence of hallux valgus: a review. Foot Ankle Clin. 2014;19:259–74.

# Chapter 6
# Midfoot Arthritis

**Christopher R. Hood Jr**

## Background

Tarsometatarsal (TMT) joint or midfoot arthritis is a common source of pain, disability, and deformity. With respect to the midfoot, two common types of arthritis are encountered, including primary osteoarthritis (OA) and secondary post-traumatic arthritis (PTA). OA includes the classic "wear and tear" degenerative joint disease that typically progresses as patients age, while PTA occurs some indeterminate time frame after a traumatizing event (e.g., fracture, crush, ligament injury). Between the two forms, PTA is reported as the more common etiology with the inciting trauma often a LisFranc complex injury, whether isolated ligamentous or fracture dislocation, resulting in complex breakdown and subsequent arthritis [1–3]. LisFranc complex injuries represent <1% of all fractures, affecting 1 in 55,000 people with an up to 20% missed diagnosis rate [4]. The age of arthritis onset is typically bimodal, with PTA patients presenting in the third-fourth decades, while OA patients present later in their sixth-seventh decades of life [5–8]. Literature regarding primary OA is sparse compared to PTA with respect to arthritis and reconstruction after onset.

Multiple treatment options exist for both conservative and surgical management of midfoot arthritis. A complete work up using the patients' past medical and trauma history, subjective complaints, physical exam with specific tests, and radiographic evaluation is collectively used to set forth an appropriate treatment plan. Based on the above findings, surgical options include procedures from a simple exostectomy or specific column arthroplasty, to more complicated fusions (isolated or multiple columns) with or without deformity correction. Additionally, there has been much debate about the appropriate treatment of the lateral column. The dispute over the lateral column is whether to include it in a concomitant medial and/or middle

C. R. Hood Jr (✉)
Hunterdon Podiatric Medicine, Hunterdon Healthcare System, Flemington, NJ, USA
e-mail: chood@hhsnj.org



D. E. Tower (ed.), *Evidence-Based Podiatry*,
https://doi.org/10.1007/978-3-030-50853-1_6

column fusion procedure, perform an arthroplasty, or refrain from surgical intervention. Here, we hope to shed light on this complicated pathology and provide direction in decision-making for treatment.

## Anatomy and Biomechanics of the Midfoot

The TMT joint was named after Jacques LisFranc de Saint-Martin based on his reported amputation through this level, despite never describing the ligament or injuries through this anatomic region [9]. However, the joint and specifically the LisFranc ligament have always been ascribed to his name.

The TMT joint, or LisFranc complex, includes the articulations between the bases of the first through fifth metatarsals (MT) distally, and the cuneiforms (e.g., medial, intermediate, lateral; metatarsocuneiform (MC) joints) and cuboid (MT-cuboid joints) proximally, representing the border between the forefoot and midfoot. There are also intercuneiform articulations as well as articulations between the lateral cuneiform and cuboid. Some will include the naviculocuneiform (NC) joint into the midfoot discussion.

There are three types (seven dorsal, five plantar, and three interosseous) of ligaments that cross the TMT joint [9, 10]. LisFranc's articulation and ligament (e.g., medial interosseous ligament) is located between the lateral aspect of the medial cuneiform and medial aspect of the second MT base. The plantar ligaments are the strongest of the three types of capsular ligaments, followed by the interosseous and dorsal ligaments. LisFranc's ligament is the strongest of the three interosseous ligaments. The intercuneiform joints contain two dorsal, two interosseous, and one plantar ligament. The dorsal ligaments join each of the three cuneiforms together, while the plantar ligament exists only between the medial and intermediate cuneiforms. Across the NC joint, each cuneiform is attached to the navicular with a dorsal and plantar ligament (medial dorsal/plantar NC ligaments are the strongest of the three pairs). Additionally, there is a medial NC ligament which receives some of its fibers from the posterior tibial tendon insertion.

The joint can be described based on two concepts: (i) columns and (ii) transverse arch.

- Columns: The foot can be broken down into medial (first MT-medial cuneiform), middle (second/third MT- intermediate/lateral cuneiform), and lateral (fourth/fifth MT-cuboid) columns, first described by Peicha et al. [9]. The second MC articulation appears to be the most important in this complex at maintaining foot stability. Across the three columns, variable sagittal plane motion exists with minimal motion at the middle column (1.5°–1.8° for second MT-middle cuneiform, >4° for third MT-lateral cuneiform) with specifically the second MC joint being recessed in comparison to the adjacent articulations. From there, motion increases at the medial (6–8 mm excursion in dorsal and plantarflexion or 1.5°–5° for first MT-medial cuneiform) and lateral (10° in both dorsal and plantarflexion and supination-pronation for fourth/fifth MT-cuboid) columns [9, 11, 12] (Fig. 6.1).

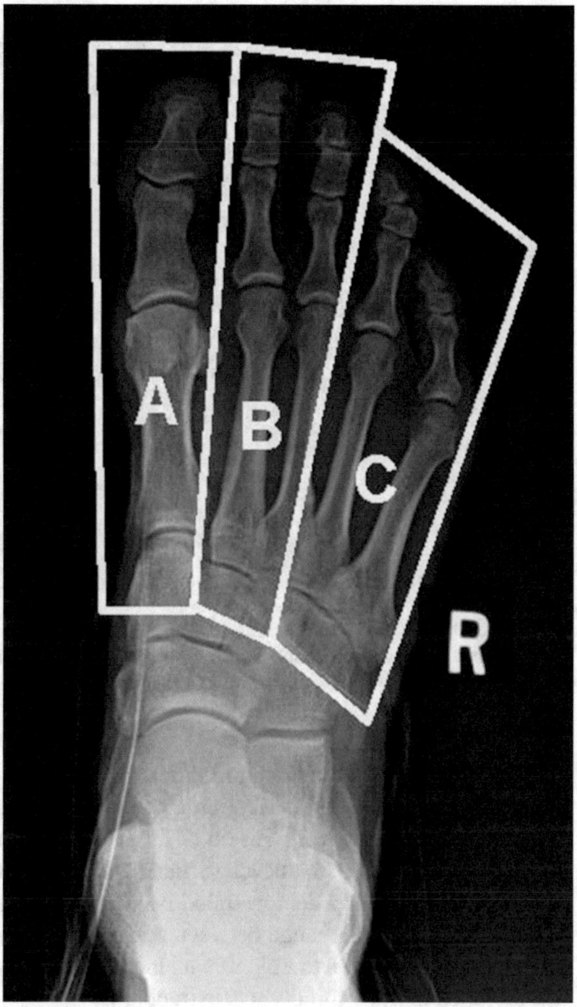


**Fig. 6.1** Weightbearing dorso-plantar x-ray (XR) of the right foot demonstrating the (**a**) medial, (**b**) middle, and (**c**) lateral columns. (Adapted from Patel et al. [4])

- Transverse Arch: In the frontal plane, the joint complex has a Roman arch configuration with the apex at the trapezoidal-shaped second MT base. Furthermore, in the transverse plane, the second MT base sits approximately 8 mm and 4 mm proximally recessed compared to the adjacent medial and lateral cuneiforms, respectively. This increases its stability and subsequent lack of motion across the middle column [4, 9, 10] (Fig. 6.2).

With the combined bony structures and ligamentous support, the medial and middle columns are fairly stiff to support the arch, while the lateral column, which has a less intimate articulation across the MT-cuboid joint, allows for triplane motion [12, 13]. As stress and load is applied to the foot, it is first transmitted to the middle column and then distributed to the medial and lateral columns. In gait, the medial column "rigid lever arm" and the flexibility of the "mobile adaptor" lateral

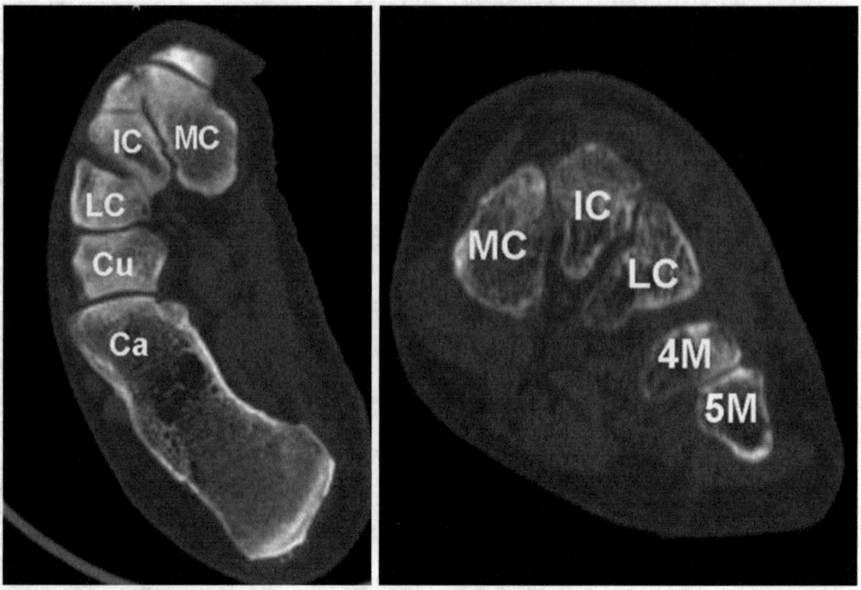


**Fig. 6.2** Computed tomography (left) axial and (right) coronal image through the midfoot demonstrating the transverse arch concept with the keystone intermediate cuneiform (IC). (MC, medial cuneiform; IC, intermediate cuneiform; LC, lateral cuneiform; 4M, 4th metatarsal; 5M, 5th metatarsal; Cu, cuboid; Ca, calcaneus)

column allow the foot to function efficiently while accommodating high or rapid changes in load. These distribution forces and adaptations collectively maintain normal foot function [1, 2]. Fusion of the lateral column can result in a stiffer foot that is less able to adapt to uneven surfaces and accommodate ground reactive forces [14]. A cadaveric study demonstrated isolated lateral forefoot, and calcaneocuboid joint pressure did not change between control (intact) and medial column arthrodesis arms in comparison to a significant increase in pressure when the lateral column was included in the arthrodesis construct [14].

Midfoot stability, whether osseous or ligamentous, provides the pillar for static stance and gait push-off mechanics. Impairment in stability can result in abnormalities in foot posture (e.g., negative lateral Meary's angle, increased plantar ligament tensile stress) and difficulties in both gait and activities that require heel rise (i.e., stairs ascent or decent) [8]. All of these factors owe to the complexity of this joint and the importance for structural integrity to prevent the development of pathology. They also play a role in surgical considerations which will be described later in this chapter.

## Causes of Midfoot Arthritis

There are many causes of midfoot arthritis. Two of the most common include OA and PTA. Additional causes include rheumatoid arthritis (RA) or other seronegative/positive inflammatory arthropathies, Charcot or diabetic neuroarthropathy, biomechanical insufficiencies (e.g., first ray hypermobility, medial column instability), and foot type (e.g., pes planus and pes cavus) [4, 6, 11].

In PTA, an injury to the LisFranc complex, the adjacent joint structures (i.e., fracture causing joint position malalignment) or the joint itself (i.e., intra-articular fracture, joint compression, subchondral marrow edema and cystic changes) results in a change at the joint interface [4, 9]. Often a LisFranc ligament or fracture dislocation is the inciting event with PTA occurring in up to 50% of cases, independent to the injury type or radiographic findings [1, 15, 16]. This high rate may be secondary to the reported staggering 20% missed or misdiagnosed injuries on initial presentation [4, 5]. Even with surgical intervention, the rates of PTA have been reported from 9.5% to 25% when treatment was performed less than 6 weeks from injury while reported at 23% with delayed (>6 weeks) treatment [16, 17]. Initial anatomic reduction is key in reducing PTA. Kuo et al. [17] noted a 16% vs. 60% rate of degenerative changes between patients who had primary anatomic vs. non-anatomic open reduction internal fixation (ORIF).

Mechanism of injury can be broken down into direct (e.g., crush, impact) or indirect causes. The indirect injury, the more common of the two mechanisms, includes abduction or plantarflexion of the forefoot on the rearfoot, or axial loading or twist on a dorsiflexed or plantarflexed foot [9]. In the real world, this translates to injuries commonly seen in high energy motor vehicle accidents (MVA) and falls from height (FFH). However, less innocuous indirect mechanism exists such as a slip, fall, and twist of the foot in the aforementioned motions. Acute treatment of these injuries is not the focus of this chapter, so we will continue with a description of the post-traumatic, degenerative findings of later stage midfoot arthritis often seen several years after the inciting trauma.

Specific to lateral column arthritis, the cause is often a LisFranc complex injury with either a concomitant compression injury to the joint or a latent instability resulting in degenerative changes. Additionally, fifth metatarsal zone 1 fractures, which have been shown to make up >50% of overall fifth metatarsal fractures, are articular and can result in altered joint mechanics and wear [18, 19].

Foot type also plays a role in the development of midfoot alterations [20] (Fig. 6.3). In pronated or flatfoot patients, subtalar pronation results in a loss of the windlass mechanism and unlocking of the midtarsal joint. This pronation can decrease the plantarflexory pull of the peroneus longus on the first ray. The resultant effect is first ray hypermobility, dorsiflexion, and jamming at the medial and middle columns with potential dorsal spur formation. Manifestation of a flatfoot can also be a result of injury, with forefoot abduction and dorsiflexion after a LisFranc complex injury [5]. Conversely, the plantarflexed first ray of a cavus foot results in excessive sub first metatarsal head loading, and as ground reactive forces push the ray into dorsiflexion during gait, similar jamming and spur formation can occur in the medial column. Moreover, a cavus or supinated foot applies greater load to the lateral column and may place this region at risk for pathology (e.g., joint instability through subluxation/dislocation, arthritis) [13]. The correlation of foot type can be seen in both stress to the foot and pain location and findings on imaging [21] (Table 6.1).

Charcot neuroarthropathy is another cause of midfoot arthritis or deformity. In the acute setting, the patient may present similar to a patient with an acute OA flare demonstrating edema and warmth over the foot. Imaging may be misleading

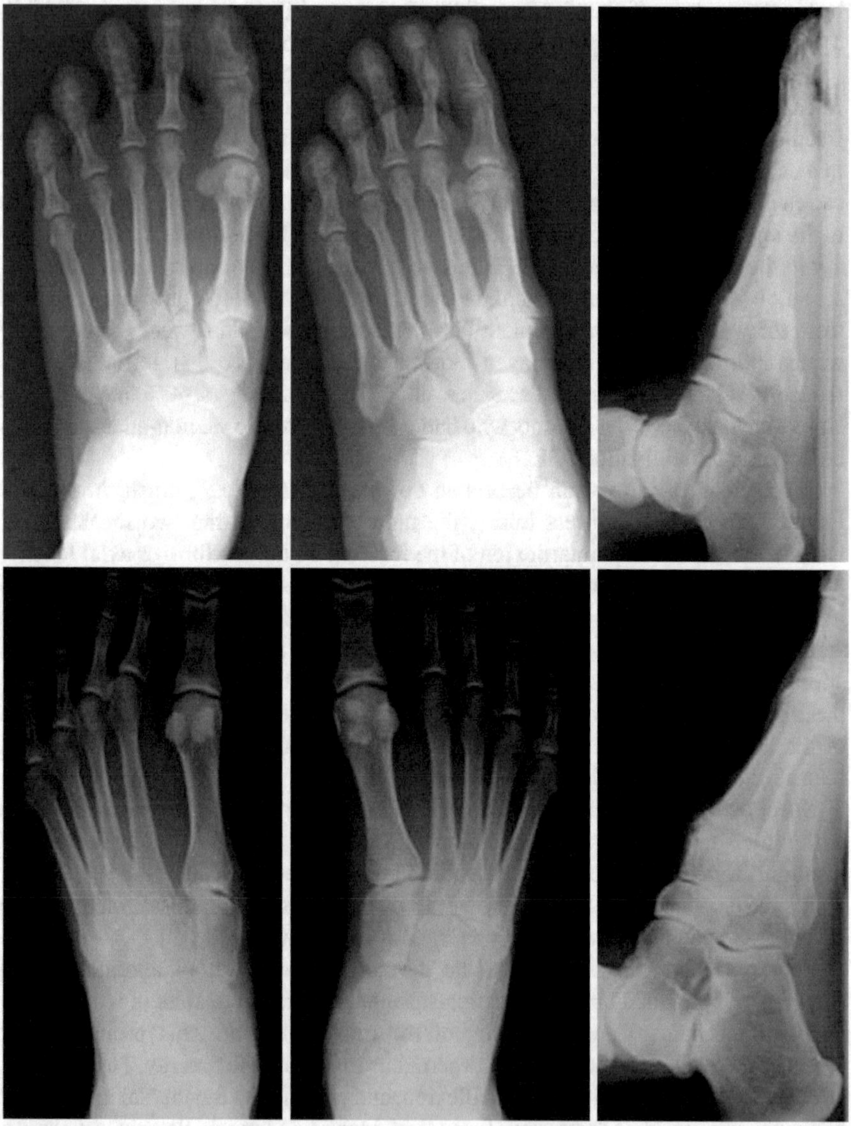

**Fig. 6.3** A 58-year-old male (top) with left foot pes planus deformity with spurring noted at the first-second MC joints. A 46-year-old female (bottom) with left foot rectus/cavus structure and history of LisFranc ligament tear 20 years prior. Comparison AP view demonstrates slight lateral translation of the second MT base with small fleck in the ligament space and dorsal spurring. Both patients with pain over the midfoot area, failed conservative treatments, and underwent medial and middle column arthrodesis

depending on the temporal presentation, from fragmentation and distortion to consolidation of the bone (Eichenholtz classification). RA and other inflammatory arthropathies may be a cause of arthrosis, although to a lesser extent. One study reviewing the radiologic pattern of pedal joint damage in patients with RA found

**Table 6.1** Foot type and exam findings

| | Stress | Imaging finding |
|---|---|---|
| Flatfoot/hindfoot valgus | Plantar aspect of medial column | XR/CT = sclerosis through NC or TMT joints |
| Cavus/cavo-varus | Lateral column or forefoot | MRI = fluid and/or marrow edema within the fourth-fifth MT-cuboid joint region |

only 20% ($n = 542$ feet) had a midfoot-predominant arthritis, which they noted can be difficult to distinguish from OA causes. Rheumatoid patients will commonly present with a collapsed flatfoot and demonstrate osseous erosions with minimal bone formation radiographically [22].

## The Patient Experience

### *Physical Exam*

On presentation, patients typically will have complaints of pain and stiffness directed to the midfoot region [4]. In the acute setting of an arthritic flare, symptoms often include local joint inflammation, swelling, and warmth. Increased pain may be elicited on palpation and attempted joint motion. In the chronic presentation, the pain will be described as a deep, dull ache with increased morning stiffness. Symptoms are aggravated by increased walking, standing, and activity, and improve with rest. Pain may be greater with activities or jobs that require heel rise or when walking up stairs. Other symptoms include local muscle loss, joint stiffness, decreased range of motion (ROM), pain with ROM (especially at end range), crepitus on ROM, and potential adjacent joint compensation and pain. Although OA may be across any combination of MC or MT-cuboid joints, anecdotally Zide et al. [23] observe primary OA most commonly in the second MC joint, followed by the third MC, medial facet of NC, and finally first MC joints.

Patients may also describe gradual foot changes over time. This includes the development of bony prominences across the midfoot that may cause rubbing and pain while wearing certain shoegear. Also, they may describe a gradual loss of arch height and/or the development of a flatfoot over time with forefoot varus, forefoot abduction, and rearfoot valgus [6]. One author noted greater abduction and dorsiflexion deformity in an OA population compared to adduction and plantarflexion in PTA patients [5].

Occasionally, sharp and radiating pain may be described, owing to irritation of the overlying nerves (e.g., superficial peroneal nerve, SPN; deep peroneal nerve, DPN). This can be attributed to the local midfoot inflamed joint environment, bone spurs, or compression from external shoegear. A Tinel's sign may be elicited across the midfoot if there is close proximity of the exostosis and the SPN (medial and intermediate dorsal cutaneous) or DPN [20, 24]. Dorsal bony exostosis may be present across the joint line with their location most often found between the first-second MC joints [20]. This can be present with or without the additional finding of arthritis [24]. Related to the presence of a dorsal exostosis, there may be accompanying skin irritation, abrasion, callus, ganglion cyst, adventitious bursae, and extensor tendinitis.

It is important to accurately diagnose the etiology of the condition. A thorough history, specifically of any past foot injuries, joint replacements, arthritic or rheumatologic conditions (e.g., rheumatoid arthritis, psoriatic arthritis, gout, pseudogout), medical conditions (e.g., hypertension, cardiovascular disease, renal or liver issues, diabetes, and Charcot), or other miscellaneous causes (e.g., lyme, sepsis/infection) may aid and guide potential future treatment options available to the patient.

In PTA, the time from injury to presentation may also play a role in treatment selection. In a review of TMT joint injuries, patients took 1.3 years post injury to reach a "stable" foot comfort level [2]. It has been theorized that with a longer time from injury to reach this "stable" point, there has been adequate time for osseous and soft tissue healing in most structures to reveal the true pathology at hand, using the below techniques to localize the pain [1].

The skin should be evaluated for any hyperkeratotic or irritation patterns, most often found in the plantar forefoot or midfoot. Often in Charcot patients (Brodsky, Type 1), thick hyperkeratotic lesions or ulcerations may be present on the plantar/lateral foot, depending on the level of advancement and lack of previous care to the foot [25].

Evaluation of gastrocnemius contracture should be performed as well, as this is a very common finding in patient with midfoot arthritis and pain [21]. This can be done through gait analysis or the Silfverskiöld test.

Physical exam tests to perform include: [3, 4, 6, 19] (Fig. 6.4)

- Joint Palpation – perform a palpation across the midfoot at each joint. Remember the second MC joint is recessed several mm.
- First Ray Stress – stabilize the middle/lateral column and translate the medial column in the sagittal plane (dorsiflexion/plantarflexion).
- Piano Key Test – isolated dorsiflexion and plantarflexion of each metatarsal head to elicit pain.
- Stress Abduction/Manipulation Test – simultaneous pronation and abduction of the forefoot onto the midfoot [3].
- Heel Rise – provocative test to induce pain at the midfoot level.
- Intra-articular Injection – differentiate pain from arthritic joint, impingement from dorsal exostosis, impingement of nerve (on exostosis). (see sections "Treatments" and "Conservative").
- Silfverskiöld Test – evaluate presence of equinus.

One should be sure to rule out potential differential diagnoses [6]. Tendinitis to the anterior tibial or posterior tibial tendons can present similar to a midfoot arthritis with local swelling and pain to the medial column region. An acute presentation of Charcot or chronic Charcot midfoot deformity is important to rule out in diabetic patients as the recommended treatment is different than the material discussed in this chapter.

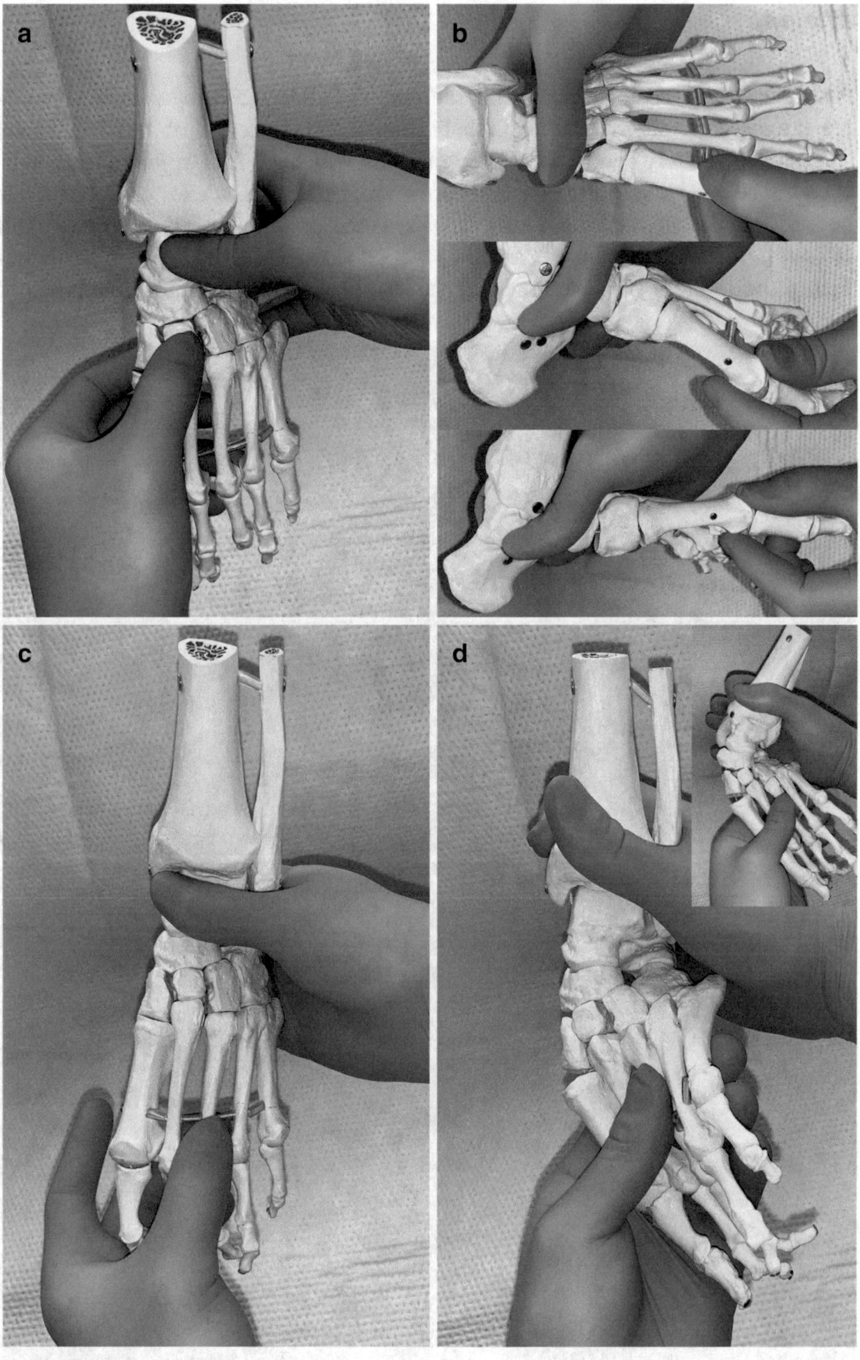


**Fig. 6.4** Clinical examples demonstrating (**a**) joint palpation, (**b**) first ray stress in dorsiflexion and plantarflexion, (**c**) piano key stress, and (**d**) stress abduction/manipulation tests

## *Imaging*

A standard three-view weightbearing radiograph (XR) series is taken first to evaluate the osseous structures, alignment, joints, and evidence of old fracture(s) (Fig. 6.5). Typically across the TMT joint, one will see a loss in joint space, subchondral sclerosis, peri-articular cyst formation, peri-articular exostoses, and loose bodies. Angular measurements may show a plantar or negative deflection (i.e., fault or "sag") in the lateral Meary's angle with apex at the TMT or NC joint, an abduction of the forefoot (i.e., increased calcaneal-fifth MT angle) and lost arch height

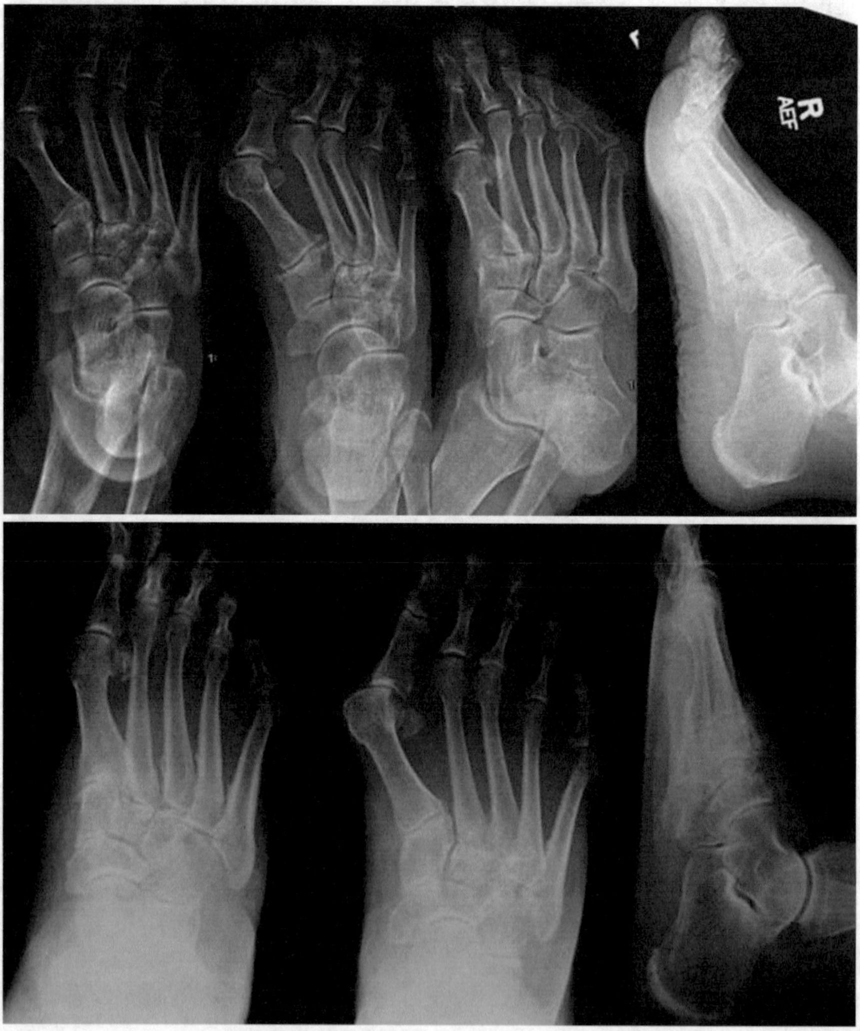


**Fig. 6.5** A 66-year-old female with history of multiple joint osteoarthritis presents with (top) midfoot arthritis (dorsal spurring, joint lipping, and subchondral sclerosis. A repeat film was taken 4 years later (bottom) noting advancement of the arthritis with loss of joint space at the second-third MC joint

[11, 26]. The anteroposterior (AP) and lateral views tend to give the most information about the level of arthritis and deformity present [26]. The second MC joint is best appreciated on the AP film while the third MC joint is best visualized on the oblique [6]. Bilateral XRs may be helpful in determining subtle differences [3] (Fig. 6.3, bottom). Attention should be paid to the adjacent joints for compensatory arthritis formation, specifically to the subtalar (STJ), talonavicular (TNJ), naviculocuneiform, intercuneiform, and first metatarsophalangeal (1st MTPJ) joints as one would evaluate in a flatfoot work up (Fig. 6.6).

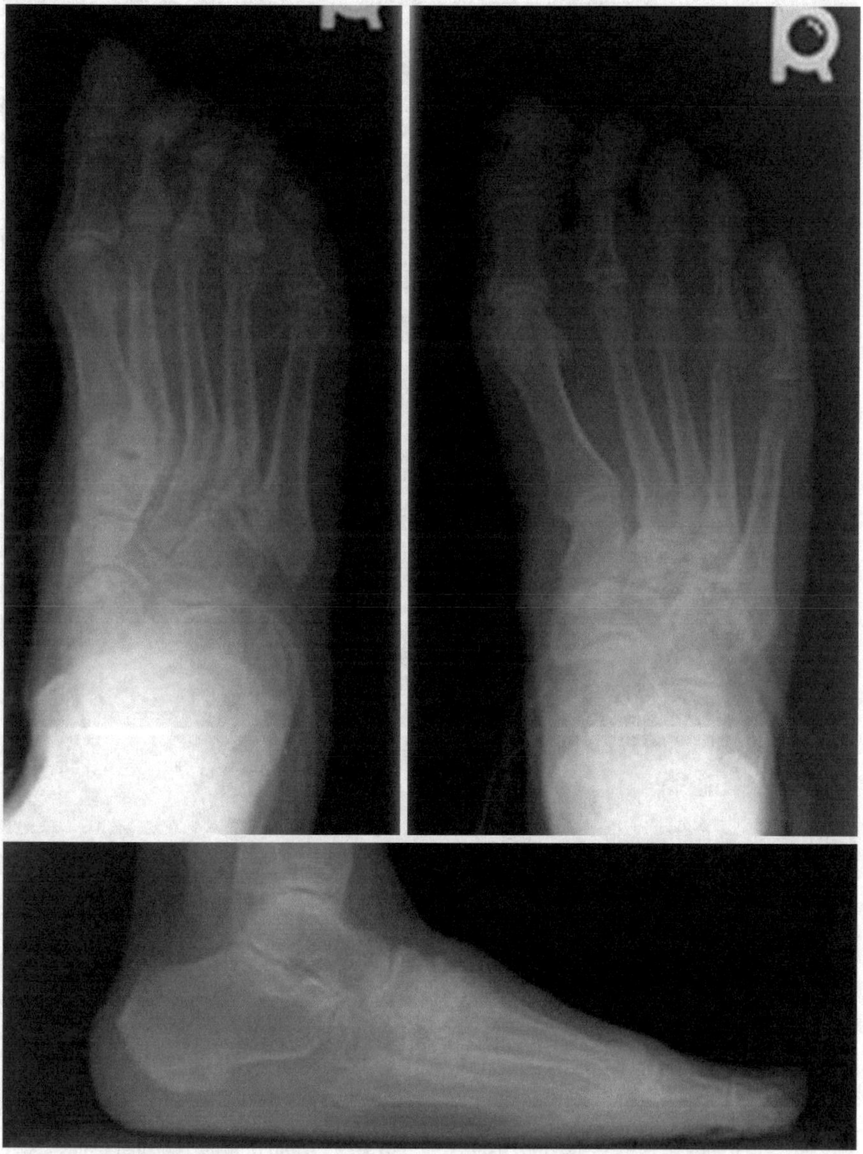

**Fig. 6.6** A 71-year-old female with arthritis noted across the first three MC joints as well as at the NC level, noted on the lateral film with joint spurring and erosion

Advanced studies such as magnetic resonance imaging (MRI) and computed tomography (CT) may also be ordered [26]. MRI will show cartilage wear, subchondral marrow edema, and cyst presentation, while CT shows greater osseous detail and cyst formation (Fig. 6.7). CT is often preferred over MRI due to its

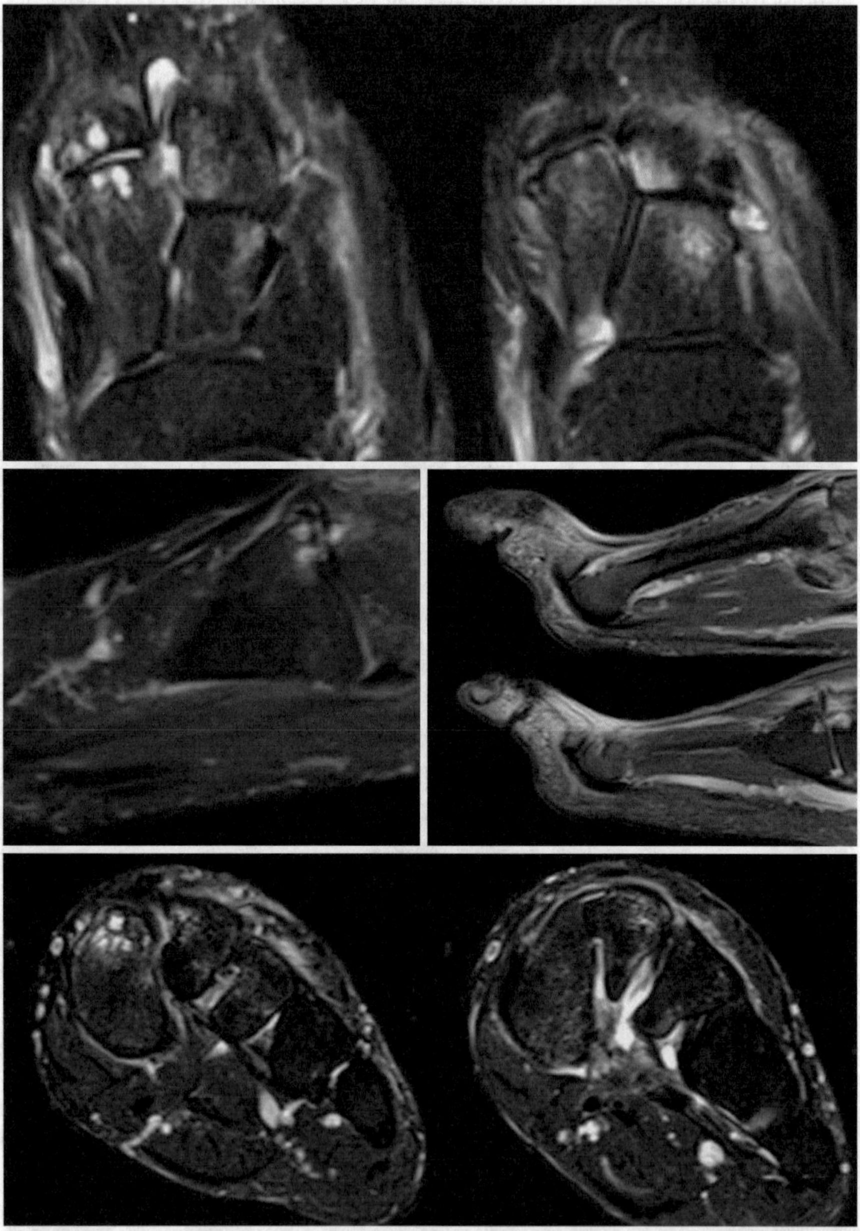

**Fig. 6.7** T2-weighted MRI in the (top) axial, (middle) sagittal, and (bottom) coronal planes. Note the cystic changes and marrow edema throughout the midfoot region, most notable at the first, second, and third MC joints

greater articular and osseous evaluation and for measuring minor joint displacements, especially in the post-traumatic setting. In long-standing arthritis, CT historically has been less helpful due to the lack of simultaneous weightbearing to evaluate deformity in stance. More recently with the creation of weightbearing CT scanners, physicians have the ability to fully understand the osseous alignment in three-dimensions and help plan when deformity correction with fusion is required [16].

Bone scans are sensitive to increased bone turnover or blood flow secondary to inflammation from arthritis. However, this does not always coincide with pain to the region being evaluated, especially the lateral column [3]. Komenda et al. [3] observed that bone scans often will show an uptake to the lateral column, but the authors rarely perform arthrodesis to this region. They feel that these advanced tests are often unnecessary in determining the painful joints. The same can be said for marrow edema signal changes on MRI.

Despite all the options, imaging should not be the main determinant in treatment. Raikin et al. [11, 15] have stated that the radiographic presence of arthritis is not an indication for a procedure. Sangeorzan et al. [15] and Komenda et al. [3] have shown that, despite the presence of lateral column arthritis on XR, true symptoms and pain were minimal to this region, not necessitating a procedure. Coetzee et al. [27] note the medial NC joint and third MC joint often trick physicians with normal XRs but visual arthrosis intraoperatively. Additionally, in a PTA population, Komenda et al. [3] found that despite the lateral column having the most motion and second MC joint having the least motion in the sagittal plane, patient pain was least in the lateral column and greatest in the second MC joint. Thus, it is important to determine the effect of the arthritis through a global approach: imaging, visual deformity, global or isolated pain, physical exam tests, and intra-operative observation when planning for surgery.

## Treatments

Treatment consists of both conservative and surgical options. In both instances, the clinician must take into account the physical exam, imaging, and patient subjective complaints in order to sequentially and appropriately treat the condition. This consists of managing pain and symptoms in an attempt to improve foot function. Furthermore, conservative treatments can be used as a tool to aid in surgical procedure selection. Conservative treatments can be attempted for 3–6 months before surgery is considered indicated. With implementing conservative measures, Mann et al. [5] demonstrated in PTA patients a 2.8-year delay between the injury and surgery and in OA patients a 10.9-year time frame between the onset of symptoms and surgery, with the chosen intervention being fusion. One exception to this includes severe deformity with potential for skin breakdown, often seen in Charcot patients, which prompts more urgent intervention.

## *Conservative*

Conservative treatment is multi-factorial (Table 6.2). Items include medication (oral, topical, injectable), activity modification, shoegear modifications, orthoses, and therapy.

One of the first line treatments with any form of arthritis includes oral medications. Non-steroidal anti-inflammatory drugs (NSAIDs) and related medications are some of the most commonly used pharmacological agents for treatment of both acute and chronic forms of arthritis. Despite their effectiveness, they each pose their own risks, and a review of the patient's medical, drug, and allergy history should always be performed.

While no studies provide evidence to their effectiveness, injection therapy comes in many forms and can act as both a therapeutic and diagnostic tool. Injections with local anesthetic and steroid have demonstrated near or complete pain relief for an average of 1.5–4.5 months [1, 19, 28]. The injection may play a role in determining appropriate surgical treatments. A diagnostic block can help differentiate pain from an intra-articular [e.g., arthritic joint(s)] vs. extra-articular [e.g., impingement from dorsal exostosis, or impingement of nerve (on exostosis)] source. It can also help to identify if a specific column is affected when intra-articular pathology is suggested based on symptomology or imaging. It has been recommended that no lateral column procedure be performed unless relief is obtained from an accurate diagnostic block under imaging (i.e., ultrasound-guided, C-arm fluoroscopy) and would make sense for this to be a guideline across the entire midfoot [19].

Others feel that the diagnostic block is unnecessary due to the small size of the joints and inaccuracy of selective injection [3]. One study showed a 21% and 28% successful joint needle placement into non-arthritic first and second MC joints,

**Table 6.2** Conservative treatments for midfoot arthritis

| Modality | Examples |
|---|---|
| Local therapies | Activity modification<br>Ice<br>Heat<br>Physical therapy/gastrocnemius stretching |
| Oral medications | NSAIDs<br>Corticosteroids |
| Topical medications | NSAIDs<br>Corticosteroids<br>Local anesthetics |
| Injection therapy | Corticosteroids<br>Viscosupplementation |
| Shoegear modifications | Custom molded orthotics<br>Carbon fiber spring plate (stiffening products)<br>Rockerbottom shoe<br>Shoelace modifications<br>Bracing |

respectively, using palpation techniques [29]. Further, even with needle placement into the joint using ultrasound guidance, successful placement was recorded at 70% and 57%, respectively, and demonstrated a 20% fluid leak to the adjacent MC joints. This was attributed to the fact that the second and third MC joints share a common joint capsule, anatomic variants, or the presence of arthritis allowing fluid leak and spread. When possible, it is preferred to perform the injection under ultrasound or fluoroscopic guidance due to greater accuracy in needle placement [19, 29].

While no studies could be found, and its use would be off-label, intra-articular viscosupplementation injections could be considered as well. There are multiple studies and case reports of its use in treatment of ankle, subtalar, and first metatarsophalangeal joint arthritis with mixed results [30].

Certain changes in the patients' shoegear type, modifications, and bracing have been effective in reducing symptoms [4, 26]. Stiffer or rockerbottom shoegear may assist in walking pain, reducing midfoot break, and bending ground reactive forces. A change in the upper material, dorsal padding or relief cutout pads, or an alteration in lacing techniques may accommodate dorsal bony prominences and reduce local pressure and neuritic symptoms [24].

Over-the-counter orthotics can provide added midfoot support to unstable areas, while a more rigid custom orthotic may provide additional arch support. Using three-quarter length custom molded inserts, Rao et al. [31] reported significant improvement in pain (17% decrease) and function after 4 weeks of use. They also noted a reduction in both magnitude (20% decrease) and duration (8.5% decrease) of load to the medial midfoot. In the setting of a Charcot deformity, cutout and relief padding may help not only support the midfoot but prevent bony prominence skin shear, breakdown, and ulceration. Carbon fiber either plated onto a custom orthotic or as a spring plate insert may provide added stiffness to the shoe preventing midfoot bending [32]. Ankle-foot orthotic bracing has shown to reduce plantar load pressures by up to 30% [4].

Finally, patients can be placed on a stretching program aimed at reducing ankle equinus and load across the forefoot and midfoot. In gait, early heel rise can transmit forces to the forefoot and midfoot (medial or lateral columns) depending on the patients gait pattern. This can be correlated to foot type and imaging findings [21].

## *Surgical*

Surgery is often reserved for intractable pain or deformity that is not relieved with the aforementioned conservative measures. Procedures include simple exostectomy, arthroplasty, arthrodesis in situ, and arthrodesis with deformity correction. No classification exists to describe the symptoms, XR findings, or recommended surgical procedures for a defined grade of deformity of midfoot arthritis. Therefore, much of the judgment in appropriate procedure selection is based on the surgeon's clinical decision-making, relying on both physical exam and plain XRs as the guide [3]. Recommendations have been made for surgical intervention after a period of 3–6 months of continued pain after implementing conservative treatments as mentioned [3, 8]. Patient expectations should be set in that they still may have a stiff foot, limited gait, and only approximately 60% of total pain relief [4].

## Exostectomy

Exostectomy for midfoot arthritis is often discussed in the setting of Charcot for the purposes of preventing or treating ulceration, but in this text will be discussed in the setting of arthritis. Often dorsal prominences are found across the first MC joint but can exist across the rest of the TMT joint. Formation of dorsal exostoses is generally the result of degeneration secondary to the high forces across the first MC joint stemming from hallux abducto valgus, first ray or midfoot hypermobility with or without a pes cavus foot type, and history of trauma [33]. A full description with etiology, classification, and treatment can be found in *McGlamry's textbook (4th Ed. Ch 38: pg. 484)* [33].

When an exostectomy is performed, it is important to evaluate the joint to confirm arthritis is minimal to non-existent. This procedure is not indicated for significant arthritic changes [24]. Limited studies have been reported on the use and effectiveness of exostectomy for treating frank arthritis in its early stages. Bawa et al. [20] were the first to describe the surgical outcomes of first-third MC joint exostectomy in 2016. In the 28 feet that underwent surgical resection after failed conservative treatments (14 feet underwent unrelated, concomitant procedures), they found a statically significant decrease in visual analog scale (VAS, 0–10) scores with a mean score of approximately 7 before surgery with improvement to <3 at 1 week, <0.2 at 3 months, and 0 at 6 and 12 months post-surgery. Their described surgical technique included not just removing the dorsal exostosis on either side of the joint, but creating a shallow depression ("saucerization") in the bone-joint interface to prevent re-growth. Of importance, the study population excluded patients with a history of trauma, Charcot, or gout.

A two-portal endoscopic technique for dorsal exostectomy has been described [24]. The procedure affords the ability to evaluate the joint and perform exostectomy with shaving and burr instrumentation through minimally invasive direct visualization. The author suggests that if upon inspection of the joint arthrodesis appears warranted, this could subsequently be performed after arthroscopic cartilage resection. One could infer that arthroplasty could too be performed using this described technique.

## Arthroplasty (Midfoot)

Arthroplasty of the midfoot will be discussed in various forms, with much of the literature being technique or case based. Gilheany et al. [34] describe a basic technique of arthroplasty to the second MC, third MC, and fourth MT-cuboid joints in isolation or combination. Once down to the joint level, joint resection is performed in a plantar apex V-shape using a 10 mm osteotome while leaving the plantar ligaments intact to retain joint stability. The procedure is not recommended for the first MC joint. While anecdotal, the paper's senior author uses this procedure for all cases of primary OA of the second-third MC and fourth MT-cuboid joints with only two patients ($n$ = 80+) in 10 years having required subsequent arthrodesis. Arthroplasty of the lateral column has also been reported for lateral column arthritis to a much greater extent which will be discussed below.

The advantages of both exostectomy and MC arthroplasty includes a shorter operative time and less demanding post-op protocol. In exostectomy, patients are often able be weightbear within 1–3 weeks of surgery, while with the arthroplasty, immediate weightbearing has been described [20, 34]. This can afford some of the more difficult patients (e.g., overweight, elderly, weak, sedentary, gait disturbances) relief without a prolonged recovery and risk for pathology like venous thromboembolism (VTE) or muscular decompensation. The addition of arthroscopic techniques affords the advantages of improved cosmetic results through small incisions, decreased tissue trauma, joint visualization and prognosis/assessment, and reduced neuritis risk [24].

## Arthrodesis

Fusion is the perceived gold standard in surgical treatment of midfoot arthritis. The surgical approach is similar whether an arthrodesis is performed directly or with deformity correction. Surgical goals include anatomic realignment, stabilization, and successful fusion [3]. Typically the first, second, and sometimes third MC joints require fusion, whereas the lateral column is debated regarding procedure type (see section "Lateral Column" below). Deformity correction attempts are preferred when there is greater than 2–3 mm of displacement or greater than 15° malalignment in either the sagittal or transverse plane [3, 16]. Otherwise, an in situ fusion will suffice. It is felt that deformity correction plays an important role in patient satisfaction post-operatively [5, 15]. Seybold et al. [16] and Zide et al. [23] discuss various techniques for deformity correction to midfoot arthritis and should be reviewed as necessary.

Of the reported results for midfoot arthritis (OA or PTA), the findings are encouraging with fusion rates >90% [5, 7, 23, 35]. Mann et al. [5] and Sangeorzan et al. [15] reported a 93% (37 of 41) satisfactory and 69% good to excellent results, respectively, with performed fusion after post-traumatic induced midfoot arthritis. In one of the few studies looking at atraumatic midfoot OA, Jung et al. [7] noted a statistically significant improvement in American Orthopaedic Foot and Ankle Society (AOFAS) Midfoot Functional test score from 34.1 to 83.9 with an improvement in gait (59.7%), pain (60.5%), and alignment (47.1%) in 59 patients ($n$ = 67 feet). Nemec et al. [35] also found statistically significant improvements in pre-operative primary OA after fusion with a reduction in VAS (mean, 6.9–2.3) and improvement in AOFAS scores (mean, 32–79). Studies suggest that recovery can take well over a year to start to appreciate the full value of the procedure(s) performed, and supportive measures (both physically and mentally/emotionally) should be performed throughout this initial recovery period.

Regardless of procedure (complete TMT fusion or optional lateral column arthroplasty), the approach is similar [11, 13, 19, 27]. The literature reports access through one, two, or three incision approaches (Fig. 6.8). In a three incision technique, placement is made medial or dorsal-medial just above the midline along the first MC joint (medial column), centered between the second/third MC joint (middle column), and centered between the fourth/fifth MT-cuboid joint (lateral column). Variable two incision techniques exist depending on the joint access required. For a global TMT joint approach, incisions are made between the first-second MC joint and third MC-fourth MT-cuboid joint [4]. For strict access to the medial and middle columns, incisions are placed medial over the first MC joint with a second incision between the second-third MC joints [23]. More recently, a one incision extended technique to access all three columns for LisFranc injuries was described and could be applied as well [36]. In isolated column surgery, a single incision can be placed directly over top of the corresponding MC joint with exception to the second MC joint where it should be biased laterally to avoid the neurovascular bundle. Incision length is typically 5 cm long. Use of intra-operative fluoroscopy can assist in appropriate incision placement through mapping out the osteology (Fig. 6.9). The appropriate incision(s) will be determined based on the work up and columns desired to fuse. A full depiction of the incision placement and dissection can be found in *Mann's Textbook (9th Ed. Ch 20: pg. 1030)* [27].

Encountered structures at risk include the distal branches of the great saphenous vein (GSV) superficially, the DPN and dorsalis pedis artery, and tendon structures

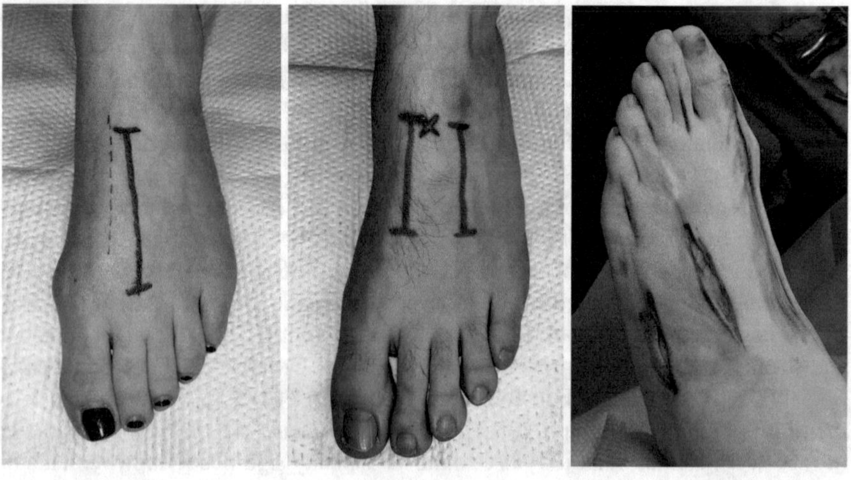

**Fig. 6.8** Approach to the midfoot with variable techniques using (left) one, (middle) two, and (right) three incisions

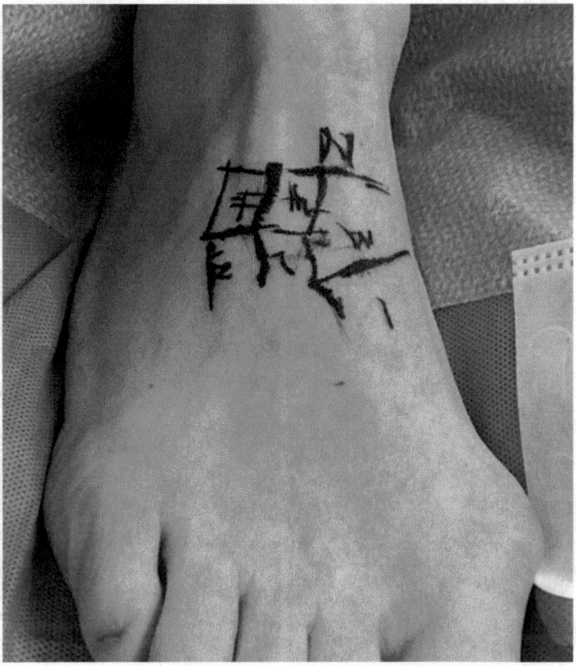

**Fig. 6.9** Fluoroscopy used pre-op to draw out the TMT joint anatomy for incision planning

deep along their anatomic routes. Dissection is carried down to the deep fascia, and the ligament and periosteum are incised to visualize the joint. All of the intervening ligaments, fibrous tissue, bony spurs and loose bodies, and most importantly articular cartilage are removed in toto, down to the bleeding subchondral base. Joint preparation should include subchondral drilling, fish-scaling, and other techniques to achieve a bleeding base at the opposing fusions sites. Use of 2.0–2.5 mm drills is preferred over K-wires due to less heat production to the subchondral bone [23]. It is important to remove the cartilage in its entirety. Remember that these joints are deep with the depth of the first through third MC joint measuring on average 32.3, 26.9, and 23.6 mm, respectively [37]. Often plantar cartilage is accidentally neglected, risking dorsal malunion or arthrodesis site nonunion.

As mentioned, at this point, the procedure can diverge specifically to the lateral column. Discussed below are various rationales as to whether a lateral column fusion, arthroplasty, or no procedure should be performed. Examples and techniques are also discussed.

Once joint preparation is complete, the fusion site is compressed with/without bone graft, and hardware is placed. Fusion can be achieved by multiple constructs, inclusive of screws, plates (e.g., straight, claw, T-plate, midfoot specific designed), screw-plate combinations (e.g., hybrid plates), staples, external fixators, or use of trephine graft [4] (Fig. 6.10). Choice of hardware is often determined based on good or poor bone quality (screw vs. plate constructs, respectively) and independent to the number of joints fused [35] (Fig. 6.11). After reduction and temporary

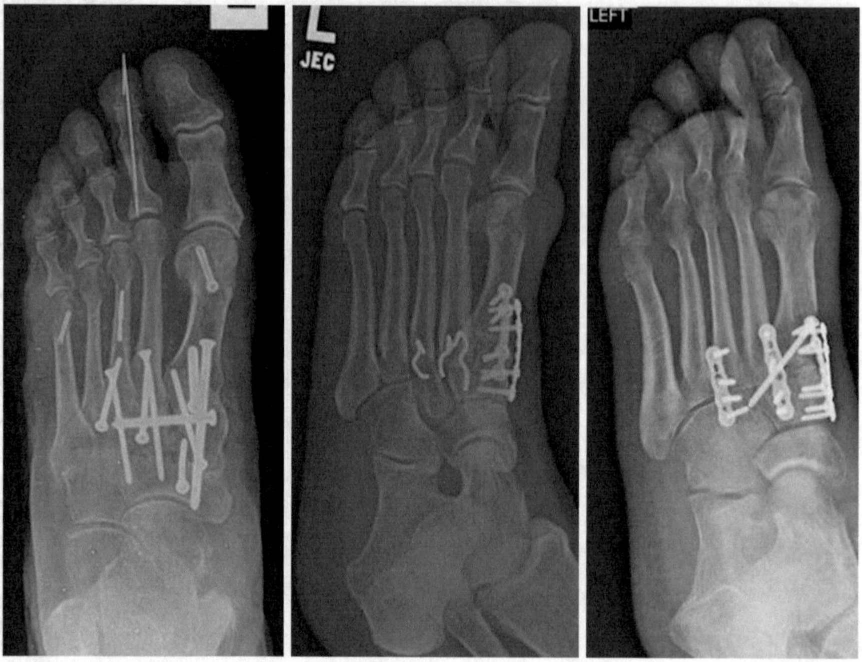


**Fig. 6.10** Multiple constructs are available for MC fusion from screws, plates, staples, or combinations

stabilization, definitive fixation is applied from medial to lateral. Standard arthrodesis principles should be applied and performed.

Most studies looking at hardware constructs across the TMT joint focus on the first MC joint in Lapidus stabilization. Due to the anatomic size of the region, multiple techniques from not only hardware constructs but position (e.g., dorsal, dorsomedial, medial, and plantar) can be employed. Barp et al. [38] retrospectively reviewed 147 patients who underwent first MC fusion for treatment of hallux valgus, demonstrating an overall nonunion rate of 6.7% with individual nonunion rates of 2%, 5%, and 9% for intra-plate compression screw, single interfragmentary screw with locking plate, and 3.5 mm crossed solid screw fixation constructs, respectively. With regard to the second and third MC joints, the options are more limited with single fixation type and a dorsal position.

In the only study to date comparing midfoot arthrodesis with screw vs. plate-screw constructs, Ahmad et al. [39] randomized patients into two groups based on fixation: 4.0 partially threaded cannulated cancellous screws (group 1) or plate-screw constructs (group 2) for varying first-third MC fusion procedures with concurrent use of calcaneal autograft ($n = 50$). While measures across all evaluated points improved (VAS, FAAM) and complication rates were low, there was no statistically significant difference between the two fixation groups. Nonunion or malunion was seen in four and two patients between groups 1 and 2, respectively. Schipper et al. [40] revealed a 95% and 100% fusion rate using staples and screw-staple constructs, respectively, with the author concluding the addition of screws did

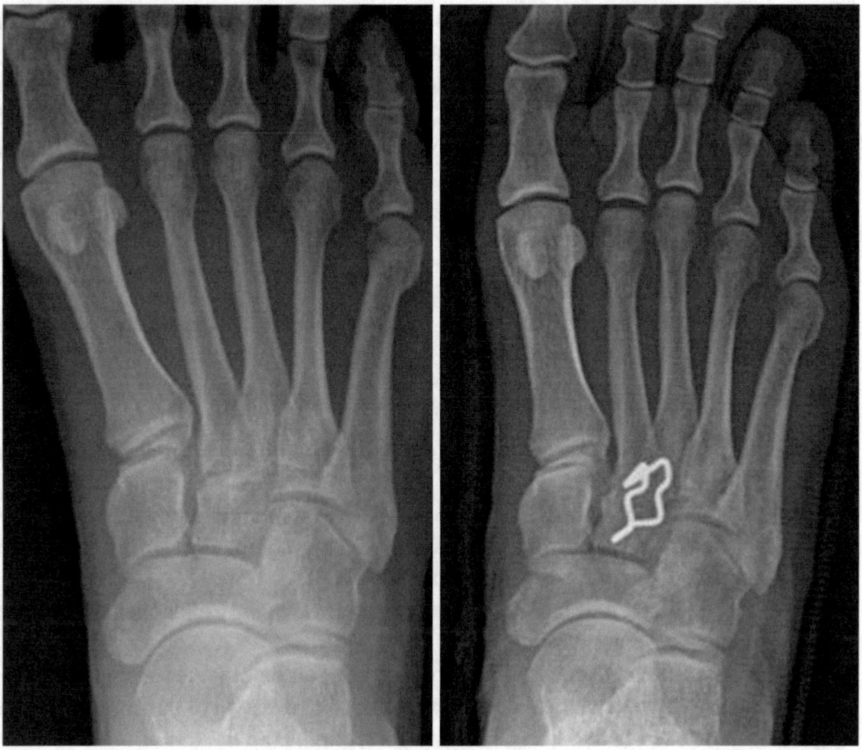

**Fig. 6.11** A 54-year-old female with a past medical history of Sjogren's and fibromyalgia presenting with medial midfoot pain and burning sensation into the medial toes. She failed conservative therapy including localized injection under ultrasound (1-week relief). XR demonstrates narrowing of the 2MC joint with musculoskeletal ultrasound revealing dorsal spurring, joint advanced arthritis, capsular thickening, and synovial hypertrophy. She underwent isolated 2MC arthrodesis with staple fixation after 9 months of conservative treatments

not help or hinder fusion. Buda et al. [41] found a higher rate of nonunion in those undergoing fusion with dorsal plating alone vs. the use of screws either independent or hybrid fixation with concurrent dorsal plating.

Some hints regarding hardware include:

- Use 4–4.5 mm crossing screws in the medial column with 3–3.5 mm single screws in the middle column. Orientation has been described in both directions [3, 16].
  - Cannulated screws afford more exact placement across the joint while solid screws provide added strength [16].
  - If screws are placed entering the metatarsal, a beveled hole should be created to countersink the screw and prevent breaking the metatarsal cortex or skin irritation [3].
  - Dorsiflexion of the hallux during stabilization of the first MC joint assists in preventing plantar gapping and ray dorsiflexion.

- A traditional "homerun" screw can add stability and restore anatomic position through drawing a laterally translated second MT medially.
- Additional fixation to the third MC joint can be recommended. Although a review of primary ORIF to the TMT joint, one study noted the highest rates of screw breakage (3.5 mm) at this joint likely due to the mobility of the lateral column [17].
- Dorsal plate contouring is important to reduce malposition of the metatarsal into a dorsiflexed position.

- Plates can be added for osteoporotic bone.
- Medial buttress plating is suggested in severe abduction deformity to achieve foot alignment [5].

Some other noted keys to arthrodesis include: [4–6, 16]

- Assistance in joint identification can be performed through sagittal plane motion at the MT head.
- Lamina or Weinraub spreaders can be used to assist in joint distraction and visualization during the joint preparation step. Many companies will include this instrument in their set in its various forms.
- Care should be taken to leave the strong plantar ligaments intact to add another point of extra-osseous stability.
- While not necessary, bone graft can be used. It can be obtained from the calcaneus, iliac crest, or even local dorsal exostosis after removal of the cortex. Wedge grafts can be used to assist in deformity correction.
- Make sure no sagittal plane deformity is created during screw placement. Continue to hold and check the metatarsal head position upon screw placement and tightening.
- In isolated second MC fusions, the LisFranc ligament articulation should be prepped as well to be included in the fusion mass. Avoid violating the first MC joint.

Closure is performed in standard layered fashion. Deflating the tourniquet prior to closure will aid in evaluating any vascular injury and reduce hematoma formation with subsequent wound healing issues. Patients are typically kept non-weightbearing for 6–8 weeks and then weightbearing as tolerated in a walking cast or fracture boot for another 4–6 weeks with serial XRs to evaluate the fusion [5, 6, 27]. Non-weightbearing has even been suggested for up to 3 months due to the risk of non-union [23]. Once adequate healing has occurred, patients are transitioned back into a stiff sole shoe or sneaker with an insert (over the counter or custom). If the procedure is part of a larger procedure that has a greater period of required osseous healing, the primary procedure will dictate the weightbearing protocol. Physical therapy can be offered for gait training, Achilles complex stretching, and limb strengthening, but is not required in a standard post-op protocol. High impact activities should be delayed until 4–6 months post-op if osseous fusion has been noted on XR with no or minimal clinical complaints of pain [6].

## Lateral Column

After the first three MC joints have been fused, the surgeon must decide if a procedure is required to address the lateral column (i.e., fourth/fifth MT-cuboid joints). A lateral column fusion or arthroplasty can be performed with concomitant procedures (e.g., medial and/or middle column fusions, talonavicular fusions, calcaneocuboid fusion, peroneal reconstruction) (Fig. 6.12). It is important to state that, conversely, a fusion or arthroplasty can be performed in isolation as well. Furthermore, some authors suggest no procedure is required at all for a good outcome with only 6–25% of patients with lateral column symptoms requiring full column TMT fusion [42].

The origin of a lateral column procedure debate is attributed to biomechanics [43]. The lateral column has defined triplane motion with the greatest total range of motion of the three columns. Furthermore, motion exists at the lateral cuneiform-cuboid articulation [12, 27]. When fusion is performed to the medial and middle columns, it places greater load on the forefoot, lateral column, and calcaneocuboid joint (CCJ) [1, 14]. Lateral fusions (i.e., in addition to the medial/middle columns or in isolation) may result in metatarsalgia (lateral, global forefoot) or CCJ arthrosis

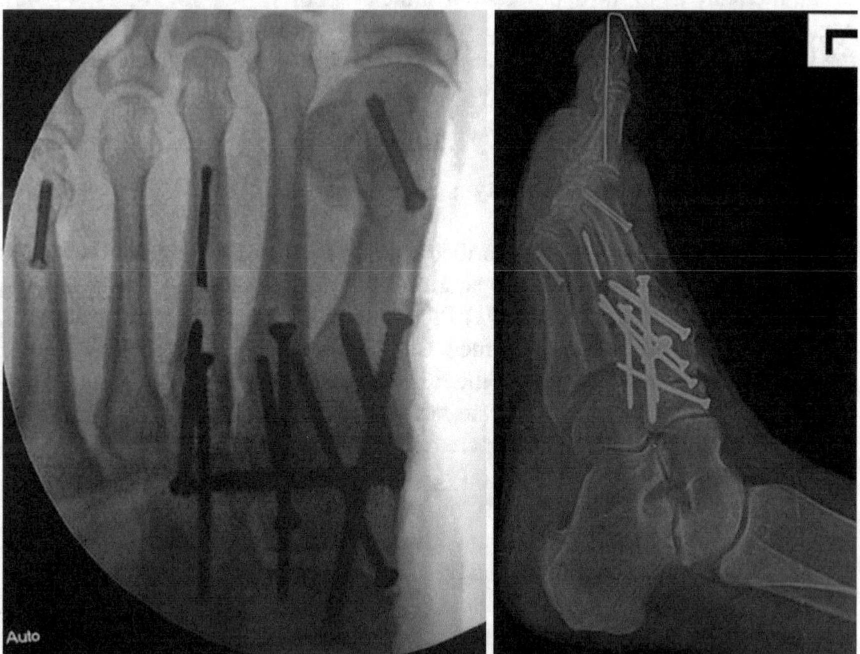


**Fig. 6.12** A 66-year-old female with 3-year history of midfoot pain, specifically to the lateral column. She failed conservative treatment and subsequently underwent a fusion of the first-third MC joints with arthroplasty of the lateral column. Note the increased space at the fourth-fifth MT-cuboid joints post resection

[14]. Because of this, it has been recommended in multiple publications to not perform a fusion across the fourth-fifth MT-cuboic joints. Instead, options include an arthroplasty [13, 19, 27] or no procedure at all [3, 15, 43], with most published studies of small case series examples with no high-level evidence to support any method of operative treatment [43].

Despite the presence of arthritis, the lateral column's tolerance to this is often high with minimal true pain. In performing a fusion, concerns include patient subjective complaints of pain and an uncomfortable, stiff foot; adjacent joint pain; lateral foot stiffness; lateral foot prominence; metatarsalgia; and stress fractures [11, 13, 19]. Additionally, there is a concern of nonunion due to too stiff of a construct across either the lateral column, medial/middle columns, or adjacent site attempted to be fused in the same surgical setting [1]. In one study looking at arthrodesis for TMT joint injuries where only two patients ($n = 32$) underwent additional lateral column fusion, both required revision by metatarsal osteotomy secondary to metatarsalgia [3]. Kuo et al. [17] also noted 50% of patients with primary lateral column ORIF ($n = 4$) developed transfer metatarsalgia and required corrective metatarsal osteotomies. Preserved lateral column motion is important for ideal foot and gait function [1].

Both examples of lateral column arthrodesis and arthroplasty (in isolation and combined with medial/middle column procedures) have been discussed and debated in the literature as to the appropriate treatment option [1, 11, 13, 15, 19, 44, 45]. Multiple authors feel that one could even get away with no procedure performed to the lateral column altogether as another option with an overall surgical tenet of preserved lateral column motion by any extent [15, 23, 27, 43, 44].

## Lateral Column: For Arthroplasty

The approach is as previously described with an incision between the fourth and fifth MT-cuboid joints. Joint preparation is typically described by removing 0.5 cm from each of the fourth and fifth MT bases, while the cuboid is debated, depending on the procedure performed. Care is taken to leave the peroneus brevis attachment intact, and resection of the fifth MT base is only required at the articulating portion, typically resecting the medial two-thirds. The plantar and medial ligaments should be retained for increased stability to the joint and spacer used with preservation of the dorsal-lateral capsule through full thickness flaps for coverage in closure.

Closure is performed in standard layered fashion. Post-operatively, for an isolated lateral column arthroplasty, the patient is non-weightbearing for 2–3 weeks and then slowly transitioned to weightbearing in a fracture boot and sneaker over the subsequent weeks. If a K-wire is used for stability purposes for either the joint and/or a biological spacer, it is often removed at 6–8 weeks post-op [3, 19]. If the procedure is part of a fusion, the fusion will dictate the weightbearing protocol.

Multiple techniques have been described in performing an arthroplasty from bone resection to resection with interpositional spacers for lateral column arthritis.

- Chang et al. [13] recommend removing 0.5 cm of bone from the bases of the fourth/fifth MT but leaving the cuboid articular surface intact to avoid bone weakening and subsidence of the biological spacer into the subchondral space. Space can be maintained with K-wire fixation for 6 weeks before removal. A full depiction of the dissection and resection is demonstrated in his chapter section "Lateral Column For Arthroplasty" in *McGlamry's Textbook (4th Ed. Ch 82: pg. 1234)* [13].
- Berlet et al. [19] discussed interposition with either sacrificing the peroneus tertius or, if not present, the corresponding extensor tendon (typically the 4th EDL slip). The tendon is released proximally, rolled into an "anchovy" (i.e., rolled disk of tendon), inserted into the resected MT base (fourth and/or fifth), and temporarily stabilized with a K-wire. In their retrospective review, eight patients underwent this procedure and felt their pain improved by 35% and 75% of the patients deemed the operation satisfactory.
- Koenis et al. [45] offer a surgical technique of resection arthroplasty with or without tendon interposition, similar to that of Chang et al. [13] and Berlet et al. [19], except a wedge resection is performed (plantar apex). In their small case series ($n = 6$), there was improvement in VAS and foot function index (FFI) scores with all but one patient satisfied with the result and willing to undergo the procedure again. There was a 50/50 split between arthroplasty and interposition procedures performed, with the authors suggesting that equal results can be achieved without the need for interposition graft.
- Shawen et al. [1] offer use of a spherical ceramic interpositional device initially used in the hand carpometacarpal joint but also has gained FDA approval for the fourth/fifth MT-cuboid joints. This technique requires removal of bone using a burr from the corresponding TMT joint surfaces with care to preserve the cortical margins and plantar ligaments. This group's retrospective review of 11 patients at final follow-up demonstrated an 87% improvement in AOFAS scores and 42% improvement in VAS scores. One patient did develop implant subsidence, but no dislocation occurred, which could be attributed to the importance of maintaining plantar ligaments on dissection.
- Hood et al. [42] described a technique of interpositional arthroplasty with a tensor fascia lata allograft, adapted from use in various other joints (e.g., jaw, elbow, subtalar, knee, thumb, and first metatarsophalangeal). Joint prep includes 0.5 cm bone resection from the cuboid and packing a fascia lata graft of 0.6–10 mm thickness into the newly created deficit. This is temporarily stabilized with an external suture button. While only a report describing a surgical technique, their case patient had a 3-year history of 10/10 VAS pain which after a combined medial/middle column fusion with lateral column arthroplasty, reduced to 3/10 at 13 months and reported approval of the procedure. The procedure could be altered with autograft or allograft (e.g., porcine, bovine, equine) use based on graft availability and patient personal or religious concerns. Tensor fascia lata was chosen by the senior author who has been performing this procedure for years due to its strong, pliable, and durable characteristics, showing minimal compression which allows it to maintain the space created after joint resection; these qualities should be evaluated in other graft materials if another graft is chosen.

### Lateral Column: For Fusion

There is also argument for fusion of the lateral column with multiple studies demonstrating improved pain and AOFAS scores post-arthrodesis. Overall, the feeling is that lateral column arthrodesis can be performed in isolation and combination for a subluxed or dislocated lateral column, painful arthritis specific to the fourth/fifth MT-cuboid joints, or failure of all appropriate conservative treatment options [11, 27]. While some of these data do not necessarily show greater results with fusion, they show no statistical significance in outcomes whether the joint is fused or motion left intact.

- Raikin et al. [11] performed one of the largest retrospective reviews on 28 feet that underwent lateral column arthrodesis with 2-year follow-up. Excluding the Charcot population, 6 feet underwent isolated lateral column arthrodesis with screw fixation, resulting in a 70.7% reduction in pain (8.2–2.4) and 82.9% improvement in functional capacity, both of which were found to be statistically significant. AOFAS midfoot scores improved from 45 to 87.6 points pre- to post-op.
- Sangeorzan et al. [15] reported no difference when fusion of the lateral column was or was not performed in their review of TMT fusion for salvage of LisFranc injuries. Of note, the author believes fusion is not needed for a good clinical result.
- Mann et al. [5] retrospectively reviewed midfoot arthrodesis procedures for an OA and PTA cohort, noting no difference in patients who did ($n$ = 8/41 feet) or did not have lateral column fusions. Of note, the author felt lateral column fusion left the patient with a stiff but tolerated foot.
- Coetzee et al. [27] do not suggest the necessity of fusion but advise if a lateral column fusion is felt to be indicated and performed, the surgeon should not perform fusion between the lateral cuneiform-cuboid joint to allow some motion between these aspects of the longitudinal arch. In a report by Mann et al. [5] where their group performed on average six articular fusions in PTA patients and four in OA patients, they encountered a total of three joint nonunions ($n$ = 41 feet), one of which was the lateral cuneiform-cuboid articulation. It is not known whether the lateral column was fused in this patient. These two points highlight the lack of need to fuse this articulation and possible added construct rigidity impacting fusion potential negatively.
- Rammelt et al. [46] reported no difference in outcomes of 20 patients with severe PTA treated with isolated medial vs. medial-lateral column arthrodesis.

### Concomitant Procedure

The typical deformity presents as a flatfoot with abduction of the forefoot and lateral and/or dorsal-angulated metatarsals due to a traumatic TMT joint injury [3]. Various other procedures include first ray realignment procedures, corrective procedures for flatfoot or cavus foot (e.g., lateral column lengthening, calcaneal slide), adjacent joint fusions, and tendon debridements, transfers, and releases [7, 16, 23]. Common procedures include:

- Naviculocuneiform joint arthritis can develop secondary to the initial trauma or from overload due to an arthritic TMT joint. With respect to the NC joint, if a sag is seen on a lateral XR, arthritis on AP/MO XR, cartilage loss on advanced imaging, a diagnostic block provides relief, or if intra-operative instability is noted with a stress exam or arthrosis is visualized, this level can be incorporated into the fusion [4]. It is recommended that at least two if not all three cuneiforms be fused to the navicular as isolated medial cuneiform-navicular fusion is difficult to achieve [27]. The NC joint along with the inter-cuneiform joints is considered "non-essential" for normal gait, and their motion is often not missed after fusion [47]. Budny et al. [47] offer a review of NC joint pathology with surgical techniques.
- Intercuneiform fusion (i.e., adjacent cuneiforms or all three) has also been recommended for increased foot stability [5, 35]. However, others recommend leaving this space alone unless marked arthritic changes are noted on XR or intra-operatively and only fusing the arthritis effected joints [7, 23, 35]. Coetzee et al. [27] suggest leaving the lateral cuneiform-cuboid articulation intact to decrease overall construct rigidity.
- Achilles complex lengthening procedures (e.g., tendo-achilles lengthening, gastrocnemius ± soleus recession) should be performed based on the results of a pre-operative Silfverskiöld test. Equinus deformity may cause an increase load on the midfoot and collapse of the arch. Addition of this procedure for treatment of primary midfoot OA is as high as 78% [35]. Technique used is based on surgeon preference as many procedures have been described from percutaneous, mini-open, open, or endoscopic methods. Tendon contracture has been noted to occur after progressing flatfoot deformity, and lengthening will allow decreased forefoot pressure as well as torque across the midfoot that can increase the risk for nonunion. If performed, active range of motion can begin 2–4 weeks post-operatively with physical therapy assistance after 6 weeks.

## Complications

Complications of midfoot fusion include wound dehiscence, infection, neuritis (e.g., traction, impingement, complex regional pain syndrome), neuroma formation (7%), nonunion (3–10%), malunion or malalignment, recurrence of deformity, exostosis re-growth, persistent pain (e.g., midfoot, metatarsalgia, lateral column, sinus tarsi), symptomatic/painful hardware (9%), and VTE [4, 6, 7, 27, 35].

Sequela complications to a midfoot fusion include metatarsalgia (6%), metatarsal stress fractures (7%), sesamoiditis, and adjacent joint arthritis [3–5]. If a lateral column fusion is performed, there is also the abovementioned foot stiffness, pain, lateral column metatarsalgia, and stress fracture of the fourth-fifth MTs that all may require a secondary corrective surgery [1, 3, 13, 19]. Mann et al. [5] found a high level of radiographic NC joint arthritis (28%) after TMT fusions. In a cadaveric biomechanical study, Nadaud et al. [14] demonstrated combined medial-lateral column fusion significantly increases lateral forefoot and CCJ pressure which in practice may result in pain and arthrosis. Jung et al. [7] noted a 7.5% ($n$ = 67 feet) rate of sinus tarsi or lateral column pain after atraumatic midfoot correction. Although a review for primary partial (e.g., first, second, and/or third MC joint) arthrodesis after TMT joint injury, Reinhardt et al. [48] reported a 12% rate of adjacent joint arthritis at 42 months (average) post fusion.

Neuritis can be multi-factorial. Pre-operative neuritis may be a result of the initial traumatic episode, evolution of local arthritis, or bone spur/shoegear irritation and compression. Intra-operative local dissection or retraction can cause neuropraxia, while post-operative tissue healing and scar formation may result in an entrapped nerve. It is important to note in your pre-op exam the presence or absence of any neuritis symptoms to determine the potential post-op cause. Post-operative neuritis has been considered a continuation of the pre-operative neuropraxia and part of the nerves healing after surgical decompression which can last 3–6 months [20]. In a non-PTA situation, Bawa et al. [20] had seven patients ($n$ = 26) with post-op neuritis after a dorsal exostectomy procedure for TMT joint spurs. Four had a continuation of their symptoms, while the remaining three experienced new neuropraxia as a result of the surgery.

Jung et al. [7] reported an overall 39% complication rate with sesamoiditis being most common in eight patients. The cause was attributed to excessive plantarflexion or loss of flexibility of the first ray upon fusion with two patients requiring corrective procedural treatments (e.g., sesamoidectomy and sesamoid shaving).

When nonunion and malalignment occur and are symptomatic, revision procedures with re-arthrodesis or correcting the alignment issue is recommended. Initial attempts to manage a nonunion can be with bone health optimization (i.e., vitamin D, calcium) and bone stimulation modalities. Malalignment issues can be corrected at the site of the initial fusion with revision, or at the site of the local deformity if appropriate. Bibbo et al. [49] provide a review with surgical techniques for correcting malunions and nonunions of the midfoot in dorsiflexion/plantarflexion, valgus, and varus positions.

Hardware complications were noted to be 9% ($n$ = 67) in one study, while another noted a 25% hardware removal rate [7, 35]. Removal of hardware should be initially managed with conservative measures with delay in removal recommended after 1 year from surgery [6].

## Special Circumstances

### *Midfoot Arthritis: Post-Traumatic Acute*

While the focus of this chapter is not acute management of LisFranc fracture dislocation, it has been shown to be a major factor in the evolution of midfoot arthritis. Depending on presentation, it may be recommended to perform a primary arthrodesis or ORIF of the joint complex to prevent the development of pain and deformity that often follows. In the acute setting of these injuries, initial management is performed through non-weightbearing, casting, and possible external fixation stabilization to allow soft tissue preservation and healing while monitoring for compartment syndrome. Fasciotomy should be performed if clinical suspicion for compartment syndrome is high.

Once the soft tissue envelope injury has had time to subside, which may take 1–3 weeks, it is then appropriate to implement definitive care through retained external fixation (pending reduction and alignment), primary fusion with internal fixation or external fixation, or joint ORIF. Factors in decision-making include the patients' age, functional demand, degree of destruction, and ligamentous vs. combined osseous-ligamentous injuries. Greater comminution results in a decreased ability to perform ORIF, and arthrodesis should be considered [50]. Kuo et al. found PTA levels at 18% vs. 40% in combined osseous-ligamentous vs. primary ligamentous injuries, respectively, suggesting (i) injury pattern over fixation methods was more responsible for the outcome and (ii) that these more subtle ligamentous injuries may do better with a primary fusion [17]. It is this variability and complexity of midfoot injuries which makes treatment difficult.

Both ORIF and arthrodesis can be performed with transarticular screws, bridge plating, staples, etc., with the key difference being joint preparation or not (Fig. 6.13). Lau et al. [51] compared transarticular screws, dorsal plating, or a combined approach and found no difference in hardware failure or removal rates with the best predictor of functional outcome (e.g., AOFAS midfoot scores, FFI scores) being a quality reduction. This point has been previously mentioned in also reducing later stage PTA development.

Multiple studies discuss primary ORIF or fusion [50]. Smith et al. [52] performed a retrospective review and meta-analysis comparing ORIF vs. primary arthrodesis with respect to patient outcomes, finding neither procedure was favored regarding patient reported outcomes, non-anatomic alignment risks, and need for revision surgery. Only hardware removal had a higher-risk ratio in the ORIF group, with its associated morbidity. While arthrodesis in this setting is the definitive procedure, ORIF may require hardware removal later to re-establish joint motion. However, hardware removal is debated as many studies have shown good results in leaving the hardware intact unless a secondary issue requires its removal. Albright et al. [53] found greater short- and long-term cost-effectiveness in purely ligamentous LisFranc (1–3 TMT) injuries with a total lifetime cost of primary arthrodesis vs. ORIF valued at $27,849 and $127,294, respectively.

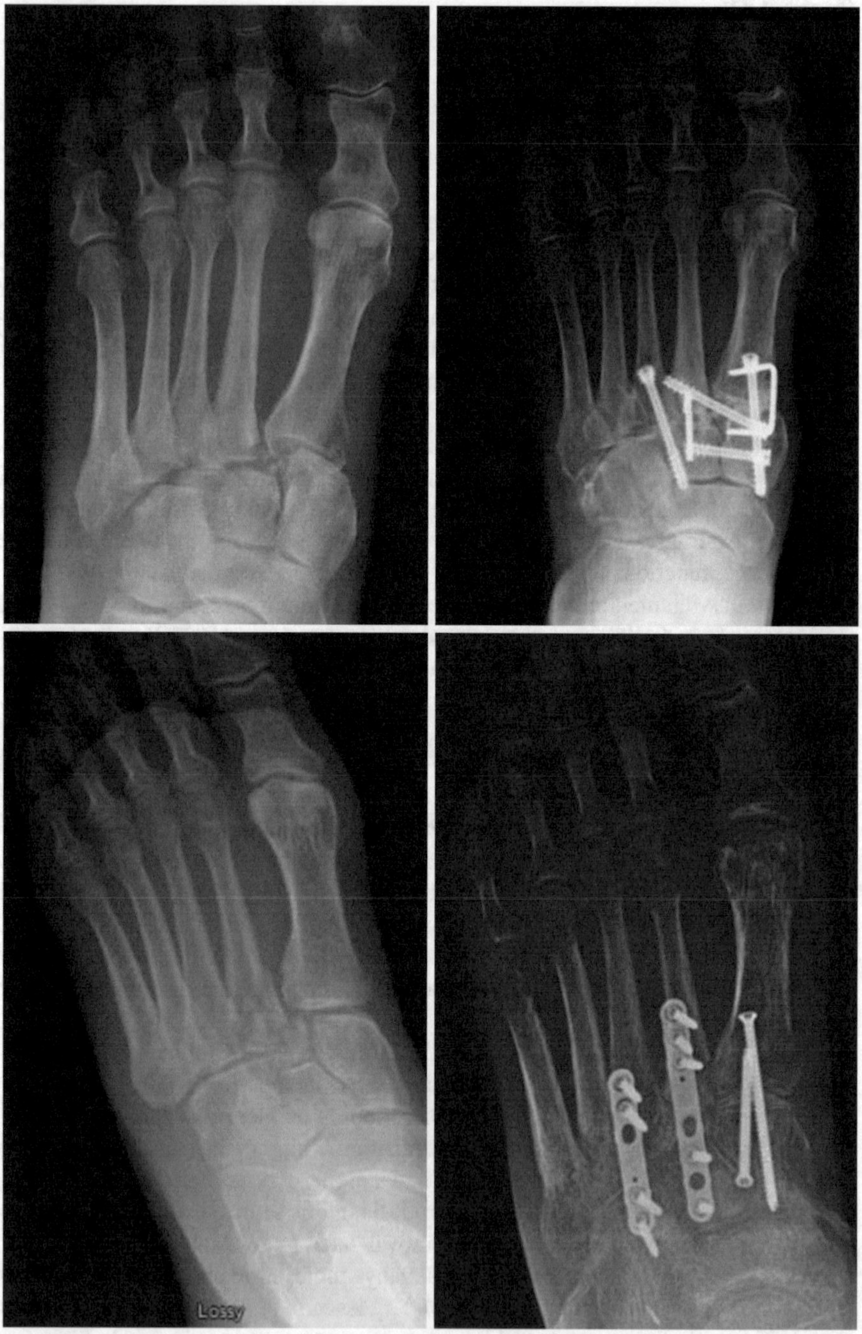


**Fig. 6.13** (Top) An 82-year-old female patient with comminuted, homolateral LisFranc fracture dislocation treated with primary fusion after falling down a short flight of stairs. (Bottom) A 49-year-old male patient with comminuted, homolateral LisFranc fracture dislocation treated after dropping a 500 pound boiler on his foot/leg. Patient sustained foot and leg compartment syndrome that underwent fasciotomy and ipsilateral tibia shaft fracture that was treated with intramedullary nailing. Due to the comminution to the 2–3 MT bases, there was an inability to perform ORIF

While no consensus has been reported on the appropriate procedure, an overlying theme for reported good outcomes is with earlier vs. delayed surgery [1, 5, 15] and better long-term results with anatomic reduction to reduce future sequela related to malalignment [51].

## *Midfoot Arthritis: Charcot Neuroarthropathy*

Discussion of Charcot has been reserved for Chap. 10 (Fig. 6.14). However, midfoot fusion is often performed in the setting of a Brodsky Type 1 midfoot breakdown with resultant rockerbottom deformity. This deformity leads to bony prominences across the midfoot, often at the cuboid, with risk for subsequent callus formation, skin breakdown, wound development, and osteomyelitis. A midfoot fusion procedure is warranted to prevent the above sequela for an "at risk" limb and/or one that is uncorrectable and unbraceable. Bevan et al. [54] noted an increased risk of ulceration when a lateral Meary's angle was greater than −27° in midfoot Charcot. Techniques differ from those described here due to the decreased bone quality, with implementation of super-constructs and beaming techniques for fusion and stabilization of the foot. Bevilacqua et al. [50] provide a comprehensive review for surgical management in these patients.

In Charcot, column fusion is also debated. The goal is to create a stable plantigrade foot without bony prominence when there is an uncorrectable/unbraceable lateral column collapse, rockerbottom deformity, or bony prominence at risk for ulceration [11]. However, other author(s) recommend leaving the lateral column alone when fusing the medial and middle columns for a Charcot reconstruction [13].

## Conclusions

The midfoot, consisting of the LisFranc ligament and multiple joint articulations, is very complex. Commonly, after an injury to this region, arthritis develops. Multiple conservative and palliative options exist to prevent surgical interventions. If failed after 3–6 months, surgery may be implemented. The various types of procedures one can perform are dependent upon a multitude of items including patient symptoms, physical exam findings, imaging, and results of diagnostic tests such as injections and stress manipulation. In lesser stage arthritis, exostectomy and arthroplasty can be performed. In end-stage arthritis, fusion is the preferred procedure across, at minimum, the medial and middle columns, whereas debate exists as to the need for lateral column procedures. While both examples exist, the literature suggests not to fuse the lateral column, either performing arthroplasty or leaving it alone. Overall, surgical intervention to the TMT joints shows good results regarding reduction in patient pain, high fusion rates, and maintaining a high function level that has left midfoot arthrodesis the gold standard in the treatment of end-stage midfoot arthritis.

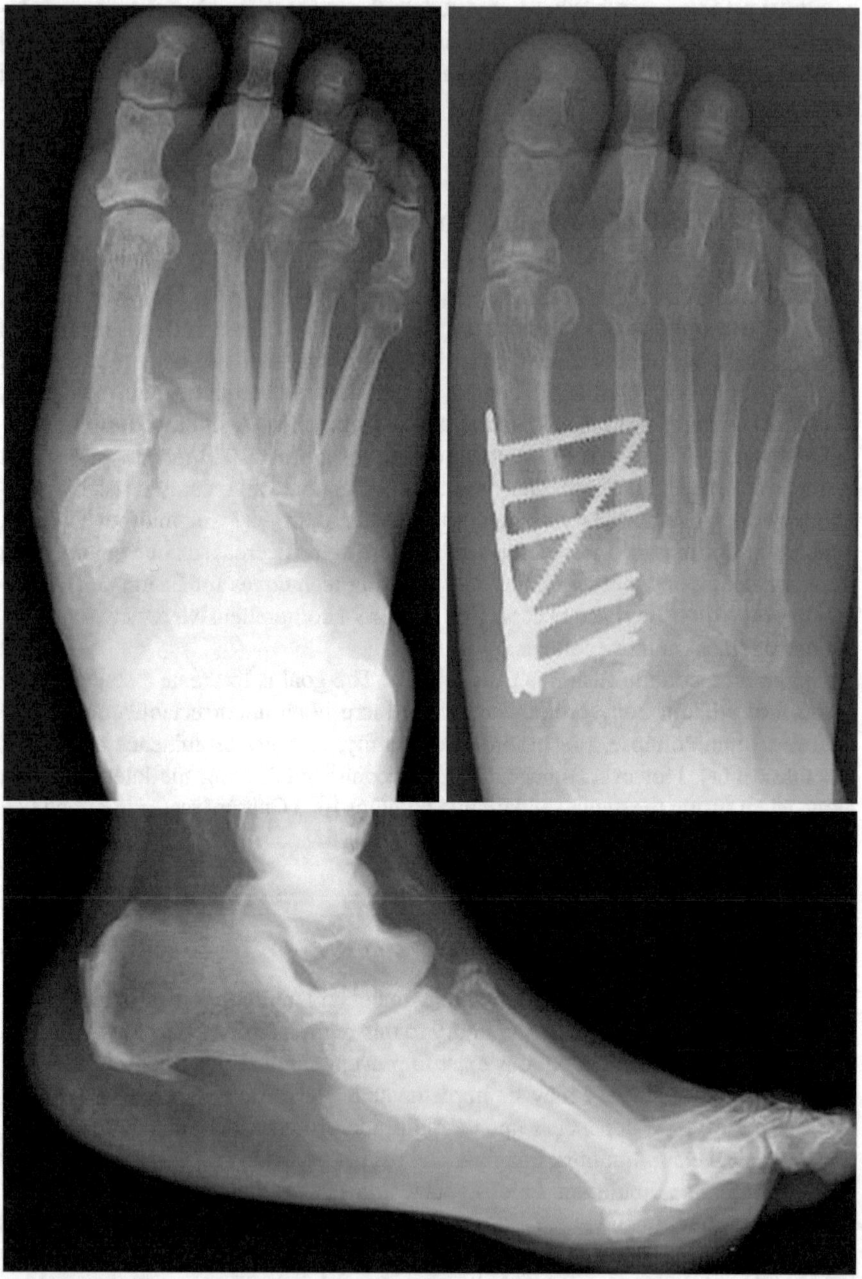

**Fig. 6.14** A 48-year-old male with right midfoot Charcot deformity with homolateral dislocation and osseous destruction. The patient underwent stabilization with a combined external and internal fixation technique with the Ilizarov frame removed at 8 weeks. At 1-year follow-up (upper right), there is maintenance of anatomic alignment without hardware failure across the arthrodesis. (Image reproduced from Capobianco CM et al; BioMed Central Ltd, Springer Link) [55]

*Dr. Hood is a fellowship-trained foot and ankle surgeon, and associate at Hunterdon Podiatric Medicine of Hunterdon Healthcare in Flemington, NJ.*

*NOTE: The authors of this chapter have no disclosures (e.g., stock, equity, or consultant status). The industry pictures/names used in this chapter were taken for representation purposes without bias. The views, opinions, and products discussed in this chapter do not reflect the views and opinions of the companies represented, but a mere representation of the published literature. Each surgeon must evaluate the appropriateness of the procedure chosen based on his or her personal medical training and experience.*

## References


1. Shawen SB, Anderson RB, Cohen BE, Hammit MD, Davis WH. Spherical ceramic interpositional arthroplasty for basal fourth and fifth metatarsal arthritis. Foot Ankle Int. 2007;28(8):896–901.
2. Brunet JA, Wiley JJ. The late results of tarsometatarsal joint injuries. J Bone Joint Surg. 1987;69-B(3):437–40.
3. Komenda GA, Myerson MS, Biddinger KR. Results of arthrodesis of the tarsometatarsal joints after traumatic injury. J Bone Joint Surg. 1996;78(11):1665–76.
4. Patel A, Rao S, Nawoczenski D, Flemister AS, DiGiovanni B, Baumhauer JF. Midfoot arthritis. J Am Acad Orthop Surg. 2010;18(7):417–25.
5. Mann RA, Prieskorn D, Sobel M. Mid-tarsal and tarsometatarsal arthrodesis for primary degenerative osteoarthrosis or osteoarthrosis after trauma. J Bone Joint Surg [Internet]. 1996;78(9):1376–85. Available from: http://jbjs.org/content/78/9/1376.abstract
6. Bariteau JT, Fantry A, Tenenbaum S. Selective fusions for primary midfoot osteoarthritis. Tech Foot Ankle Surg. 2016;15(2):74–8.
7. Jung HG, Myerson MS, Schon LC. Spectrum of operative treatments and clinical outcomes for atraumatic osteoarthritis of the tarsometatarsal joint. Foot Ankle Int. 2007;28(4):482–9.
8. Rao S, Nawoczenski DA, Baumhauer JF. Midfoot arthritis: nonoperative options and decision making for fusion. Tech Foot Ankle Surg. 2008;7(3):188–95.
9. Desmond EA, Chou LB. Current concepts review: lisfranc injuries. Foot Ankle Int. 2006;27(8):653–60.
10. Sarrafian SK, Kelikian AS. Syndesmology. In: Kelikian AS, editor. Sarrafian's anatomy of the foot and ankle. 3rd ed. Philadelphia: Lippincott Williams & Wilkins; 2011. p. 208.
11. Raikin SM, Schon LC. Arthrodesis of the fourth and fifth tarsometatarsal joints of the midfoot. Foot Ankle Int. 2003;24(8):584–90.
12. Ouzounian TJ, Shereff MJ. In vitro determination of midfoot motion. Foot Ankle [Internet]. 1989;17(3):140–6. Available from: http://www.ncbi.nlm.nih.gov/pubmed/15237199.
13. Chang TJ. Lateral column arthroplasty. In: Southerland JT, editor. McGlamry's comprehensive textbook of foot and ankle surgery. 4th ed. Philadelphia: Lippincott Williams & Wilkins; 2013. p. 1234.
14. Nadaud JP, Parks BG, Schon LC. Plantar and calcaneocuboid joint pressure after isolated medial column fusion versus medial and lateral column fusion: a biomechanical study. Foot Ankle Int. 2011;32(11):1069–74.
15. Sangeorzan BJ, Veith RG, Hansen ST. Salvage of lisfranc's tarsometararsal joint by arthrodesis. Foot Ankle Int. 1990;19(4):193–200.
16. Seybold JD, Coetzee JC. Surgical management of posttraumatic midfoot deformity and arthritis. Tech Foot Ankle Surg. 2016;15(2):79–86.

17. Kuo RS, Tejwani NC, DiGiovanni CW. Outcome after open reduction and internal fixation of lisfranc joint injuries. J Bone Joint Surg. 2000;82-A(11):1609–18.
18. Kane JM, Sandrowski K, Saffel H, Albanese A, Raikin SM, Pedowitz DI. The epidemiology of fifth metatarsal fracture. Foot Ankle Spec. 2015;8(5):354–9.
19. Berlet GC, Anderson RB. Tendon arthroplasty of basal fourth and fifth metatarsal arthritis. Foot Ankle Int. 2002;23(5):440–6.
20. Bawa V, Fallat LM, Kish JP. Surgical outcomes for resection of the dorsal exostosis of the metatarsocuneiform joints. J Foot Ankle Surg [Internet]. 2016;55(3):496–9. https://doi.org/10.1053/j.jfas.2015.12.004.
21. Bowers AL, Castro MD. The mechanics behind the image: foot and ankle pathology associated with gastrocnemius contracture. Semin Musculoskelet Radiol. 2007;11(1):83–90.
22. Matsumoto T, Nakamura I, Miura A. Radiologic patterning of joint damage to the foot in rheumatoid arthritis. Arthrit Care. 2014;66(4):499–507.
23. Zide JR, Brodsky JW. Surgical approaches to arthritis and deformity of the midfoot. Tech Foot Ankle Surg. 2016;15(2):87–92.
24. Lui TH. Endoscopic resection of dorsal boss of the second and third tarsometatarsal joints. Arthrosc Tech [Internet]. 2017;6(1):e1–5. https://doi.org/10.1016/j.eats.2016.08.028.
25. Bevilacqua NJ, Rogers LC. Surgical management of Charcot midfoot deformities. Clin Podiatr Med Surg [Internet]. 2008 [Cited 2013 Nov 24];25(1):81–94. Available from: http://www.ncbi.nlm.nih.gov/pubmed/18165114.
26. Hirose CB, Coughlin MJ, Stevens FR. Arthritis of the foot and ankle. In: Mann's surgery of the foot and ankle. 9th ed. Philadelphia: Elsevier Saunders; 2014. p. 867.
27. Coetzee JC. Treatment of hindfoot and midfoot arthritis. In: Mann's surgery of the foot and ankle. 9th ed. Philadelphia: Elsevier Saunders; 2014. p. 1030.
28. Protheroe D, Gadgil A. Guided intra-articular corticosteroid injections in the midfoot. Foot Ankle Int. 2018;39(8):1001–4.
29. Khosla S, Thiele R, Baumhauer JF. Ultrasound guidance for intra-articular injections of the foot and ankle. Foot Ankle Int [Internet]. 2009;30(9):886–90. Available from: http://journals.sagepub.com/doi/10.3113/FAI.2009.0886
30. Grogan KA, Chang TJ, Salk RS. Update on viscosupplementation in the treatment of osteoarthritis of the foot and ankle. Clin Podiatr Med Surg [Internet]. 2018;26(2):199–204. https://doi.org/10.1016/j.cpm.2009.03.001.
31. Rao S, Baumhauer JF. Shoe inserts alter plantar loading and function in patients with midfoot arthritis. J Orthop Sport Phys Ther. 2009;39(7):522–31.
32. Yi T, Kim JH, Oh-Park M, Hwang JH. Effect of full-length carbon fiber insoles on lower limb kinetics in patients with midfoot arthritis. Am J Phys Med Rehabil. 2018;97(3):192–9.
33. Smith TF, Dowling LB. Common pedal prominences. In: Southerland JT, editor. McGlamry's comprehensive textbook of foot and ankle surgery. 4th ed. Philadelphia: Lippincott Williams & Wilkins; 2013. p. 484–92.
34. Gilheany MF, Amir OT. Metatarsocuneiform joint resection arthroplasty for atraumatic osteoarthrosis: an alternative to arthrodesis. J Foot Ankle Surg [Internet]. 2013;52(1):122–4. https://doi.org/10.1053/j.jfas.2012.09.005.
35. Nemec SA, Habbu RA, Anderson JG, Bohay DR. Outcomes following midfoot arthrodesis for primary arthritis. Foot Ankle Int. 2011;32(4):355–61.
36. Philpott A, Lawford C, Lau SC, Chambers S, Bozin M, Oppy A. Modified dorsal approach in the management of lisfranc injuries. Foot Ankle Int. 2018;39(5):573–84.
37. Ryan JD, Timpano ED, Brosky TA II. Average depth of tarsometatarsal joint for trephine arthrodesis. J Foot Ankle Surg Ankle Surg [Internet]. 2012;51(2):168–71. https://doi.org/10.1053/j.jfas.2011.10.028.
38. Barp EA, Erickson JG, Smith HL, Almeida K, Millonig K. Evaluation of fixation techniques for metatarsocuneiform arthrodesis. J Foot Ankle Surg [Internet]. 2017;56(3):468–73. https://doi.org/10.1053/j.jfas.2017.01.012.

39. Ahmad J, Lynch M-K, Maltenfort M. Comparison of screws to plate-and-screw constructs for midfoot arthrodesis. Foot Ankle Int. 2018;epub:1–8.
40. Schipper ON, Ford SE, Moody PW, Van Doren B, Ellington JK. Radiographic results of nitinol compression staples for hindfoot and midfoot arthrodesis. Foot Ankle Int. 2018;39(2):172–9.
41. Buda M, Hagemeijer NC, Kink S, Johnson AH, Guss D, Digiovanni CW. Effect of fixation type and bone graft on tarsometatarsal fusion. Foot Ankle Int. 2018;39(12):1394–402.
42. Hood JRCR, Hoffman SM, Miller JM. Lateral column of the foot arthroplasty with interpositional fascia lata graft: a new technique. Tech Foot Ankle Surg. 2017;16(1):34–40.
43. Russell DF, Ferdinand RD. Review of the evidence: surgical management of 4th and 5th tarsometatarsal joint osteoarthritis. Foot Ankle Surg [Internet]. 2013;19(4):207–11. https://doi.org/10.1016/j.fas.2013.06.002.
44. Sangeorzan BJ, Hansen ST. Early and late posttraumatic foot reconstruction. Clin Orthop Relat Res [Internet]. 1989;243(June):86–91. Available from: http://www.ncbi.nlm.nih.gov/pubmed/2566404.
45. Koenis MJJ, Louwerens JW. Simple resection arthroplasty for treatment of 4th and 5th tarsometatarsal joint problems. A technical tip and small case series. Foot Ankle Surg [Internet]. 2018;21(1):70–2. https://doi.org/10.1016/j.fas.2014.05.006.
46. Rammelt S, Schneiders W. Primary open reduction and fixation compared with delayed corrective arthrodesis in the treatment of tarsometatarsal (lisfranc) fracture dislocation. J Bone Joint Surg. 2008;90-B(11):1499–506.
47. Budny AM, Grossman JP. Naviculocuneiform arthrodesis. Clin Podiatr Med Surg. 2007;24:753–63.
48. Reinhardt KR, Oh LS, Schottel P, Roberts MM, Levine D. Treatment of lisfranc fracture-dislocations with primary partial arthrodesis. Foot Ankle Int [Internet]. 2012;33(1):50–6. Available from: http://journals.sagepub.com/doi/10.3113/FAI.2012.0050
49. Bibbo C, Anderson RB, Davis WH. Complications of midfoot and hindfoot arthrodesis. Clin Orthop Relat Res. 2001;391:45–58.
50. Bevilacqua NJ. Tarsometatarsal arthrodesis for lisfranc injuries. Clin Podiatr Med Surg [Internet]. 2017;34(3):315–25. https://doi.org/10.1016/j.cpm.2017.02.003.
51. Lau S, Guest C, Hall M, Tacey M, Joseph S, Oppy A. Functional outcomes post lisfranc injury – transarticular screws, dorsal bridge plating or combination treatment? J Orthop Trauma. 2017;31(8):447–52.
52. Smith N, Stone C, Furey A. Does open reduction and internal fixation versus primary arthrodesis improve patient outcomes for lisfranc trauma? A systematic review and meta-analysis. Clin Orthop Relat Res. 2016;474(6):1445–52.
53. Albright RH, Haller S, Klein E, Baker JR, Weil LW Jr, Weil LSW Sr, et al. Cost-effectiveness analysis of primary arthrodesis versus open reduction internal fixation for primary ligamentous lisfranc injuries. J Foot Ankle Surg [Internet]. 2018;57(2):325–31. https://doi.org/10.1053/j.jfas.2017.10.016.
54. Bevan WPC, Tomlinson MPW. Radiographic measures as a predictor of ulcer formation in diabetic charcot midfoot. Foot Ankle Int [Internet]. 2008 [Cited 2013 Nov 24];29(6):568–73. Available from: http://www.ncbi.nlm.nih.gov/pubmed/18549751.
55. Capobianco CM, Ramanujam CL, Zgonis T. Charcot foot reconstruction with combined internal and external fixation: case report. J Orthop Surg Res. 2010;5(1):1–9.

# Chapter 7
# Flatfoot Deformity

**Andrew J. Meyr and Laura E. Sansosti**

## Introduction

Any meaningful discussion into a specific pathology should begin with an attempt to clarify an objective and broadly accepted definition. With respect to the so-called "flatfoot" deformity, this represents a surprisingly qualitative, subjective, and variable task considering the amount of time, energy, resources, and scientific literature that have historically been dedicated to the complaint. This challenge might be best considered within three specific limitations.

The first limitation is the relatively ambiguous terminology used to describe what is likely a wide range of clinical pathologies. Some nomenclature seems to refer to the structural nature and general appearance of the complaint (i.e., flatfoot, pes valgus, pes planus, pes planovalgus, collapsed arch, fallen arch, etc.). Other languages seem to refer to the dynamic aspects associated with the conditions (i.e., pronation syndrome, overpronation, pronating foot type, etc.). And further wording still more specifically refers to some of the involved anatomic structures (i.e., peritalar subluxation, posterior tibial tendon dysfunction, spring ligament failure, sinus tarsi impingement, etc.). For the purposes of this chapter, we chose to utilize the admittedly broad term "flatfoot," with specification and differentiation as necessary utilized throughout.

The second limitation is the general clinical practice to consider the deformity as a categorical outcome. In other words, our profession has a tendency to broadly

A. J. Meyr (✉)
Department of Surgery, Temple University School of Podiatric Medicine,
Philadelphia, PA, USA
e-mail: ajmeyr@gmail.com

L. E. Sansosti
Departments of Surgery and Biomechanics, Temple University School of Podiatric Medicine,
Philadelphia, PA, USA
e-mail: laura.sansosti@temple.edu



D. E. Tower (ed.), *Evidence-Based Podiatry*,
https://doi.org/10.1007/978-3-030-50853-1_7

group foot types into one of three boxes: "rectus," "flat," or "cavus." Conceptually, this might initially represent a problem as it implies the presence of dysfunction and deformity in the "flat" and "cavus" groups, when in actuality structure is not always related to symptomatology. Further, one might argue that this categorization is not consistent with clinical experience. In reality, a range of foot types are encountered more closely representing a continuous spectrum than distinct categories. And it is difficult, if not impossible, to draw definitive lines within this spectrum to signify where a "rectus foot" ends and a "flatfoot" begins when considering the examination of the complaint from a clinical or radiographic perspective. These lines are blurred if present at all.

Complicating this matter further is that these categories also likely represent the foot in a static position, and not the dynamic and mobile positioning in which the musculoskeletal structure of the foot would be expected to take throughout the course of a single step. In fact, most believe that the foot progresses through a normal, relatively fluid range of neutral positioning, relative pronation, and relative supination over the course of the gait cycle. Based on this assumption, we might clarify our definition of "flatfoot" a bit further within this chapter to involve a foot that does not function appropriately through this range of pronation to supination, with a tendency toward overpronation in the setting of associated clinical symptomatology.

And the third limitation is perhaps the most challenging of all, particularly with respect to the "evidence-based" theme of this text. Although the biomechanical and pathomechanical function of the foot has been historically and is currently investigated with established scientific principles and many dedicated and appropriately celebrated tomes on the subject have served as the basis of podiatric education for decades, these primarily represent theory. This statement might be a difficult pill for many to swallow but for better or worse is a state of affairs that we would do well to accept. It is again difficult, if not impossible, to study this topic within the strict confines of a contemporary evidence-based medicine paradigm. This is a model that is primarily designed for comparative and interventional analyses, and not necessarily for more descriptive ones. And, although it would be easy to dichotomize this as a negative, your authors would argue that this represents a flaw within evidence-based medicine itself and not the topic of podiatric biomechanics. In fact, a lack of high powered clinical evidence implies neither inaccuracy nor a lack of knowledge.

When considering this point, the authors are reminded of a quote from the nineteenth-century French physicist and mathematician Henri Poincaré who said: "There isn't one way of measuring science that is more true than another; that which is generally adopted is only more convenient. Most science is not absolute truth; it is advantageous" [1]. On the surface this might seem rather unscientific, but in fact it represents an effective blend of evidence-based practice, scientific theory, and clinical experience. We might all have slightly different views and theories of the specific biomechanical function of the lower extremity, but that which is most effective for a specific clinician in practice is that which is most advantageous to their patient's care. And while our profession might never agree on all of the finite details, individual clinicians making treatment decisions based on their individual interpretation of evidence-based practice, scientific theory, and clinical experience do represent an inherently scientific approach to diagnosis and treatment.

Interestingly, Poincaré is also considered one of the founding parents of the scientific concept known as "chaos theory" [1]. Although this name implies somewhat of an anarchy without rules or guiding principles, in fact chaos theory relates quite closely to our discussion of flatfoot and the inherent limitations therein. Chaos theory actually rejects concepts of randomness and instead attempts to elucidate and describe the underlying patterns of a complex system that simply hasn't yet been well understood, observed, or measured. It also proposes that small changes to the initial conditions of the system are likely to lead to substantially different long-term outcomes.

How does this not describe the complex system known as a flatfoot! Even though there are certainly some accepted patterns that are observed relative to the flatfoot deformity, structure, and function alone, do not completely describe the complexities of patient symptoms nor their responses to treatment interventions. And, although all human feet have theoretically evolved to a similar morphology and function, most experienced practitioners would agree that most feet do not function in exactly the same manner nor will they respond in exactly the same way to standard treatment interventions or protocols.

This accurately represents the philosophic objective of this chapter. In line with chaos theory, we will attempt to elucidate the common underlying patterns of the complex tissue structure known as the flatfoot deformity and attempt to describe how seemingly small changes to the structure and function of the foot might lead to different clinical situations of patient symptoms requiring individual physician prescription. This will be attempted by posing and answering five presumably basic questions.

## Question 1: What Is the Pathoanatomy of the Flatfoot Deformity?

To utilize another analogy from the history of science, consider the motion of a simple pendulum. Thomas Kuhn described a pendulum in *The Structure of Scientific Revolutions* as a "heavy body falling with difficulty" [2]. In other words, the natural path for the object is for it to fall straight toward the ground in a direct line. But the string attached to the body impedes this motion and passively "pulls" the object on a consistent, cyclical, and arcing path, almost in opposition to the natural will of the object.

Perhaps the human gait cycle is not too different from this seemingly elementary example. When a human takes even a single step forward, it actually represents a rather precarious proprioceptive position for the body to be placed in. All of the subject's body weight and momentum are advanced in a forward direction, and in effect the person is falling anteriorly. But we implicitly trust from experience that we will not fall and that our leading lower extremity will instead effectively impede this action.

Of course this act of "fall impeding" is a complicated neuromuscular and skeletal event driven by centuries of evolutionary morphology [3–6]. First, the hip flexes and the knee extends to place the foot in a mechanically advantageous position to strike the ground and oppose the weight of the falling body. And instead of the foot striking the ground as an inert stationary object, it does so in a specific way to first effectively absorb the shock of the body's force.

Pressure is defined as force divided by area. During the gait cycle, the "force" is a relative constant defined by the weight and pace of the subject. The "area" is also relatively constant in that the plantar foot has a certain fixed anatomic surface, but it is able to maneuver in such a way as to provide a relative increase in the functional area. First, the entire surface of the plantar foot does not normally strike the ground simultaneously but instead in a relative posterior-to-anterior (i.e., heel-to-toe) direction [7–9]. This spreads the constant force out over a relatively greater period of time and thus decreases the peak pressure experienced at any specific point. The longer the time (even on the order of fractions of a second), the lower the peak pressure experienced. And the osseous and ligamentous anatomy of the medial and lateral longitudinal arches arranged in this posterior-to-anterior direction provides a degree of intrinsic stability for accepting this force as opposed to a static block of bone. Second, the posterior aspect of the foot normally strikes the ground in a relatively inverted position and immediately transitions through a range of inversion to eversion to further spread out the constant force over a relatively greater time period in a lateral-to-medial orientation [7–9]. Again, the peak pressure experienced at any given point from the fall is decreased as the force is spread out over a relatively wide area and time frame.

At this point it is fair to say that the leading foot is in a relatively flattened position. And what we have just generally described above as a controlled fall is commonly referred to as foot "pronation" in contemporary practice and is commonly taught as the ability of the foot to function as a so-called mobile adapter [7–9].

With this broad understanding, we can now return to the beginning and further discuss the specific anatomy of this series of events. As the hip flexes and the knee extends, the leg and foot also move more subtly to put the posterior calcaneal tuber in a mechanically advantageous position to strike the ground. The ankle dorsiflexes, and the subtalar joint inverts to situate the calcaneus in relative dorsiflexion and inversion for the initial shock of heel strike [7–9]. This is unquestionably a harsh force but is intrinsically supported by the specialized compartmentalization of the calcaneal fat pad and the rounded cortical morphology of the posterior calcaneus [10, 11]. Immediately, the joints of the posterior foot initiate relative pronation in order to spread out this force both relatively laterally and anteriorly. The calcaneus will subsequently move from a position of relative inversion/supination to neutral positioning and through a range of relative eversion/pronation.

Although clinically and surgically the ankle, subtalar, calcaneocuboid, and talonavicular joints are considered individually, the functional anatomic configuration of these joints might be considered a bit more basic. In fact, it might be easier for this particular exercise to conceptualize the talus as a functional part of the leg instead of the foot during gait. In other words, as the calcaneus starts relative eversion following heel strike, the structural and ligamentous anatomy dictate that the cuboid and the navicular follow the motion of the calcaneus essentially independently of the talus [7–9]. The talus is almost "left behind" in the ankle mortise and relatively plantarflexes and adducts toward the midline of the body throughout this process. These combined motions give "pronation" of the foot. The calcaneus (and subsequently the remainder of the foot) is relatively dorsiflexed, abducted, and everted relative to the talus. Hansen termed this conceptualization of foot function "peritalar subluxation" as the entire foot almost appears to "swing off" of the talar head during pronation [12]. This view is reinforced by common radiographic measurements of the flatfoot including talar head uncovering, the cuboid abduction angle, Kite's angle, and Meary's angle [13] (Figs. 7.1 and 7.2).

At this point it might be worth pausing to consider that although the foot is in a distinctly "pronated" position through this arthrologic maneuvering, this represents a perfectly normal and accepted aspect of foot function. Pronation is often dichotomized as "bad" or "negative" when considering the flatfoot deformity, but this mechanism is the means by which the human body is able to "fall with difficulty" during the gait cycle. Without this combination of movements, it is likely that we would either clumsily fall forward as we try and take a step or injure soft tissue and bone structures by absorbing too much pressure as the body weight abruptly strikes the ground. Pronation is an essential, normal part of human gait.

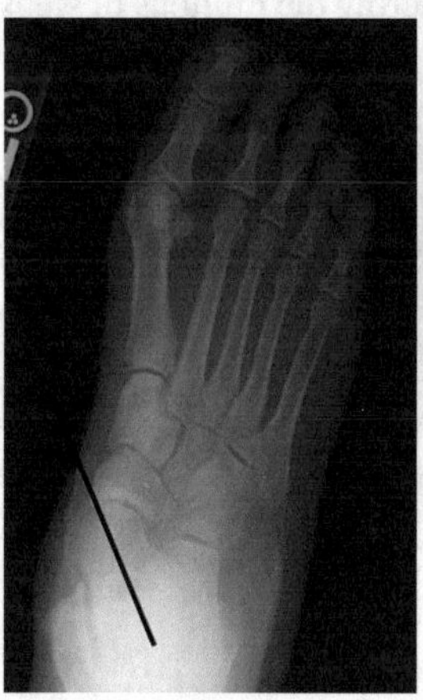
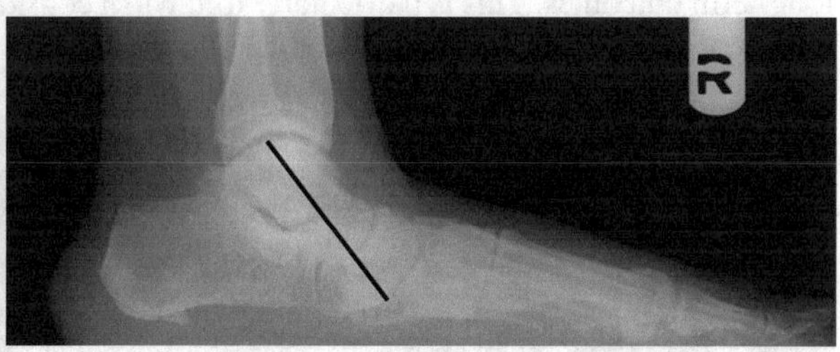


**Figs. 7.1 and 7.2** Radiographic appearance of the foot in a pronated position. Figure 7.1 (an AP weight-bearing projection) and Fig. 7.2 (a lateral weight-bearing projection) demonstrate the common radiographic appearance of a pronated foot in line with the peritalar subluxation paradigm. Note how the midfoot and forefoot have pronated off of the longitudinal axis of the talus into relative abduction on the AP projection and relative dorsiflexion on the lateral projection. This might be further objectified with measurement of talar head uncovering, the cuboid abduction angle, Kite's angle, the talar declination angle, and Meary's angle among others

Of course, however, this only represents about half of normal foot function. We have taken that brave initial step forward and effectively fallen with difficulty. But in order to keep forward momentum going, we have to now reverse track and relatively supinate as the center of pressure traverses distally. At this point the foot has accepted the brunt of body weight posteriorly and moved it in a relatively lateral direction as it courses anteriorly toward the midfoot and forefoot. To perhaps simplify this action conceptually while staying within a peritalar subluxation paradigm, the actions of supination now "pull" the remainder of the foot back on top of the relatively stationary talar head and transform the medial column into a "rigid lever" for forward propulsion [7–9]. And it might be most simple to visualize this by means of the posterior tibial tendon "pulling" on the navicular/midfoot from a relatively abducted position into a relatively adducted position on the talar head (Figs. 7.3 and 7.4). The talus relatively dorsiflexes and abducts, while the calcaneus/cuboid/navicular complex relatively inverts, adducts, and plantarflexes. Through these actions and others, the center of pressure travels lateral to medial as it courses proximal to distal into the forefoot, eventually driving out the medial rays to propel the body into another step forward (Fig. 7.5).

So if "pronation" is a natural and necessary part of the human gait cycle, why is the pathologic flatfoot deformity so often associated with the term? The reasons are, of course, multifactorial. But it might be easiest to visualize that it starts with a relatively simple breakdown or multiple simple breakdowns that occur somewhere within this complex process involving the coordination of multiple bones, joints, muscles, tendons, and ligaments. And in line with chaos theory, a relatively small change to the initial conditions might have the potential to drastically affect the long-term outcomes. This is particularly true when considering the millions of steps that are thought to occur over the course of a lifetime.

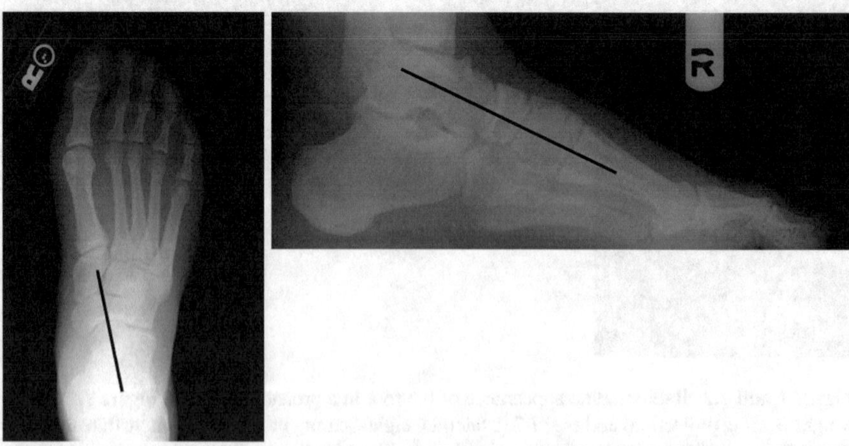


**Figs. 7.3 and 7.4** Radiographic appearance of the foot in a neutral position. Contrast Fig. 7.3 (an AP weight-bearing projection) and Fig. 7.4 (a lateral weight-bearing projection) with Figs. 7.1 and 7.2. In this neutral or even supinated position, the midfoot and forefoot are now directly in line with the longitudinal axis of the talus in both the transverse and sagittal planes

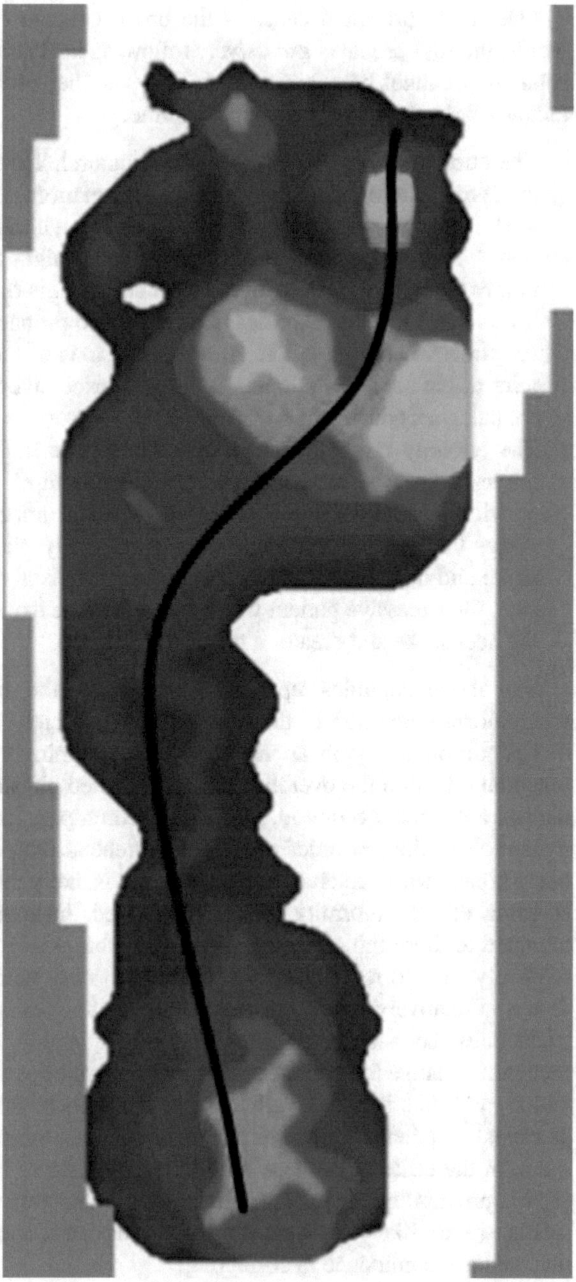

**Fig. 7.5** Pedobarographic depiction of the stance phase of gait in a left foot. This pedobarograph demonstrates a relatively normal progression of the center of pressure in a posterior-to-anterior direction during gait initiating with heel strike in the central calcaneus, traversing laterally through the midfoot and then medially through the forefoot and out the hallux

One likely prevalent cause is the broad concept of "overpronation." In other words, the foot pronates *excessively* following heel strike to the point that effective supination cannot be achieved. And, any number of relatively small contributing factors might cause this to occur over time:

- The etiology might be static and/or structural. This might come in the form of excessive external rotation or valgus orientation of the hip, femur, knee, tibia, ankle, talus, subtalar joint, calcaneus, etc. As a common example, a tarsal coalition of the middle facet of the subtalar joint might position the articulation in a relatively everted orientation for heel strike. This disrupts the expected cycle of inversion to eversion and leads to excessive pronation without the opportunity for effective compensation. An abnormal axis of the subtalar joint or midtarsal joint might achieve a similar effect with excessive initial valgus positioning of the calcaneus during heel strike.
- The etiology might be more dynamic and/or functional. Ligamentous laxity might be present, particularly of medial structures, leading to excessive valgus positioning following heel strike. Or, equinus deformity of the Achilles tendon places the forefoot and midfoot in a relatively plantarflexed position for heel strike and disrupts the expected proximal-to-distal course of the center of pressure. Or, excessive patient weight increases the expected force experienced during heel strike and creates a relative imbalance.

The above examples represent just a few of the dozens of possible scenarios where normal function of the foot might be affected. The diagnostic challenge of this condition comes in appreciating these seemingly minor variations and their potential effect on the overall complex. Detailed physical and radiographic examinations are usually required, involving the complex in both static positioning and dynamic function, in order to fully comprehend the pathogenesis. And, if we are being honest with ourselves as physicians, it is likely that a complete clinical understanding of the deformity is rarely achieved. Instead, it is human nature to be attracted to those things which we have an ability to correct. So, for example, it is relatively easy to recognize an equinus deformity with the Silfverskiöld test, and thus it is relatively easy to recommend stretching exercises and/or perform a gastrocnemius recession or Achilles tendon lengthening. And, it is relatively easy to recognize relative forefoot abduction during a radiographic, stance, and gait examination, and thus it is relatively easy to recommend and perform an Evans lateral calcaneal lengthening procedure. This point is not meant in any way to denigrate or question the efficacy of these time-tested procedures but might speak to a certain pretest probability of deformity recognition and treatment intervention. In other words, we are likely to be more naturally drawn to those aspects of the deformity that we have confidence in correcting.

In line with this thinking, one final consideration with respect to pathoanatomy is that our clinical interventional response often does not necessarily address the underlying pathology and instead is directed at patient symptoms. In fact, the majority of the symptomatology associated with the flatfoot might be better considered as the "effect" as opposed to the "cause." Posterior tibial tendon dysfunction provides a hallmark example of this. Certainly an acutely ruptured posterior tibial tendon could lead to a flatfoot deformity as the body loses one of the primary agents of supination [7–9]. But in most situations, the pathology associated with the posterior tibial tendon represents the chronic consequence of a separate primary etiology. For whatever reason, overpronation following heel strike has occurred, and the posterior tibial tendon begins firing earlier, harder, and longer in an attempt to compensate and effectively supinate the foot [7–9, 12]. This might work temporarily, but eventually microtrauma and chronic inflammation cause the tendon to weaken, stretch, tear, and become symptomatic. Simply repairing the damaged tendon as an isolated procedure is unlikely to have substantial effect except in early stages of the disease process as it does not necessarily address the underlying cause of the increased workload in the first place [14–16].

The subsequent questions in this chapter will attempt to more specifically define this pathogenesis and symptomatology and discuss the direct and indirect aspects of treatment prescription.

## Question 2: What Dictates the Symptomatology of a Flatfoot?

As discussed in the previous section, the flatfoot deformity is one that is often complex and multifactorial potentially involving multiple tendons, ligaments, joints, and bones. And while some patients might remain asymptomatic even in the setting of substantial clinical deformity, many experience a variety of complaints. Soft tissue structures, and the posterior tibial tendon in particular, seem to have the largest potential for producing symptoms consistent with chronic inflammation and damage. However these structures might also include the plantar calcaneonavicular (spring) ligament, deltoid ligament, interosseous ligaments of the subtalar joint, lateral ankle ligaments, and other extrinsic tendons of the ankle including the Achilles tendon, tibialis anterior tendon, and peroneal tendons [17–19]. Similarly, depending on the progression and severity of the deformity, pain might originate from the affected joints of the midfoot (particularly through the medial column), rearfoot, and ankle [20].

A thorough physical examination is critical in order to properly evaluate the origin of these symptoms as subjective complaints might be somewhat generalized. Simple active and passive range of motion exercises will initially help to determine if the deformity is rigid versus flexible in nature. Rigid deformities are typically at either end of the deformity spectrum meaning that they present relatively early (usually in the form of a tarsal coalition at the talocalcaneal or calcaneonavicular joints) or late (usually in the form of end-stage degenerative arthrosis) [17, 21]. The age of the patient should be considered if a coalition is suspected, as well as an association of symptoms with activity and/or peroneal tendon spasm [21]. In addition to radiographs, particularly the Salter-Harris view, a common peroneal nerve block might be of some diagnostic value.

Symptoms associated with the adult presentation are likely related to the stage of deformity and disease progression. In addition, age, obesity, and other medical comorbidities may play a role in symptom development. These symptoms often begin near the medial rearfoot and specifically along the course of the posterior tibial tendon. They might be focal to the insertion of this tendon, as is often the case in a Kidner foot type or gorilliform navicular, or may extend along the distal course of the tendon at the medial malleolus. Degeneration and chronic damage to the tendon most commonly occur at the retromalleolar watershed region approximately 2–4 cm proximal to the insertion [18]. Initially, pain related to the tendon will most likely be reported as occurring primarily with activity or standing but may occur at rest with longstanding disease. Patients with severe posterior tibial tendon involvement will be limited or unable to perform single/double heel raises [21, 22]. Weakness against resisted inversion is also a hallmark of posterior tibial tendon involvement or potentially even complete rupture of the tendon [17]. Several clinical classification systems have been proposed to specifically describe the posterior tibial tendon involvement within this deformity including the Johnson and Strom [14, 15], Funk [23], and Janis [24] classifications.

Medial symptoms might also result as a consequence of spring ligament attenuation or tear, which in some cases might even be present independent of symptoms of the posterior tibial tendon. The deltoid ligament might also subsequently attenuate as the deformity progresses leading to medial ankle symptoms and relative instability. All of these in concert are likely to cause abnormal rearfoot/ankle joint position and function, leading to the development of degenerative changes [18, 20]. Once the medial tendinous and ligamentous structures have failed, the ankle will shift into a valgus position with the lateral talar dome opposing the ankle mortise [22]. These patients are likely to present with crepitus and pain with ankle range of motion.

Lateral symptoms might also be expected in the midfoot and rearfoot as the foot progressively abducts and the Achilles tendon moves into a relatively lateral orientation. This specifically presents in the form of sinus tarsi syndrome and inferior fibular impingement [17, 18]. A study by Martus and colleagues reported on the presence of an accessory anterolateral talar facet as a source of impingement symptoms in the flatfoot deformity [21]. Although only a small study cohort, all 7 feet were found on MRI to have bone marrow edema signifying impingement between an accessory facet and anterior calcaneus. Malicky et al. [25] reported on talocalcaneal and subfibular impingement in a group of 19 patients who underwent weight-bearing simulated CT scans. They noted sinus tarsi impingement in 92% of this cohort and calcaneofibular impingement in 66%.

Degenerative arthritic changes, which may eventually develop, can result in beaking or exostosis formation, particularly at the dorsal midfoot. In addition to the direct arthritic pain, this might additionally produce nerve symptoms in line with a compression neuritis. Further, compensation for the flatfoot deformity might also lead to forefoot deformity and symptomatic callus formation related to the underlying pathomechanics [22].

## Question 3: Can Flatfoot Be Effectively Treated Conservatively?

The initial management of the flatfoot deformity is nearly always through conservative means. Physical examination techniques and an understanding of the specific contributing anatomic aspects of the deformity are paramount in order to determine how to most directly address the primary deforming force or forces with these measures. For example, in considering patients with flexible posterior tibial tendon symptoms versus rigid coalitions, orthoses would be fabricated differently to provide more corrective versus accommodative function, respectively [26].

The literature with respect to conservative management in pediatric patients is generally supportive, and several data reviews are available. A 2011 Cochrane review found that most children are initially placed in a variety of insoles or orthotic devices [27]. Although no definitive conclusions could be reached with respect to the potential superiority of individual specific devices, a consistent improvement in foot posture and forefoot abduction was noted. The authors also commented that the performance of physical modalities including therapy was found to be beneficial, despite some inherent shortcomings of the included investigations. And interestingly, the authors also describe that progressive development should be considered a confounding variable when considering this topic. In other words, it is difficult to determine exactly what role "outgrowing the deformity" through skeletal maturity plays, but it likely has some influence. MacKenzie and colleagues further performed a systematic literature review regarding the conservative management of pediatric flatfoot and noted similar findings to the Cochrane review [28].

Most of the data, however, is somewhat limited in that the provided interventions are relatively poorly controlled compared to higher levels of evidence. It is simply difficult to control for confounding variables when considering this pathology. Additionally, a number of different outcome measurements are utilized making comparisons between studies challenging. For example, Riccio et al. performed a comparative study examining differences between physical therapy and orthotics [29]. They utilized static foot posture as an outcome measure and noted that therapy was more effective in increasing the number of normal footprints long term. Somewhat similarly, Capasso evaluated a dynamic varus heel cup and found it to be more effective than a simple insole but utilized four different footprint methods [30]. And then in another example of a relatively structural outcome measure, Leung and colleagues found decreased eversion of the calcaneus through gait with the exception of heel strike with the use of an UCBL insert [31].

In terms of more functional outcome measures, Whitford and Esterman compared pain and function between groups treated with over-the-counter and custom orthoses. A significant reduction in pain was noted over time; however, there was no difference in function between the two groups [32]. Mereday et al. found similar reduction in pain with use of UCBL inserts [33].

When considering the conservative management of the adult flexible flatfoot deformity, the initial approach is also usually with shoegear modification and accommodative inserts. Patients with a flexible flatfoot would theoretically benefit from a lace-up straight last shoe with a firm heel counter to prevent relative valgus positioning of the calcaneus [26]. Medial counter reinforcements support the arch and prevent medial shoe collapse, and this has the potential to reduce symptoms of posterior tibial tendon strain. And, rocker bottomed soles might also be beneficial in those with rigid deformities [26].

The specific literature relating to this, however, has a similar list of limitations to the pediatric data including relatively small sample sizes, a general lack of control groups and randomization, variable outcome measures, and relatively short follow-up periods. With that being said, some comparative investigations are available. Imhauser and colleagues examined the efficacy of external support on the flatfoot deformity through a cadaveric study in which the main support structures of the medial longitudinal arch were sectioned [34]. Six different braces were then tested including in-shoe orthoses, ankle braces, and a molded ankle-foot orthosis. The authors noted the in-shoe orthoses stabilized the medial longitudinal arch and hindfoot, whereas the ankle braces did not, leading to the recommendation that an in-shoe orthosis should be incorporated as a first-line conservative intervention. In a study by Alvarez et al., conservative management of stage I and II posterior tibial tendon dysfunction with orthoses and physical therapy was assessed [35]. Following a median of 10 therapy sessions over 4 months, 83% of patients demonstrated improvement in subjective and functional outcomes with an 89% satisfaction rate. Notably 11% of their study cohort went on to operative intervention due to failure of the conservative protocol. Chao et al. studied 49 patients with posterior tibial tendon dysfunction managed with orthoses which subjects wore for a mean time of 12.3 hours/day [36]. Good to excellent results were reported in 67% of patients based on a functional scoring system accounting for pain, function, use of an assistive device, distance of ambulation, and patient satisfaction.

Nielsen et al. performed a retrospective cohort study on 64 consecutive patients evaluating the efficacy of bracing, physical therapy, and anti-inflammatory medications [37]. Patients were assessed over a 27-month period with a success rate of 87.5% reported. Although they noted a prevalence rate of obesity of 78.1% in their cohort and 62.5% of the patients who failed conservative treatment measures were obese, body mass index was not a statistically significant predictor for treatment failure. The use of bracing did yield a statistically significant association with successful nonoperative treatment. And interestingly, patients with any form of specific tearing of the posterior tibial tendon, as noted on MRI, were statistically more likely to fail nonoperative treatment.

For patients with more progressive and/or arthritic symptoms, more aggressive bracing above the ankle might be warranted to decrease or eliminate motion. Symptom relief has been reported in the range of 50–90% of patients with this form of management [15, 36, 38].

In summary, it seems reasonable to conclude that conservative interventions in the form of external support and physical modalities have the potential to provide some relief of patient symptoms without substantial risk or complication. However, the specific expectations related to these interventions and which specific patient factors are associated with benefit from specific interventions remain inconclusive.

## Question 4: What Is the Effectiveness of a Single Surgical Procedure?

For those patients who fail conservative treatment or for whom conservative treatment is not an option, many different surgical interventions have been described for deformity correction and symptom relief. These range from soft tissue procedures such as tendon transfers and direct ligament repairs to major joint arthrodeses. And, while it is possible that some procedures might be performed on an individual basis (such as an isolated subtalar joint arthrodesis), more often multiple procedures are performed in combination where each individual procedure is intended to serve a specific purpose or address a specific anatomic aspect of the overall reconstruction. This makes measuring the effect of any single surgical procedure challenging.

Perhaps the individual procedure that has been most studied in isolation is the arthroereisis, although even this is often combined with at least an Achilles tendon lengthening or gastrocnemius recession. This is a relatively minimally invasive procedure used to treat flexible deformities by internally restricting pronation at the subtalar joint. A broad review of the literature demonstrates a trend toward positive results with this intervention when considering radiographic and functional outcomes. However, it should be noted that this is a common conclusion when reviewing the literature of any surgical procedure from any surgical specialty. First of all, surgeon scientists have a tendency to publish positive results as opposed to negative ones. This is simply human nature. Second, by definition an intervention is performed in all patients in all of these studies, and thus some effect should be expected. In other words, this is not a clinical complaint that is amenable to a study that utilizes a placebo or sham intervention for comparison. All patients underwent an intervention that would be expected to produce at least some effect.

A few other inherent limitations are commonly observed in studies investigating the effect of a surgical procedure. Most investigations of this form are retrospective cohort analyses where the only comparison is preoperative to postoperative outcomes. Because of this, it is difficult to examine the comparative effectiveness of similar procedures. Additionally, as most are retrospective, a certain degree of selection bias is inherent. Although comparisons might be calculated between differing surgical procedures, unless randomization was performed, there must have been some reason that the surgeon made the specific surgical recommendation in the first place, even if they were not consciously aware of it.

With that said, however, there are some examples of investigations that invoke a direct comparison. Paolo and colleagues performed a prospective study on 13 children undergoing bilateral arthroereisis with two different implant types [39]. At the 1-year postoperative mark, both implant groups demonstrated similar improvement in rearfoot frontal plane alignment and radiographic parameters, as well as more physiologic firing of the tibialis anterior tendon. Chong and colleagues sought to compare the efficacy of subtalar arthroereisis in comparison to the Evans lateral column lengthening osteotomy [40]. Twenty-four feet with a mean age of 12.8 years were prospectively compared utilizing kinematic motion analysis, pedobarometry, radiography, and the Oxford Ankle-Foot Questionnaire for Children. At the 1-year postoperative mark, significant differences were noted in both groups compared to preoperative measures; however, no differences between the groups were observed. And, in a meta-analysis allowing for pooled data of individual outcomes, complication rates ranging between 4.8% and 18.6%, unplanned removal rates of 7.1–19.3%, and patient satisfaction rates ranged from 79% to 100% were reported [41].

The Cotton osteotomy within the medial cuneiform is primarily described as an adjunctive procedure addressing the sagittal plane component of the flatfoot deformity. As it is one of the few osseous procedures specifically addressing the sagittal plane, some limited data is available with respect to the procedure in isolation. Kunas and colleagues attempted to measure the direct effect of the Cotton osteotomy utilizing a specific radiographic measurement at the 40-week follow-up [42]. Notably, incremental changes in graft size were found to be associated with progressive angular correction. And then in a retrospective comparative study examining flatfoot reconstructions with and without a Cotton osteotomy, Aiyer et al. found that patients who underwent the Cotton procedure had statistically significant changes in articular surface angles and arch height [43].

Osteotomies in and around the calcaneus are more challenging to review individually. Although performed within the same anatomic area, each has a specific indication. For example, the Evans lateral calcaneal osteotomy produces a predominantly transverse plane correction but is able to provide deformity correction in all three cardinal body planes. Whereas the medial calcaneal slide osteotomy is primarily considered a frontal plane procedure. Very few studies have produced meaningful data with respect to a comparison between these and other procedures. Saunders and colleagues compared a step-cut lengthening calcaneal osteotomy (SLCO) to the Evans, noting the requirement for a significantly larger graft size in the Evans group as well as a higher rate of return for hardware removal in the Evans group [44]. FAOS scores, lateral column pain, exercise tolerance, and ambulation distance were equivalent between groups. Smith, Adelaar, and Wayne studied combinations of flatfoot corrective procedures in an attempt to determine which was the most efficacious [45]. All procedures included a tendon transfer, a medializing calcaneal osteotomy (MCO), and one of the three lateral column procedures – Evans osteotomy, calcaneocuboid distraction arthrodesis, or Z-calcaneal osteotomy. While the combinations of Evans or Z-lengthening with the MCO produced the greatest decrease in rearfoot valgus and forefoot abduction, they significantly increased lateral column ground reaction forces and joint contact forces. Wadehra and colleagues similarly, retrospectively, reviewed a combination of 56 pediatric and adult feet undergoing flatfoot reconstruction with gastrocnemius recession and varying combinations of MCO, Evans osteotomy, and Cotton osteotomy [46]. Radiographic parameters improved with all combinations of the procedures leading the authors to conclude that a plantigrade foot can be recreated in any number of ways.

## Question 5: What Should Be the Expectations of Patients and Physicians with Respect to Surgical Treatment?

By way of conclusion, readers should appreciate that the inherent value to any discussion about this deformity comes if it results in a means to improve patient care. And while radiographic and pedobarographic outcome measures provide some clinical evidence in the assessment of the correction of the flatfoot deformity, patient-centered and functional outcome measures might be argued to be of greater clinical importance. This might be particularly true in contemporary practice because of an increasing emphasis on outcomes-based and value-based reimbursement strategies by healthcare institutions and insurance providers. And, in line with the data previously reported in this chapter, this has been primarily positive in the literature when considering commonly performed interventions for this condition.

Faldini et al. performed a study with the purpose of evaluating patient-perceived quality of life following subtalar arthroereisis [47]. Results showed an Italian Modified Foot Function Index mean score of 4.5 with excellent results for the perception of quality of life and self-reported foot and ankle scores. Chong and colleagues reported on 1-year postoperative results of the arthroereisis with the Oxford Ankle-Foot Questionnaire, demonstrating improvements in the score of both pediatric patients and their parents [40]. Similar score improvements were noted in the lateral column lengthening group, although this did not reach statistical significance. Yontar et al. examined pediatric flatfoot reconstruction results in 21 feet with a mean follow-up of 39.2 months [48]. All cases included a lateral column lengthening and a percutaneous lengthening of the Achilles or gastrocnemius recession. AOFAS scores showed a statistically significant increase from 56.76 to 95.29, with all parents indicating that they would elect to undergo operative intervention again.

Walley and colleagues compared outcomes between 2 cohorts of patients: 30 treated with medial displacement calcaneal osteotomy, posterior tibial tendon resection, flexor digitorum longus transfer, spring ligament reefing, and Achilles lengthening and 15 treated with the above plus an arthroereisis [49]. Final SF-36 scores were 77.1 and 75.4 in the control and experimental groups, while VAS scores decreased significantly in both groups from 8.10 to 3.20 in the control group and 8.83 to 2.44 in those who underwent the addition of the arthroereisis.

Conti et al. investigated the effect of talonavicular joint position on clinical outcomes following flatfoot reconstruction [50]. In comparing postoperative outcomes in a position of adduction or abduction, those who were overcorrected into a slight adduction had lower improvement in FAOS daily activities, quality of life, pain, and sports activity scores. However, no statistically significant differences were noted between the two groups. In a separate investigation, Conti and colleagues studied the optimal heel position following reconstruction [51]. Fifty-five patients were classified postoperatively into groups of valgus ($n$ = 18), mild varus ($n$ = 17), and moderate varus ($n$ = 20). Those who had a mild varus postoperatively demonstrated significantly greater improvement in FAOS pain scores and symptoms scores compared to those in valgus and moderate varus, respectively. And, in a final investigation by this group, the relationship of age and outcomes was evaluated [52]. Conti et al. examined 140 feet in groups of <45 years ($n = 21$), 45–65 years ($n = 87$), and >65 years ($n = 32$). Although the authors had initially hypothesized inferior clinical outcomes in the older group, no significant differences were observed.

None of these studies are or should be considered definitive with respect to the flatfoot deformity, but a trend toward positive patient-centered outcomes seems clear in both pediatric and adult patients. The real gaps in our current knowledge base that should be investigated by future generations include examining the relationship between structural deformity and patient symptoms, determining specific indications for conservative vs. surgical interventions, identifying specific indications for individual and combination surgical procedures, and developing clear expectations of intervention for both conservative and surgical treatments.

## References

1. Gray J. Henri Poincare: a scientific biography. Princeton: Princeton University Press; 2012.
2. Kuhn TS. The structure of scientific revolutions. 3rd ed. Chicago, London: University of Chicago Press; 1996.
3. Harcourt-Smith WE, Aiello LC. Fossils, feet and the evolution of human bipedal locomotion. J Anat. 2004;204(5):403–16.
4. Niemitz C. The evolution of the upright posture and gait – a review and a new synthesis. Naturwissenschaften. 2010;97(3):241–63.
5. Wang W, Abboud RJ, Gunther MM, Crompton RH. Analysis of joint force and torque for the human and non-human ape foot during bipedal walking with implications for the evolution of the foot. J Anat. 2014;225(2):152–66.
6. Wang WJ, Crompton RH. Analysis of the human and ape foot during bipedal standing with implications for the evolution of the foot. J Biomech. 2004;37(12):1831–6.
7. Root ML, Orien WP, Weed JH. Normal and abnormal function of the foot. Clinical biomechanics volume II. Clinical Biomechanics Corporation. Los Angeles; 1977. p. 127–64.
8. Inman VT. Human locomotion. Can Med Assoc J. 1966;94(20):1047–54.
9. Sgarlato TE. Pathomechanics of various developmental abnormalities. In: Sgarlato TE, editor. A compendium of podiatric biomechanics. San Francisco: California College of Podiatric Medicine; 1971. p. 78–151.
10. Snow SW, Bohne WH. Observations on the fibrous retinacula of the heel pad. Foot Ankle Int. 2006;27(8):632–5.
11. Campanelli V, Fantini M, Faccioli N, Cangemi A, Pozzo A, Sbarbati A. Three-dimensional morphology of heel fat pad: an in vivo computed tomography study. J Anat. 2011;219(5):622–31.
12. Hansen ST. Functional reconstruction of the foot and ankle. Philadelphia: Lippincott, Williams & Wilkins; 2000. p. 17–34.
13. Sanner WH (2003) Foot segmental relationships and bone morphology. Foot and ankle radiology, p 272–302, RA Christman, Churchill Livingstone, St. Louis, Missouri.
14. Johnson KA, Strom DE. Tibialis posterior tendon dysfunction. Clin Orthop Relat Res. 1989;239:196–206.
15. Myerson MS. Adult acquired-flatfoot deformity: treatment of dysfunction of the posterior tibial tendon. Instr Course Lect. 1997;46:393–405.
16. Weinraub GM, Saraiya MJ. Adult flatfoot/posterior tibial tendon dysfunction: classification and treatment. Clin Podiatr Med Surg. 2002;19(3):345–70.

17. Abousayed MM, Alley MC, Shakked R, Rosenbaum AJ. Adult-acquired flatfoot deformity. J Bone Joint Surg. 2017;5(8):e7.
18. Smyth NA, Aiyer AA, Kaplan JR, Carmody CA, Kadakia AR. Adult-acquired flatfoot deformity. Eur J Orthop Surg Traumatol. 2017;27:433–9.
19. Spratley EM, Matheis EA, Hayes CW, Adelaar RS, Wayne JS. Validation of a population of patient-specific adult acquired flatfoot deformity models. J Orthop Res. 2013;31(12):1861–8.
20. Greisberg J, Hansen ST Jr, Sangeorzan B. Deformity and degeneration in the hindfoot and midfoot joints of the adult acquired flatfoot. Foot Ankle Int. 2003;24(7):530–4.
21. Martus JE, Femino JE, Caird MS, Kuhns LR, Craig CL, Farley FA. Accessory anterolateral talar facet as an etiology of painful talocalcaneal impingement in the rigid flatfoot: a new diagnosis. Iowa Orthop J. 2008;28:1–8.
22. Toullec E. Adult flatfoot. Orthop Traumatol Surg Res. 2015;101:S11–7.
23. Funk DA, Cass JR, Johnson KA. Acquired adult flatfoot secondary to posterior tibial tendon pathology. J Bone Joint Surg Am. 1986;68(1):95–102.
24. Janis LR, Wagner JT, Kravitz RD, Greenberg JJ. Posterior tibial tendon rupture: classification, modified surgical repair, and retrospective study. J Foot Ankle Surg. 1993;32(1):2–13.
25. Malicky ES, Crary JL, Houghton MJ, Agel J, Hansen ST, Sangeorzan BJ. Talocalcaneal and subfibular impingement in symptomatic flatfoot in adults. J Bone Joint Surg. 2002;84A(11):2005–9.
26. Marzano R. Nonoperative management of adult flatfoot deformities. Clin Podiatr Med Surg. 2014;31:337–47.
27. Evans AM, Rome K. A Cochrane review of the evidence for non-surgical interventions for flexible pediatric flatfeet. Eur J Phys Rehabil Med. 2011;47:69–89.
28. MacKenzie AJ, Rome K, Evans AM. The efficacy of nonsurgical interventions for pediatric flexible flatfoot: a critical review. J Pediatr Orthop. 2012;32:830–4.
29. Riccio I, Gimigliano F, Gimigliano R, Porpora G, Iolascon G. Rehabilitative treatment in flexible flatfoot: a perspective cohort study. Musculoskelet Surg. 2009;93:101–7.
30. Capasso G. Dynamic varus heel cup: a new orthosis for treating pes planovalgus. Ital J Orthop Traumatol. 1993;19:113–23.
31. Leung AK, Mak AF, Evans JH. Biomedical gait evaluation of the immediate effect of orthotic treatment for flexible flat foot. Prosthet Orthot Int. 1998;22:25–34.
32. Whitford D, Esterman AA. Randomized controlled trial of two types of in-shoe orthoses in children with flexible excess pronation of the feet. Foot Ankle Int. 2007;28:715–23.
33. Mereday C, Dolan CM, Lusskin R. Evaluation of the University of California Biomechanics Laboratory shoe insert in "flexible" pes planus. Clin Orthop Relat Res. 1972;82:45–58.
34. Imhauser CW, Abidi NA, Frankel DZ, Gavin K, Siegler S. Biomechanical evaluation of the efficacy of external shoe stabilizers in the conservative treatment acquired flat foot deformity. Foot Ankle Int. 2002;23(8):727–37.
35. Alvarez RG, Marini A, Schmitt C, Saltzman CL. Stage I and II posterior tibial tendon dysfunction treated by a structured nonoperative management protocol: an orthosis and exercise program. Foot Ankle Int. 2006;27(1):2–8.
36. Chao W, Wapner KL, Lee TH, Adams J, Hecht PJ. Non-operative management of posterior tibial tendon dysfunction. Foot Ankle Int. 1996;17(12):736–41.
37. Nielsen MD, Dodson EE, Shadrick DL, Catanzariti AR, Mendicino RW, Malay DS. Nonoperative care for the treatment of adult-acquired flatfoot deformity. J Foot Ankle Surg. 2011;50(3):311–4.
38. Augustyn JF, Lin SS, Berberian WS, Johnson JE. Non operative treatment of adult acquired flat foot with the Arizona brace. Foot Ankle Clin. 2003;8(3):491–502.
39. Paolo C, Giada L, Lisa B, Sandro G, Alberto L. Functional evaluation of bilateral subtalar arthroereisis for the correction of flexible flatfoot in children: 1-year follow-up. Gait Posture. 2018;64:152–8.

40. Chong DY, Macwilliams BA, Hennessey TA, Teske N, Stevens PM. Prospective comparison of subtalar arthroereisis with lateral column lengthening for painful flatfeet. J Pediatr Orthop B. 2015;24:345–53.
41. Fernandez de Retana P, Alvarez F, Bacca G. Is there a role for subtalar arthroereisis in the management of adult acquired flatfoot? Foot Ankle Clin N Am. 2012;17:271–81.
42. Kunas GC, Do HT, Aiyer A, Deland JT, Ellis SJ. Contribution of medial cuneiform osteotomy to correction of longitudinal arch collapse in stage IIb adult-acquired flatfoot deformity. Foot Ankle Int. 2018;39(8):885–93.
43. Aiyer A, Dall GF, Shub J, Myerson MS. Radiographic correction following reconstruction of adult acquired flat foot deformity using the Cotton medial cuneiform osteotomy. Foot Ankle Int. 2016;37(5):508–13.
44. Saunders SM, Ellis SJ, Demetracopoulos CA, Marinescu A, Burkett J, Deland JT. Comparative outcomes between step-cut lengthening calcaneal osteotomy vs traditional Evans osteotomy for stage IIb adult-acquired flatfoot deformity. Foot Ankle Int. 2018;39(1):18–27.
45. Smith BA, Adelaar RS, Wayne JS. Patient specific computational models to optimize surgical correction for flatfoot deformity. J Orthop Res. 2017;35(7):1523–31.
46. Wadehra A, Fallat LM, Jarski R. Surgical management of stage 2 adult and pediatric acquired flatfoot without tendon transfer or arthrodesis: a retrospective study. J Foot Ankle Surg. 2018;57(4):658–63.
47. Faldini C, Mazzotti A, Panciera A, Persiani V, Pardo F, Perna F, Giannini S. Patient-perceived outcomes after subtalar arthroereisis with bioabsorbable implants for flexible flatfoot in growing age: a 4-year follow-up study. Eur J Orthop Surg Traumatol. 2018;28(4):707–12.
48. Yontar NS, Ogut T, Guven MF, Botanlioglu H, Kaynak G, Can A. Surgical treatment results for flexible flatfoot in adolescents. Acta Orthop Traumatol Turc. 2016;50:655–9.
49. Walley KC, Greene G, Hallam J, Juliano PJ, Aynardi MC. Short- to mid-term outcomes following the use of an arthroereisis implant as an adjunct for correction of flexible, acquired flatfoot deformity in adults. Foot Ankle Spec. 2019;12(2):122–30. https://doi.org/10.1177/1938640018770242.
50. Conti MS, Chan JY, Do HT, Ellis SJ, Deland JT. Correlation of postoperative midfoot position with outcome following reconstruction of the stage II adult acquired flatfoot deformity. Foot Ankle Int. 2015;36(3):239–47.
51. Conti MS, Ellis SJ, Chan JY, Do HT, Deland JT. Optimal position of the heel following reconstruction of the stage II adult-acquired flatfoot deformity. Foot Ankle Int. 2015;36(8):919–27.
52. Conti MS, Jones MT, Savenkov O, Deland JT, Ellis SJ. Outcomes of reconstruction of the stage II adult-acquired flatfoot deformity in older patients. Foot Ankle Int. 2018;39(9):1019–27.

# Chapter 8
# Ankle Arthroscopy

**Daniel J. Hatch and Stephen A. Mariash**

## History

Early pioneers in arthroscopy were motivated to succeed with their desire to examine the human body with minimal trauma. The genesis of this art form started in the viscera and genitourinary areas of the body. Philipp Bozzini developed the first endoscope in 1806 [1]. His device, called the "Lichtleiter," or light conductor, utilized a candle as a light source.

On October 21, 1879, Thomas Alva Edison invented an incandescent lamp called the "mignon." The success of the mignon filament and light source enabled other pioneers to advance their devices [2].

Severin Nordentoft (1866–1922) from Denmark first used an endoscope in the knee joint in 1912 and also coined the term "arthroscopy" [2]. The start of the twentieth century brought us the "Father of Arthroscopy," Kenji Takagi (1888–1963). In 1918, Takagi examined the knee joint, albeit in a cadaveric specimen. Takagi was motivated to diagnose tuberculosis of the knee, a condition that prevented kneeling, which would have been considered a social disgrace at that time. Takagi went on to develop 11 optical instruments after his first one (called "#1") in 1931 [3].

In 1931, Michael S. Burman (1896–1974) reported on the examination of joints including the ankle [4]. It was his conclusion that the ankle was not conducive to

D. J. Hatch (✉)
Clinical Instructor: Scholl College of Podiatric Medicine, North Chicago, IL, USA

Director of Surgery: North Colorado Podiatric Surgical Residency, Greeley, CO, USA

Private Practice: Foot and Ankle Center of the Rockies, Denver, CO, USA
e-mail: dhatch@facrockies.com

S. A. Mariash
International Foot and Ankle Foundation for Education and Research, Everett, WA, USA

Practice: St Cloud Orthopedic Associates, St Cloud, MN, USA



D. E. Tower (ed.), *Evidence-Based Podiatry*,
https://doi.org/10.1007/978-3-030-50853-1_8

arthroscopic examination. Thankfully, his observations were eventually challenged. Examination of "live" joints was first performed in 1939 by Takagi [5]. His protégé, Masaki Watanabe (1911–1994), carried on the tradition of numbering his new devices starting with #13. The Watanabe #14 was produced in 1955. The #21 was the first production arthroscope in 1959. It was also the last to use an incandescent light source. The first fiber-optic (cold light) scope, #22, was developed in 1967. In 1970, Watanabe developed #25, which later formed the basis for the Dyonics "needlescope." Watanabe also originated the concept of "triangulation" and wrote the first *Atlas of Arthroscopy* published in English in 1957 [2].

Arthroscopic instrumentation evolved from simple probes and forceps to the retrograde knife developed by O'Connor, who collaborated with The Richard Wolf Corporation in Rosemont, IL [6]. In 1975, Lanny Johnson, in cooperation with the Dyonics Corporation, developed the first motorized intra-articular shaver [2]. Power instrumentation dramatically improved operative arthroscopy. As a result of the increased interest, the International Arthroscopy Association was formed in 1972, and in 1982 the Arthroscopic Association of North America (AANA) was formed. Further operative developments were achieved with the use of Holmium-YAG lasers for debridement and repair of lesions. However, this mode of treatment has given way to radiofrequency devices primarily due to cost containment issues.

Ankle arthroscopy reports in the American literature began with Drez et al. in 1982 and also Heller and Vogler in the same year [7, 8]. This was followed by Richard Lundeen (1951–2011) in 1985 with articles on anatomy and lateral ankle stabilization [9, 10]. James Guhl (1928–2008), the third president of the AANA, was noted for his pioneering work in ankle arthroscopy and his textbook on foot and ankle arthroscopy. There was enough interest in the topic that a journal was established in 1985, *Arthroscopy: The Journal of Arthroscopy and Related Research* [2].

Presently, ankle arthroscopy articles and textbooks are in the mainstream of surgical approaches for ankle joint pathology. Notable authors of current textbooks include Richard Ferkel and Niek van Dijk.

## Indications

The indications for ankle arthroscopy have expanded with enhanced fiber optics and instrumentation. Historically, arthroscopy was only utilized for diagnostic purposes. Presently, there are many forms of pathology that are amenable to surgical arthroscopy.

In 2009, Glazebrook et al. published a systematic review of evidence-based indications for ankle arthroscopy [11]. While the authors graded the levels of evidence, arthroscopy was recommended as a treatment modality for the following conditions: synovitis, anterior joint impingement, osteochondral defects of the talus (OLT), ankle arthrodesis, removal of loose bodies, ankle instability, septic arthritis, arthrofibrosis, and fracture reduction assistance (see Table 8.1).

**Table 8.1** Indications of arthroscopy per Glazebrook et al.

| Procedure | Grade of recommendation | Recommendation |
|---|---|---|
| Anterior impingement (osseous or soft tissue) | B | For intervention |
| Osteochondral defects <1.5 cm | B | For intervention |
| Ankle arthrodesis | B | For intervention |
| Loose bodies | C | For intervention |
| Ankle instability | C | For intervention |
| Septic arthritis | C | For intervention |
| Arthrofibrosis | C | For intervention |
| Ankle arthrosis (severe) | C | Against intervention |
| Fractures | I | For intervention |
| Synovitis | I | For intervention |

## Contraindications

Contraindications for ankle arthroscopy include poor vascular perfusion, venous congestion of the lower extremity, and poorly or unmanaged complex regional pain syndrome (CRPS). Local skin infection, significant edema, and cellulitis are also considered contraindications.

## Anatomy

The fundamentals of arthroscopy require a thorough understanding of the anatomy. Paul Golano and his colleagues published a pictorial essay in 2016 [12] (see Fig. 8.1). This essay provides a detailed understanding of the intricate ankle anatomy pertinent to ankle arthroscopy. When the anatomical understanding is combined with Ferkel and Fischer's [13] systematic evaluation of the ankle joint, successful ankle arthroscopy can be performed (see Fig. 8.2). Arthroscopic portals are utilized to pass instrumentation into the ankle joint while safely avoiding neurovascular structures. Standard portals are the anterior lateral, anterior medial, and posterior lateral. Other portals may be placed depending on the pathology being treated (Fig. 8.3). Additional portals include posterior medial, transmalleolar, and accessory portals.

## Instrumentation

There are specific instruments utilized for ankle arthroscopy. The instruments for small joint arthroscopy have evolved from large joint arthroscopy, i.e., the knee. The newer, specialized instruments for ankle arthroscopy have made the procedure

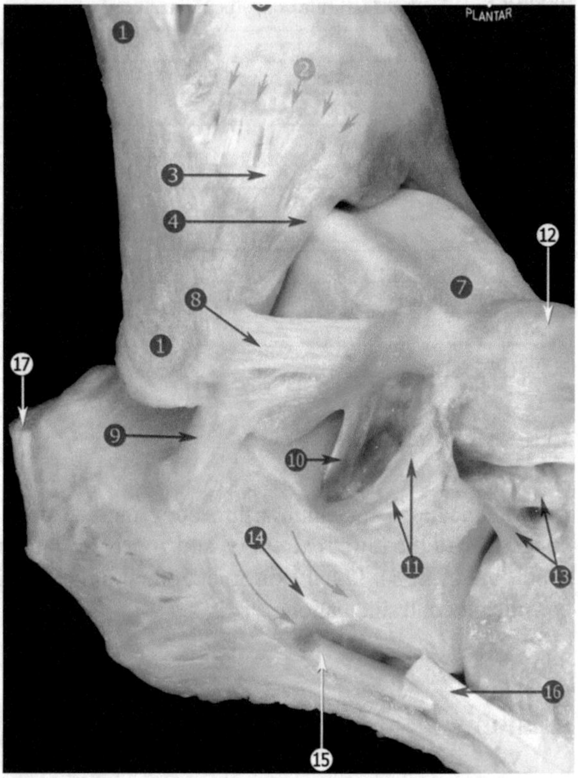


**Fig. 8.1** Lateral ankle anatomy (reprinted with permission from Golano et al.)

| **Anterior Ankle** | **Central Ankle** | **Posterior Ankle** |
|---|---|---|
| Deltoid | Mediocentral tibiotalus | Medial Gutter |
| Medial Gutter | Middle tibiotalus | Medial Talus |
| Medial Talus | Lateral tibiotalus | Central Talus |
| Central Talus | Capsular reflection of FHL | Lateral Talus |
| Lateral Talus | Transverse Tib-Fib ligament | Tib-Fib Articulation |
| Tibial-Fibular Trification | Post Inf Tib Fib Lig | Lateral Gutter |
| Lateral Gutter | | Posterior Gutter |
| Anterior Gutter | | |

**Fig. 8.2** Ferkel's 21-point examination

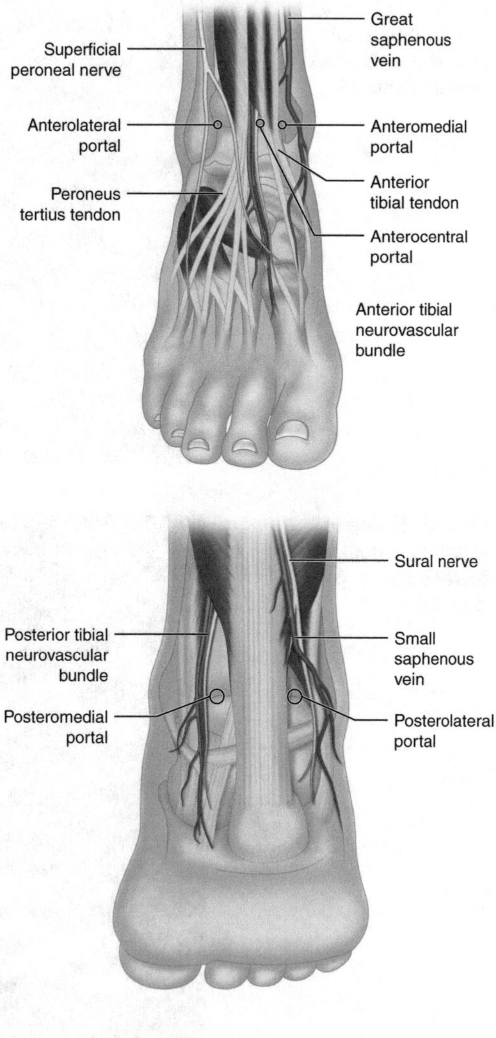


**Fig. 8.3** Standard arthroscopic portals

easier and more efficient. These instruments may be divided into four categories: (1) instruments for viewing, (2) excisional instruments, (3) instruments for reconstruction, and (4) accessory instruments.

## *Instruments for Viewing*

The arthroscope may vary in size from 1.9 to 2.7 mm in diameter (Fig. 8.4). The tip of the arthroscope may be angulated 30 degrees or 70 degrees (Fig. 8.5). The 30-degree arthroscope is most commonly used, while the 70-degree arthroscope may offer superior visualization in certain situations such as visualizing over the medial and lateral dome of the talus (Fig. 8.6).

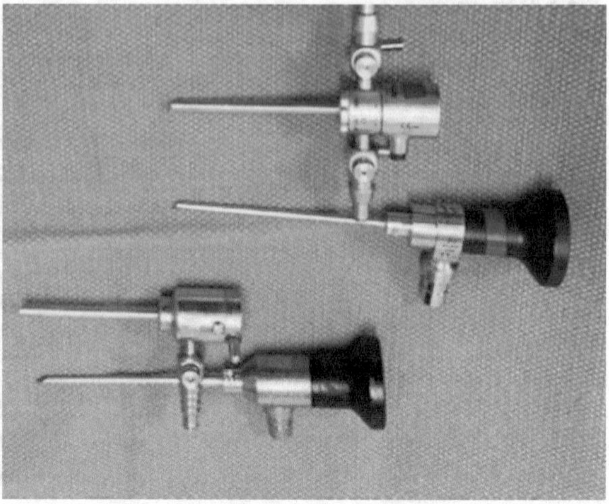

**Fig. 8.4** Arthroscopes with dual-port cannula (top) and single-port cannula (bottom)

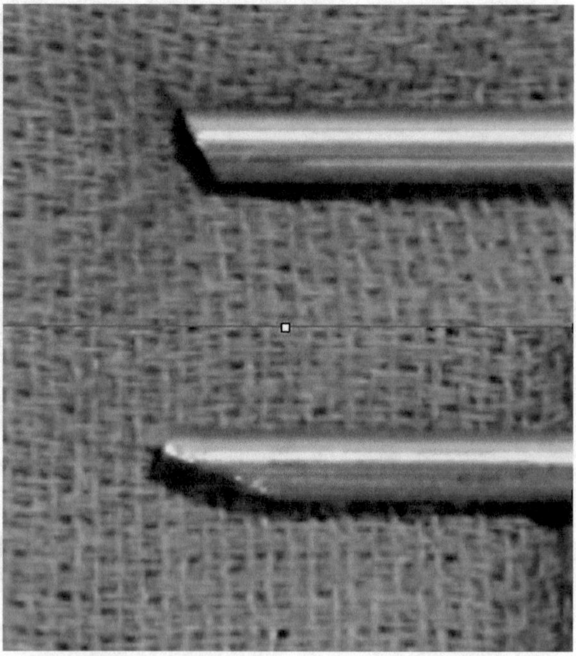

**Fig. 8.5** 30 degree arthroscope (top) and 70 degree arthroscope (bottom)

The camera is a high-definition solid-state device (Fig. 8.7). Each manufacturer has its own coupling system that links the arthroscopic lens to the camera.

The cannula is a hollow tube used to accept the camera lens. The cannula will protect the surrounding soft tissues and, at the same time, maintain the portal for the arthroscope and allow access for the inflow and/or outflow ports. The cannula may have one or two ports used for ingress and egress. An obturator (blunt probe) is inserted through the cannula to gain access to the joint. The light cable connects the illumination source to the camera lens and permits the transmission of light.

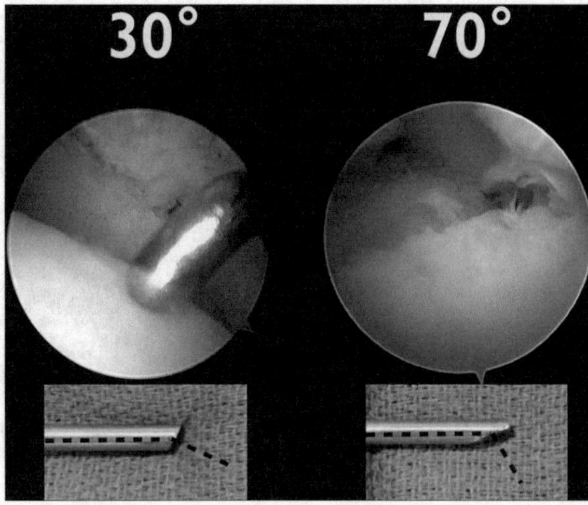


**Fig. 8.6** 30 degree versus 70 degree visualization of the lateral talar dome. Note how the 70 degree scope allows viewing over the dome in order to appreciate the talar dome lesion

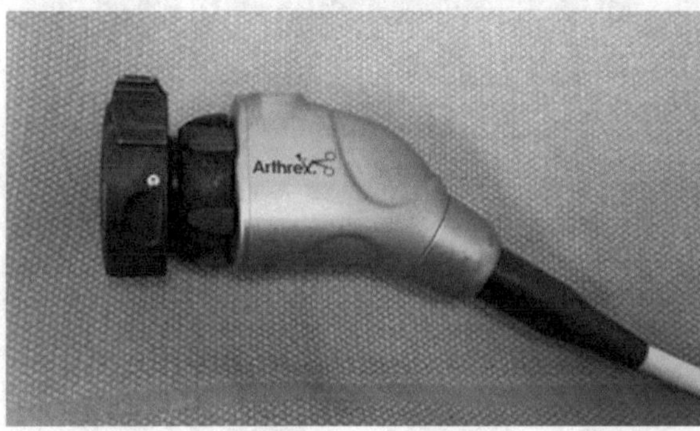


**Fig. 8.7** Arthroscopic camera

## *Excisional Instruments*

Excisional instruments may be subdivided into hand instruments and motorized instruments.

Hand instruments consist of needles and syringes, probes, cutting instruments, grasping instruments (forceps), suction punches, and motorized instrumentation.

A needle and syringe filled with saline is utilized to insufflate the joint prior to establishing the portals. A larger diameter needle, such as #22 gauge, may be used (Fig. 8.8).

Probes have a blunt tip and may be employed to palpate or maneuver structures and determine the consistency of cartilage. In addition, a probe that contains gradient markings may be used to determine dimensions and depth (Fig. 8.9a, b).

A cutting instrument includes retractable knives and scissors and other various shaped and angled sharp curettes and osteotomes which are utilized to incise structures (Fig. 8.10).

Grasping instruments, such as basket forceps and pituitary forceps, are used to grab onto structures, including loose bodies in order to excise them from the ankle joint.

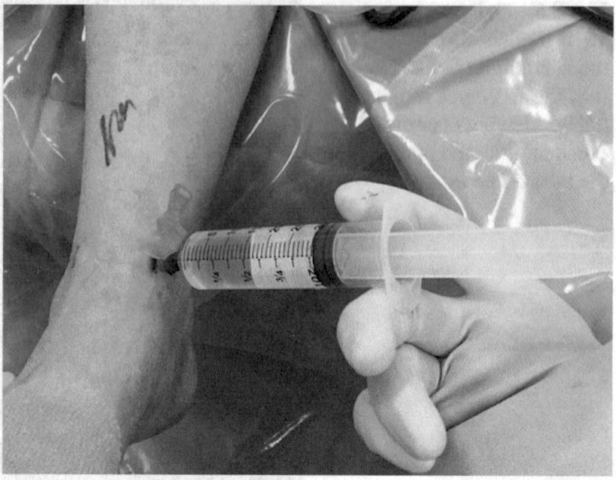

**Fig. 8.8** Needle and syringe filled with saline is used to insufflate the ankle joint

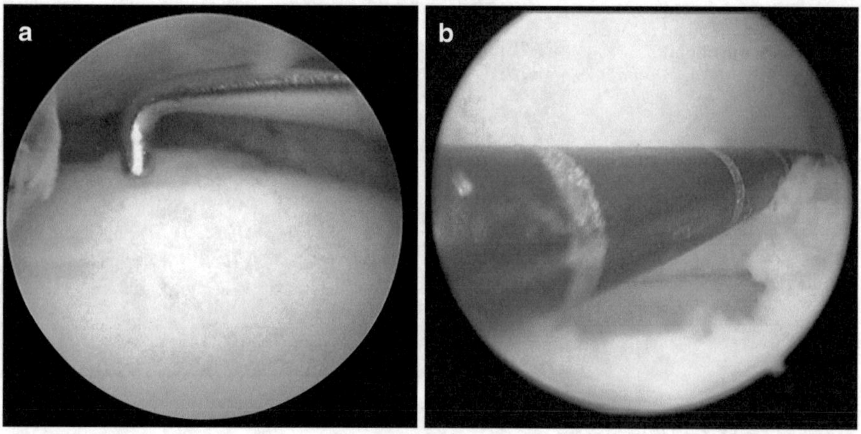


**Fig. 8.9** (**a**) Blunt probe used to palpate the consistency of the cartilage of the talar dome. (**b**) Gradient markings on the probe to determine measurements

Suction punches are grasping instruments with sharp jaws that have the outflow tubing attached. The suction aids in maneuvering the structure into the jaws. The jaws may be opened and closed in order to incise the grasped object. The outflow suction will then remove the pathologic tissue from the ankle joint.

Motorized instrumentation includes shavers and burrs of varying diameters. The rotation of the instrumentation may be set via buttons on the handpiece or foot pedal to be clockwise, counterclockwise, or oscillate. The speed may also be manually controlled up to about 8,000 RPM.

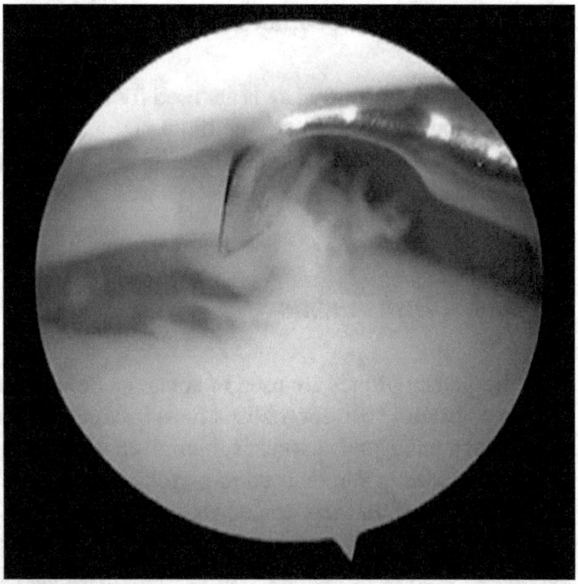

**Fig. 8.10** Angulated cutting instrument utilized to incise a cartilage lesion

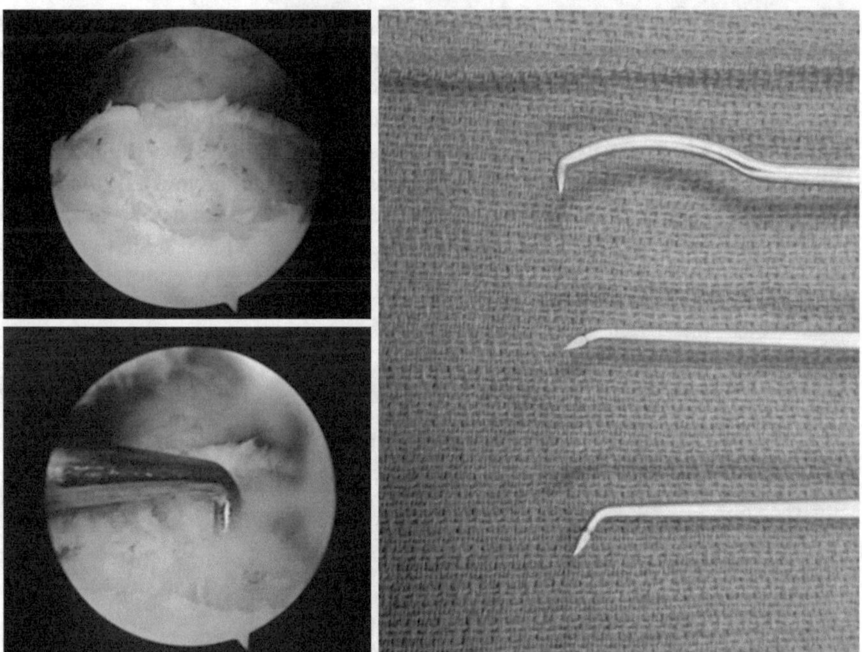

**Fig. 8.11** Awls used for microfracture technique of an osteochondral lesion of the talus

## Instruments for Reconstruction

Various angled and shaped awls are used for manual microfracture of osteochondral lesions of the talar dome or distal tibial plafond (Fig. 8.11). Likewise, manufacturers supply power instrumentation for microfracture technique such as flexible fluted drills with different angled cannulas, as well as retractable trocar pins.

## Accessory Instruments

Radiofrequency probes are used to ablate pathologic tissue by way of medium frequency alternating current (radio waves) between 350 and 500 kHz. Collateral damage to surrounding soft tissues is minimized with this technique.

Aiming devices can be used to perform retrograde or antegrade drilling of subchondral cysts of the talar dome. Also, this method can be utilized to guide the formation of a transmedial malleolar portal in order to gain access to a more posteriorly positioned osteochondral lesion of the medial aspect of the talus (Fig. 8.12).

Leg holders maintain stability of the limb during the operative procedure (Fig. 8.13). Distractors are not always required, but they may be employed to widen the joint space in order to facilitate access to pathology that otherwise may not be appreciated. In the early days of ankle arthroscopy, distraction was attained by driving a Steinmann pin into the tuberosity of the calcaneus and applying manual traction to the pin which was exposed medially and laterally at the level of the calcaneus. This invasive method was replaced by several noninvasive techniques. Manufacturers have various strap systems that are applied to a fixed distraction device attached to the operating table. It is set to a predetermined distraction force which is usually between 22 and 25 lbs. Prolonged distraction over 30 lbs may lead to damage to

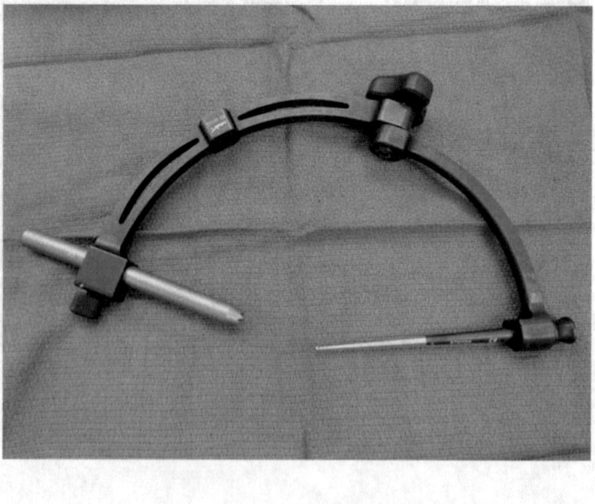

**Fig. 8.12** Aiming device

Fig. 8.13 Leg holder

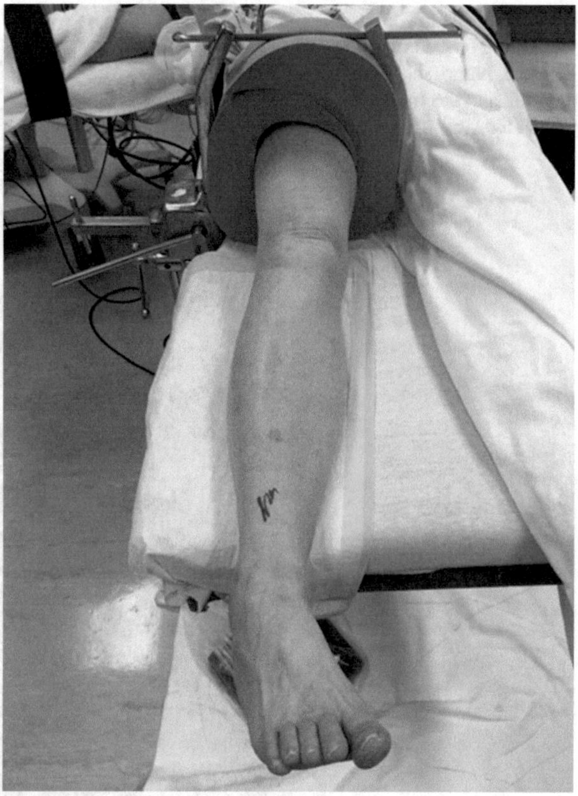

neurovascular structures [14]. Contraindications for distraction are CRPS, open epiphysis, and pyarthrosis.

## Standard Setup and Patient Positioning

For standard ankle arthroscopy, the patient is placed in the supine position. A padded leg holder is placed around the thigh and is used to attain countertraction. The monitor and associated equipment (console, pump, shaver control, electrosurgical generator) are arranged in a stacked, tower configuration (Fig. 8.14). The tower is positioned on either side of the patient. In some operating rooms, the monitor may be suspended from the ceiling in direct view of the surgeon.

The procedure begins by marking out the standard anteromedial and anterolateral portals. A needle and syringe filled with saline or lactated Ringer's solution is employed to insufflate the ankle joint through the anteromedial portal, typically, approximately 15–20 cc's. The anteromedial portal is then established by incising the skin with a blade and then using a hemostat to spread the underlying soft tissues.

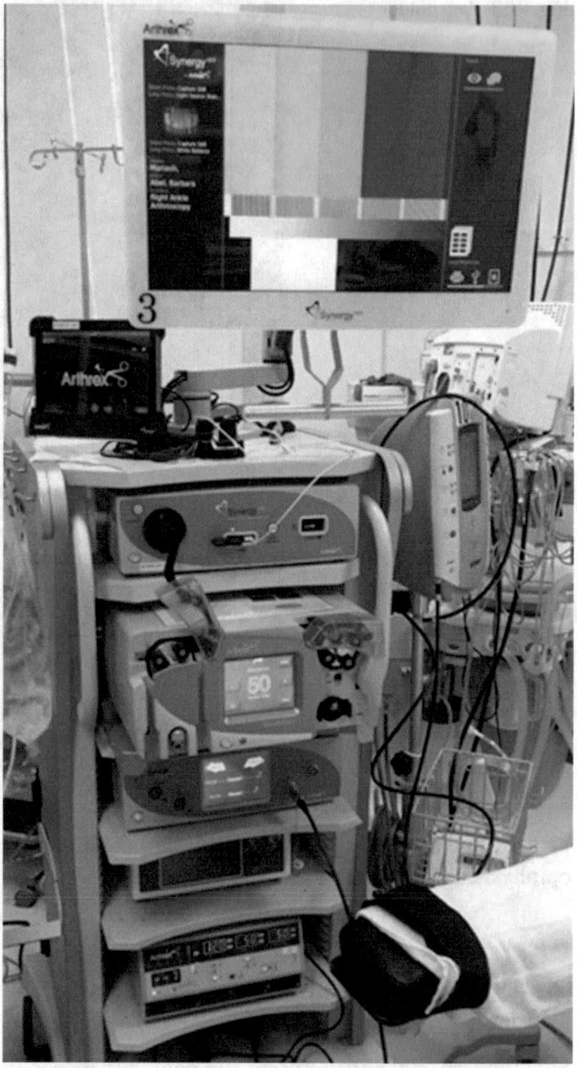


**Fig. 8.14** The tower consisting of the monitor, console, pump, shaver control, and electrosurgical generator

The obturator (blunt probe) is placed into the cannula, and the ankle joint capsule is penetrated in order to access the ankle joint. The obturator is then removed and replaced by the arthroscope, and the joint is visualized. In order to maintain sufficient hydrostatic pressure and continuous flow for distention of the ankle joint, a plastic bag filled with saline or lactated Ringer's solution is placed above the patient on an IV pole, and the fluid is delivered by way of gravity. Alternatively, the inflow tubing may be connected to a pump which controls the intra-articular pressure.

Likewise, the anterolateral portal is established, and appropriate instrumentation is placed into the anterolateral portal. The outflow tubing is connected to a cannula in the second portal or to the accessory connector in the same cannula that houses the arthroscopic lens. The outflow may be managed through the arthroscopic pump as well. By increasing the flow of fluid, the field of view can be cleared of blood and soft tissue extravasation. In this manner, visualization is improved, and hemostasis is maintained. Hemostasis can also be improved by use of a thigh tourniquet and/or injecting an ampule of epinephrine into the bag of normal saline or lactated Ringer's solution.

The technique of identifying the instrumentation and associated landmarks of the ankle joint is referred to as triangulation and involves a combination of pistoning, rotation, and translation of the arthroscope within the ankle joint.

## Commonly Treated Conditions

Synovitis of the ankle is commonly observed and may be acute with red injected villi or chronic with white fibrous tissue [9] (Fig. 8.15a, b). Acute and chronic synovitis are usually treated by use of a synovial shaver or radiofrequency instrumentation.

Anterior ankle joint impingement is most commonly caused by direct trauma most common in soccer players [15]. Classification systems exist that describe the extent of spurring (Scranton and McDermott 1992) [16], amount of arthrosis of the joint (van Dijk 1997) [17], or a combination of both spurring and arthrosis (Parma et al. 2014) [18]. The pain associated with anterior spurring is usually related to soft tissue impingement (Fig. 8.16). Spurring and arthrosis are treated by resection with small osteotomes and mallet followed by abrasion with rotary burrs.

Soft tissue lesions that are frequently encountered in the ankle joint are meniscoid bodies, fibrous bands, and Bassett's lesion. Wolin et al. described meniscoid bodies as a soft tissue, hyalinized, impingement lesion in 1950 [19] (Fig. 8.17) that is believed to be formed by compressive forces on synovial tissue in the anterior

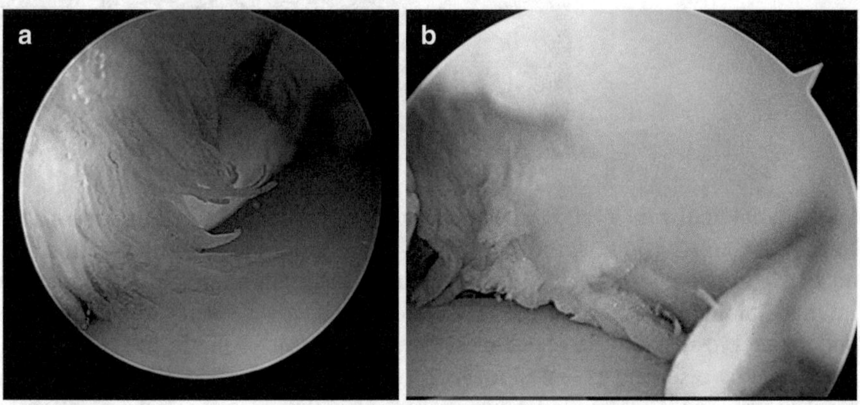


**Fig. 8.15** (**a**) Acute synovitis. (**b**) Chronic synovitis

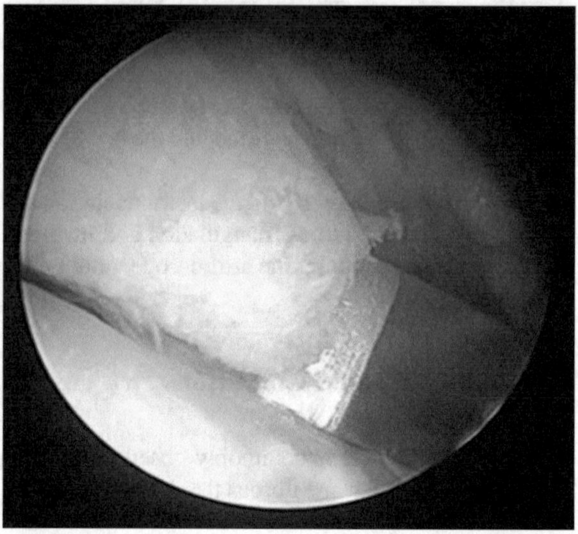

**Fig. 8.16** Anterior osseous impingement with osteotome resection

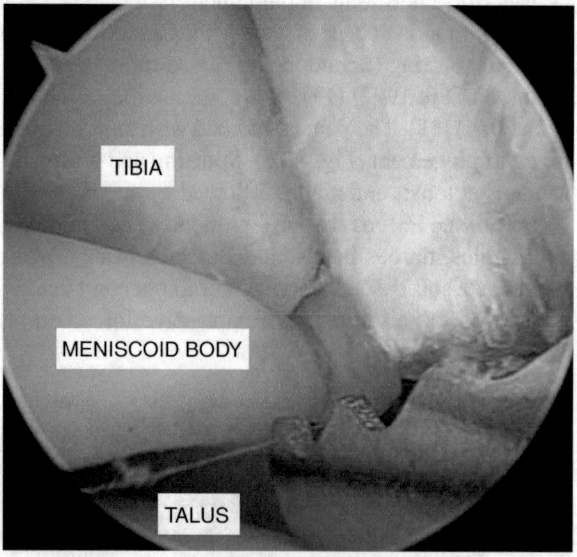


**Fig. 8.17** Miniscoid body. (Photo courtesy of Meagan Jennings, DPM, FACFAS)

lateral tibial fibular interval. Fibrous bands may be encountered and impinge structures in the anterior joint space (Fig. 8.18). These lesions are readily resected and ablated to clear the joint space. Bassett's lesion is the inferior fascicle of the anterior inferior tibiofibular ligament (Fig. 8.19). This ligament may abrade the talar dome and create erosions on the chondral surface. Treatment of the resultant lesion is performed by resecting the inferior aspect of the anterior inferior tibiofibular ligament and repairing the chondral defect on the anterior lateral aspect of the talar dome.

Fig. 8.18 Fibrous band

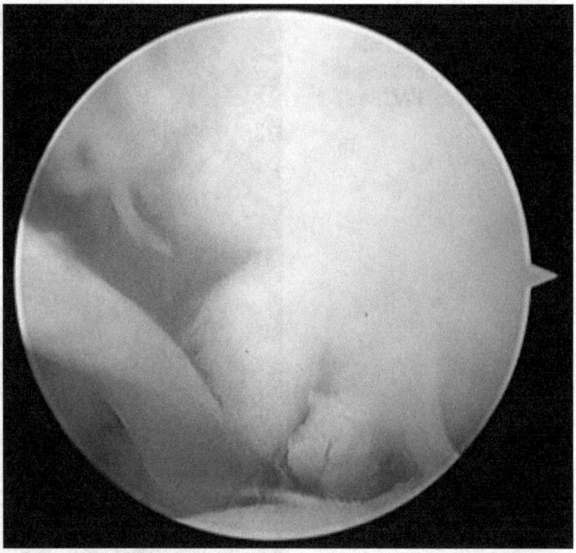

Fig. 8.19 Bassett's lesion. (Photo courtesy of Meagan Jennings, DPM, FACFAS)

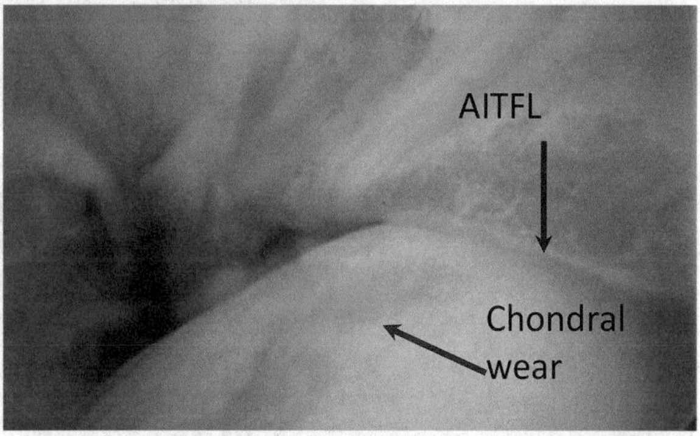


Posterior ankle joint impingement involves soft tissue and, more commonly, an os trigonum (Fig. 8.20). An os trigonum may be approached either by a lateral subtalar approach or direct posterior approach as advocated by Van Dijk [20, 21]. Pau Golano et al. published a detailed anatomic description of this approach in 2006 [22]. Smyth et al. described the technique and outcomes of the posterior approach [23].

Osteochondral defects (OCD) were originally described by Kappis in 1922 [24]. OCDs were known at that time as osteochondritis dissecans. Presently, the more commonly utilized term to describe the condition is osteochondral lesion of the talus (OLT). In 1959, Berndt and Harty published their classic paper on transchondral fractures of the talus that included their staging system 1–4 [25]. The lesion is treated by a variety of methods depending on lesion size and location. Lesions under 1.5 $cm^3$ are commonly treated with a microfracture technique that may also utilize

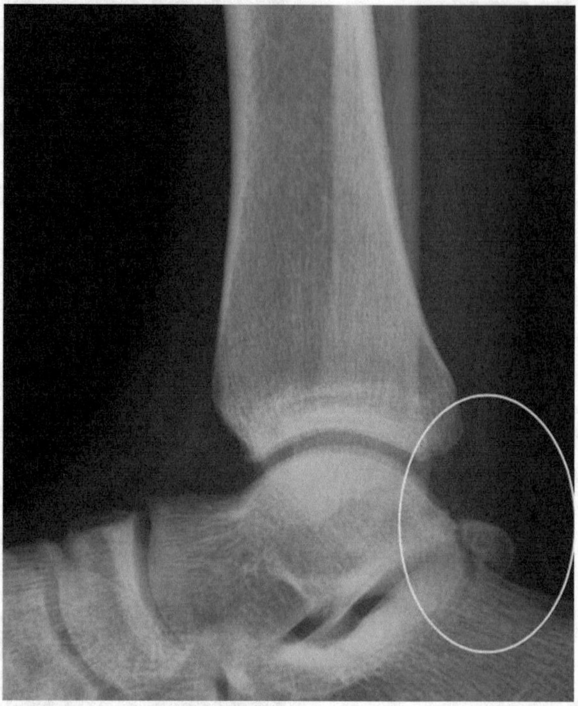

**Fig. 8.20** Radiograph revealing an os trigonum. (Photo courtesy of Meagan Jennings, DPM, FACFAS)

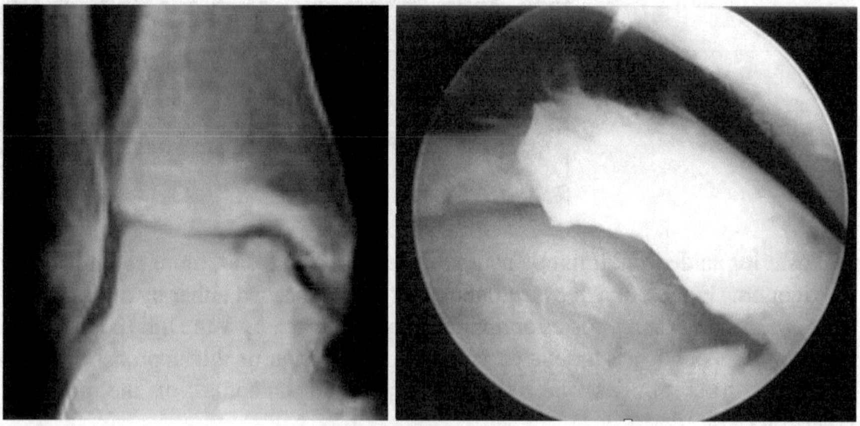

**Fig. 8.21** Osteochondral lesion of the talus on X-ray and arthroscopically

layering of a cartilage substrate over the lesion with fibrin glue (Fig. 8.21). Subchondral lesions may be filled directly or backfilled with an injected calcium phosphate into the void to allow osseous ingrowth (Fig. 8.22). Lesions larger than 1.5 $cm^3$ may be best treated by en bloc resection of the lesion and replacement with a talar allograft (Fig. 8.23).

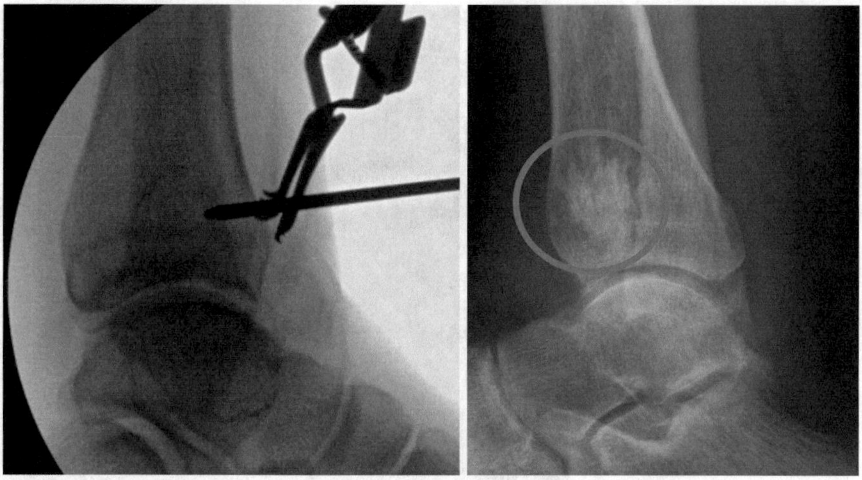

**Fig. 8.22** Intraoperative injection of calcium phosphate and subsequent radiographic appearance. (Photo courtesy of Meagan Jennings, DPM, FACFAS)

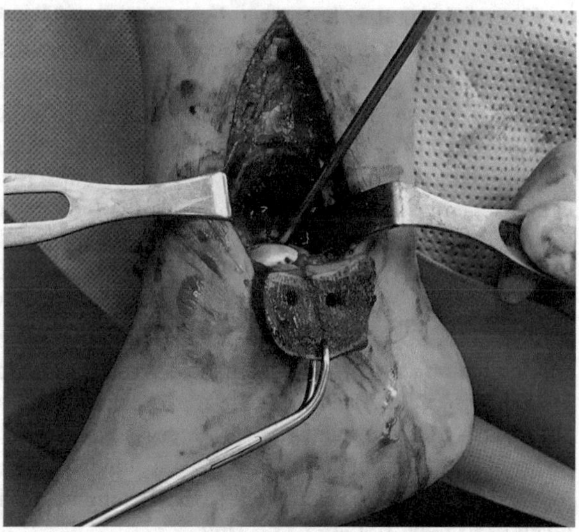

**Fig. 8.23** Medial malleolar exposure to insert talar allograft in a large medial dome lesion

Loose bodies are often encountered during arthroscopic procedures (Fig. 8.24). These are readily treated by direct extraction. Sometimes the bodies are so large they need to be pulverized prior to removal.

Arthroscopic ankle arthrodesis has evolved into a successful method of treating ankle arthrosis. Studies have demonstrated faster osseous consolidation and less morbidity with an arthroscopic approach when compared to traditional open techniques [26, 27]. One option for fixation is utilizing cannulated screws in a tripod technique as advocated by Schuberth et al. [28] (Fig. 8.25).

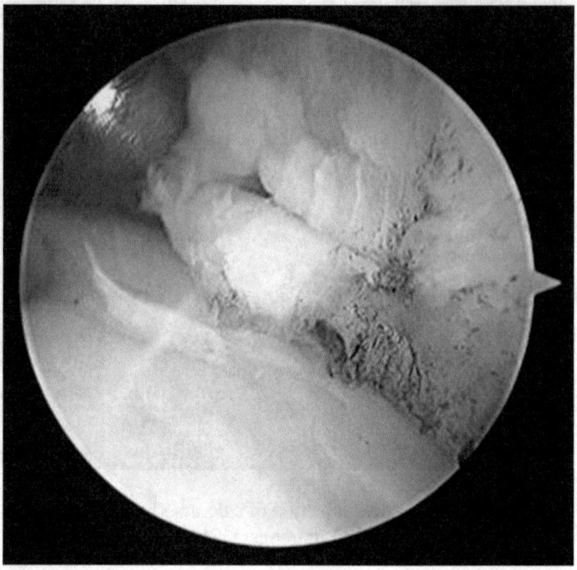

**Fig. 8.24** Osteochondral loose bodies

One of the first arthroscopically assisted ankle stabilizations was reported by Hawkins in 1994 [29]. He introduced a staple over the anterior talofibular ligament then plicated the ligament onto the talar neck. Suture anchors and thermal shrinkage of ligaments were then explored as techniques [30]. The current trend is to perform an anatomic arthroscopic Broström. The most common method of fixation is the use of bone anchors in the fibula (Fig. 8.26). Advocates for this technique include Vega et al. [33] and Acevedo and Mangone [34]. It has been documented in the literature that anatomic repairs are more functional than nonanatomic [31, 32]. The search for the easiest, most reproducible, and reliable stabilization procedure continues. There have been favorable comparisons of arthroscopic stabilization to standard open methods [35, 36]. Additionally, it was found by Hua et al. that in 84 ankles with chronic lateral ankle instability that most had intra-articular pathology [37].

Arthroscopic assistance for the repair of traumatic injuries may provide a valuable tool in fracture management. Internal assessment of fracture lines and alignment provides optimal reduction. This technique may also be utilized in reduction of latent syndesmotic injuries [38]. Another area of utilization is in the reduction of juvenile articular fractures [39] (Fig. 8.27).

## Complications

The complication rate in ankle arthroscopy is relatively low ranging from 0.7% to 17% [40–43]. Ferkel et al. did a large study in 1993 of 518 cases and found a complication rate of 9.8% [43]. Neurologic sequelae are the most commonly

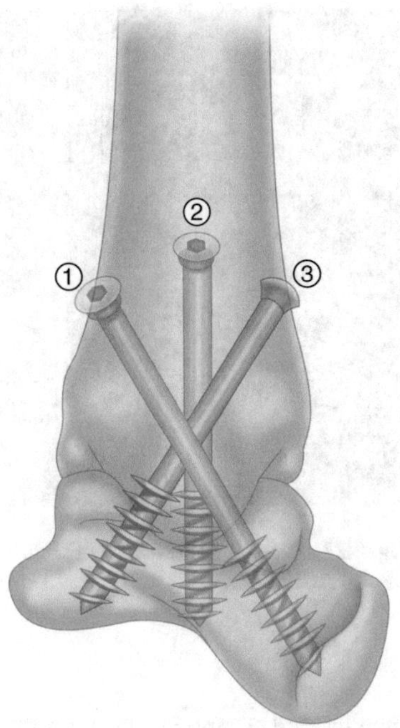


**Fig. 8.25** Tripod technique for fixation of ankle arthrodesis

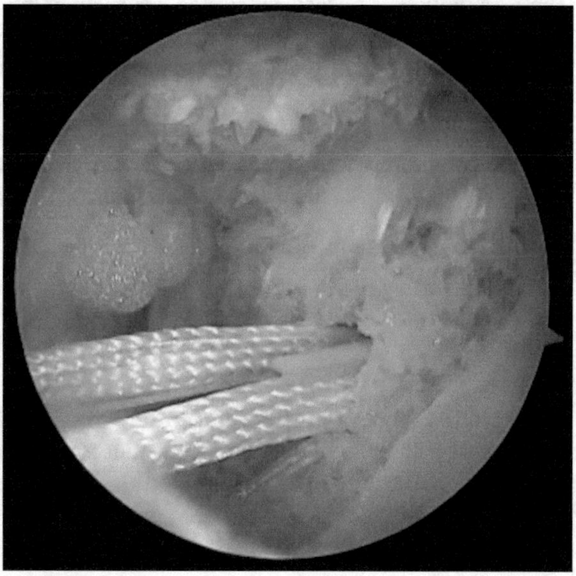

**Fig. 8.26** Use of a bone anchor for lateral ankle stabilization

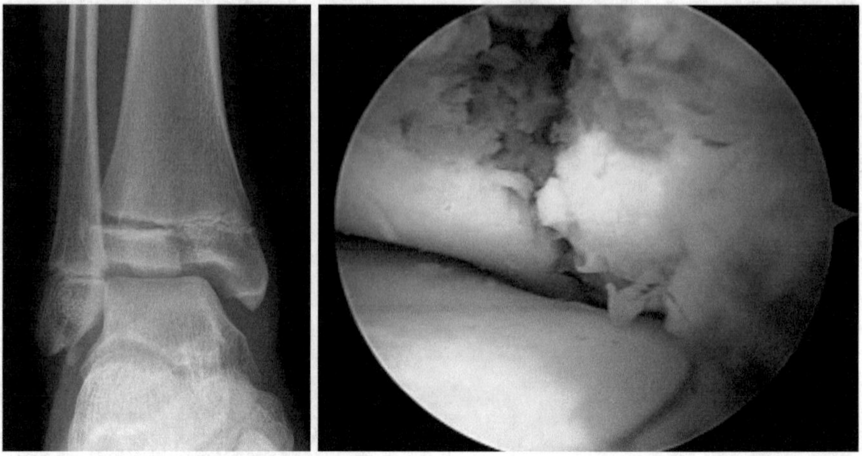

**Fig. 8.27** Type III Salter–Harris Fracture of tibial plafond. (Photo courtesy of Meagan Jennings, DPM, FACFAS)

encountered complications with the superficial peroneal nerve being the most commonly injured. Superficial peroneal nerve injury may be due to poor portal placement, instrument injury to surrounding soft tissues, or prolonged use of a tourniquet. These conditions are also supported by a study by Deng et al. in 2012 [44]. Extravasation of arthroscopy fluid into the surrounding soft tissue is also commonly encountered and is due to a lack of balance of fluid management. If the ingress and egress are not in sync, excessive fluid may build in the subcutaneous layers of tissue around the ankle. Hemarthrosis and pseudoaneurysm have also been reported due to vascular compromise/damage. Aggressive debridement in the anterior lateral ankle can easily expose the peroneus tertius muscle causing intra-articular bleeding (Fig. 8.28).

## Summary

Ankle arthroscopy is a valuable diagnostic and surgical tool that may be applied to a variety of pathological conditions inherent to the joint and surrounding soft tissues. Further advances in optics and instrumentation will continue to progress this surgical modality. Complications may be avoided with proper patient selection, knowledge of anatomy, and experience.

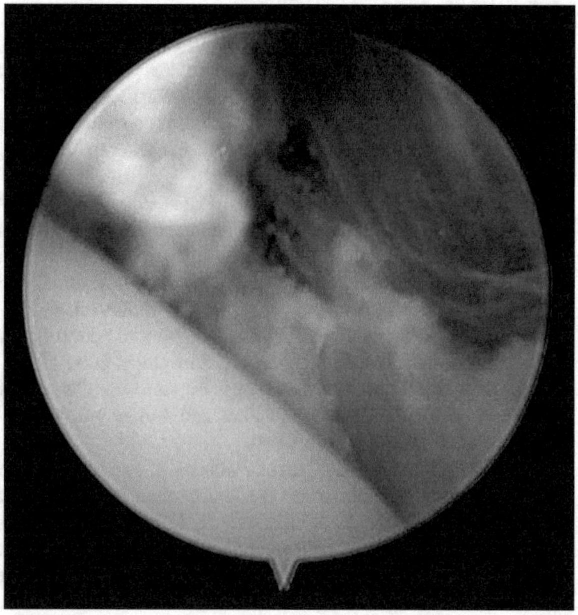

**Fig. 8.28** Aggressive debridement exposing the peroneus tertius muscle that can easily bleed into the joint

# References


1. Bozzini VP. Der Lichtleiter, oder Beschreibung einer einfachen Vorrichtung, und ihrer Anwendung zur Erleuchtung innerer Hohlen, und Zwischenraume des Lebenden animalischen Korpers. u.s.w. 23 Seiten in Fol.geheftet. Weimer; 1807.
2. Jackson RW. A history of arthroscopy. Arthroscopy. 2010;26:91–103.
3. Jackson RW. Arthroscopy of the knee. New York: Grune and Stratton; 1976.
4. Burman MS. Arthroscopic or direct visualization of joints: experimental cadaver study. J Bone Joint Surg. 1931;13:669.
5. Wantanbe M. Arthroscopy of small joints. Tokyo, New York: Igaku- Shoin; 1982.
6. Bechtol RC. The O'Connor years. Textbook of arthroscopic surgery. JB Lippincott: Philadelphia; 1984.
7. Drez D, Guhl JF, Gollehan DL. Ankle arthroscopy- technique and indications. Clin Sports Med. 1982;1:35–45.
8. Heller AS, Vogler HW. Ankle joint arthroscopy. J Foot Surg. 1982;21:23–9.
9. Lundeen RO. Arthroscopic anatomy of the anterior aspect of the ankle. J Am Podiatr Med Assoc. 1985;75:367–71.
10. Lundeen RO, Hawkins RB. Arthroscopic lateral ankle stabilization. J Am Podiatr Med Assoc. 1985;75:372–6.
11. Glazebrook MA, Ganapathy V, Bridge MA, Stone JW, Allard J-P. Evidence-based indications for ankle arthroscopy. Arthroscopy. 2009;25:1478–90.
12. Golanó P, Vega J, de Leeuw PAJ, Malagelada F, Manzanares MC, Götzens V, van Dijk CN. Anatomy of the ankle ligaments: a pictorial essay. Knee Surg Sports Traumatol Arthrosc. 2016;24:944–56.
13. Ferkel RD, Fischer SP. Progress in ankle arthroscopy. Clin Orthop Relat Res. 1989:210–20.
14. Dowdy PA, Watson BV, Amendola A, Brown JD. Noninvasive ankle distraction: relationship between force, magnitude of distraction, and nerve conduction abnormalities. Arthroscopy. 1996;12:64–9.

15. Tol JL, Verheyen C, Van Dijk CN. Arthroscopic treatment of anterior impingement in the ankle. J Bone Joint Surg Br. 2001;83:9–13.
16. Scranton PE Jr, McDermott JE. Anterior tibiotalar spurs: a comparison of open versus arthroscopic debridement. Foot Ankle. 1992;13:125–9.
17. van Dijk CN, Tol JL, Verheyen CC. A prospective study of prognostic factors concerning the outcome of arthroscopic surgery for anterior ankle impingement. Am J Sports Med. 1997;25:737–45.
18. Parma A, Buda R, Vannini F, Ruffilli A, Cavallo M, Ferruzzi A, Giannini S. Arthroscopic treatment of ankle anterior bony impingement: the long-term clinical outcome. Foot Ankle Int. 2014;35:148–55.
19. Wolin I, Glassman F, Sideman S, Levinthal DH. Internal derangement of the talofibular component of the ankle. Surg Gynecol Obstet. 1950;91:193–200.
20. van Dijk CN, Scholten PE, Krips R. A 2-portal endoscopic approach for diagnosis and treatment of posterior ankle pathology. Arthroscopy. 2000;16:871–6.
21. van Dijk CN. Subtalar arthroscopy. In: van Dijk CN, editor. Ankle arthroscopy: techniques developed by the Amsterdam Foot and Ankle School. Berlin, Heidelberg: Springer Berlin Heidelberg; 2014. p. 295–308.
22. Golanó P, Vega J, Pérez-Carro L, Götzens V. Ankle anatomy for the arthroscopist. Part II: role of the ankle ligaments in soft tissue impingement. Foot Ankle Clin. 2006;11:275–96, v–vi.
23. Smyth NA, Zwiers R, Wiegerinck JI, Hannon CP, Murawski CD, van Dijk CN, Kennedy JG. Posterior hindfoot arthroscopy: a review. Am J Sports Med. 2014;42:225–34.
24. Kappis M. Weitere Beiträge zur traumatisch-mechanischen Entstehung der "spontanen" Knorpelablösungen (sogen. Osteochondritis dissecans). Langenbecks Arch Klin Chir Ver Dtsch Z Chir. 1922;171:13–29.
25. Berndt AL, Harty M. Transchondral fractures (osteochondritis dissecans) of the talus. J Bone Joint Surg Am. 1959;41-A:988–1020.
26. Myerson MS, Quill G. Ankle arthrodesis. A comparison of an arthroscopic and an open method of treatment. Clin Orthop Relat Res. 1991:84–95.
27. Ferkel RD, Hewitt M. Long-term results of arthroscopic ankle arthrodesis. Foot Ankle Int. 2005;26:275–80.
28. Schuberth JM, Ruch JA, Hansen ST Jr. The tripod fixation technique for ankle arthrodesis. J Foot Ankle Surg. 2009;48:93–6.
29. Hawkins RB. Arthroscopic stapling repair for chronic lateral instability. Clin Podiatr Med Surg. 1987;4:875–83.
30. Nery C, Raduan F, Del Buono A, Asaumi ID, Cohen M, Maffulli N. Arthroscopic-assisted Broström-Gould for chronic ankle instability: a long-term follow-up. Am J Sports Med. 2011;39:2381–8.
31. Liu SH, Baker CL. Comparison of lateral ankle ligamentous reconstruction procedures. Am J Sports Med. 1994;22:313–7.
32. Schmidt R, Cordier E, Bertsch C, Eils E, Neller S, Benesch S, Herbst A, Rosenbaum D, Claes L. Reconstruction of the lateral ligaments: do the anatomical procedures restore physiologic ankle kinematics? Foot Ankle Int. 2004;25:31–6.
33. Vega J, Golanó P, Pellegrino A, Rabat E, Peña F. All-inside arthroscopic lateral collateral ligament repair for ankle instability with a knotless suture anchor technique. Foot Ankle Int. 2013;34:1701–9.
34. Acevedo JI, Mangone P. Arthroscopic Brostrom technique. Foot Ankle Int. 2015;36:465–73.
35. Labib SA, Slone HS. Ankle arthroscopy for lateral ankle instability. Tech Foot Ankle Surg. 2015;14:25–7.
36. Yeo ED, Lee K-T, Sung I-H, Lee SG, Lee YK. Comparison of all-inside arthroscopic and open techniques for the modified Broström procedure for ankle instability. Foot Ankle Int. 2016;37:1037–45.
37. Hua Y, Chen S, Yunxia L, Chen J, Li H. Combination of modified Brostrom procedure with ankle arthroscopy for chronic ankle instability accompanied by intra articular symptoms. Arthroscopy. 2010;26:524–8.

38. Schuberth JM, Jennings MM, Lau AC. Arthroscopy assisted repair of latent syndesmotic instability of the ankle. Arthroscopy. 2008;24:868–74.
39. Jennings MM, Lagaay P, Schuberth JM. Arthroscopic assisted fixation of juvenile intra-articular epiphyseal ankle fractures. J Foot Ankle Surg. 2007;46:376–86.
40. Small NC. Complications in arthroscopic surgery performed by experienced arthroscopists. Arthroscopy. 1988;4:215–21.
41. Martin DF, Baker CL, Curl WW, Andrews JR, Robie DB, Haas AF. Operative ankle arthroscopy. Long-term follow-up. Am J Sports Med. 1989;17:16–23; discussion 23
42. Barber FA, Click J, Britt BT. Complications of ankle arthroscopy. Foot Ankle. 1990;10:263–6.
43. Ferkel RD, Heath DD, Guhl JF. Neurological complications of ankle arthroscopy. Arthroscopy. 1996;12:200–8.
44. Deng DF, Hamilton GA, Lee M, Rush S, Ford LA, Patel S. Complications associated with foot and ankle arthroscopy. J Foot Ankle Surg. 2012;51:281–4.

# Chapter 9
# Achilles Tendon Ruptures

**Roya Mirmiran**

## Case Presentation

MG is a 31-year-old male with no known medical comorbidities, except for his love of sports, who sustained an acute pain to the posterior aspect of his left ankle in the midst of playing basketball. He heard a loud snap and thought another player hit his ankle from behind. He was not able to move his ankle and was limping due to weakness of his ankle. The physical examination noted localized edema at the posteromedial ankle. He was unable to flex his ankle, and there was a dell at the posterior aspect of his ankle (Fig. 9.1), approximately 3 cm above the Achilles tendon insertion site. The Achilles tendon was soft and spongy 3 cm above its insertion site. Homan's test was negative, but there was a positive Simmonds-Thompson test [1–3].

Intraoperatively, MG was found to have complete disruption of the Achilles tendon (Fig. 9.2). The tendon was repaired using the Krackow stitch [4]. Postoperatively, active range of motion was started at 3 weeks, followed by formal physical therapy at 4 weeks. At 3 months postoperatively, MG was able to walk without use of any assistive devices, and he gained all function back except he continued to have difficulty with single heel rise on the left leg.

R. Mirmiran (✉)
Department of Podiatry, Sutter Medical Group, Sacramento, CA, USA



D. E. Tower (ed.), *Evidence-Based Podiatry*,
https://doi.org/10.1007/978-3-030-50853-1_9

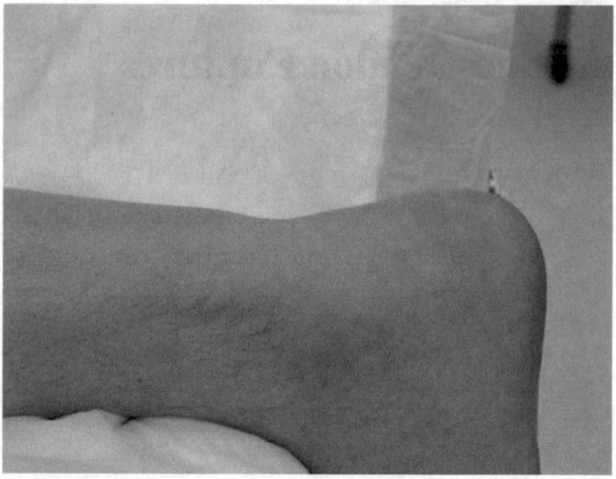

**Fig. 9.1** The clinical picture shows a "dell" on the posterior ankle which is a hallmark sign for a complete Achilles tendon rupture

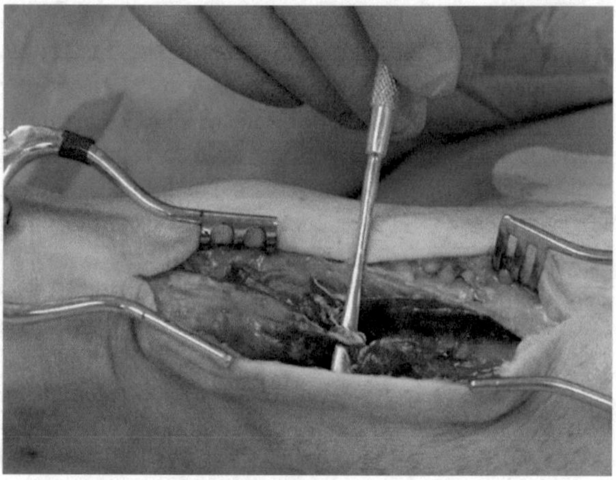

**Fig. 9.2** Patient noted to have complete rupture of his Achilles tendon with only a few strands holding the two ends of the ruptured tendon

## The Science Behind Achilles Tendon Rupture

It is well recognized that the "watershed" area of the Achilles tendon is the common site of rupture. The assumption is that inadequate blood flow in this region results in weakness of the tendon and subsequent tear. Recent studies have shown that in addition to insufficient blood flow, history of prior tendinopathy and tendon degeneration may also place a patient at higher risk of rupture when compared to patients with healthy Achilles tendons. A study comparing histological findings of acutely ruptured Achilles tendons ($N = 35$), to intact but symptomatic tendons ($N = 13$), versus control tendons with no known tendon pathology ($N = 16$) showed ruptured and tendinopathic tendons to have similar histological findings and were significantly more degenerated than control tendons [5]. Similar findings were also reported by Hansen et al. where in their study, tissue biopsy specimens of an acutely ruptured site were compared to healthy portions of the tendon in the same patient revealing a lower collagen content in the ruptured portion of the tendons [6]. The authors concluded that reduced collagen content may have placed the tendon at risk of a mechanical weakening [6].

The waves noted within tendon fibers are called crimps. The angle of fibril cramps can vary based on how stretched or relaxed a tendon may be [7, 8]. In a study reviewing the size of tendon fibrils and crimp angle in 10 patients, the authors noted that the number of fibrils, rather than size of the tendon fibrils, has a higher impact in the ruptured portion of the tendon. Fewer fibrils were seen in the ruptured rather than the intact portion of the tendon. There were no differences in the crimp angle [7]. Jarvinen et al. reported decreased collagen fiber thickness and presence of crimp angle in ruptured tendons [8]. Ruptured tendons have also been shown to have increased lectin with different histological presentations when compared to healthy tendons [9]. In a study by Saxena, the presence of a fascial band, covering the "watershed" region, was found to be crucial to the integrity of the Achilles tendon [10]. The fascial band was absent in three patients who had sustained an Achilles tendon rupture [10]. The authors concluded that the risk of Achilles tendon rupture may not necessarily be related to the degree of blood flow in the "watershed" zone of the tendon but rather histological integrity and composition of the tendon itself [10].

## Treatment Goal

The Achilles tendon is the largest and thickest tendon in the lower leg. As such, it provides significant function, and its loss may result in great disability and gait disturbance. The common demographics for patients sustaining an Achilles tendon rupture are male gender in the mid-fourth to fifth decades of life [11]. Male to female ratio is reported to range from 2:1 to 12:1 [11]. The rupture is recognized to be mainly related to an acute trauma in most patients [11, 12]. Other etiologies, such as certain medication use, have also been linked to Achilles tendon rupture [13–15]. Aging further degenerates the tendon and places it at higher risk of subsequent tear.

The ultimate goal of treatment is to regain tendon strength and function. When treating the tendon, one must consider the patient's functional goals, medical comorbidities, location of tear (midsubstance vs insertional), chronicity of the rupture, and the patient's age. The decision for surgical or nonsurgical treatment may vary based on such non-modifiable factors. Patients must be educated on the possibility of not achieving full pre-injury function regardless of chosen treatment. Among 559 NFL players with a sports injury, players with Achilles tendon tear (when compared to other injuries) demonstrated significant decline in a number of games performed at 1 year [16]. Although most were able to recover 2–3 years after surgery, a full recovery was not achieved among all athletes post-Achilles tendon injury [16]. In a level III study involving 348 basketball players, those with an Achilles tendon rupture had the lowest rate of return to play [17].

## Treatment Options: Cut or Cast

Surgical and conservative treatment outcomes for Achilles tendon rupture have been compared and/or reviewed in a number of studies. In a retrospective study of 47 patients, 23 had nonsurgical treatment, whereas the remainder of the patients underwent surgical repair [18]. Nonsurgical treatment included use of an ankle equinus cast and boot. Conservatively treated patients had better results regarding reduction of pain, return to unaided walking, and return to work. Patient satisfaction, return to sports, and strength were similar for both groups. Complication rates were similar except there were four re-ruptures in the nonoperative group with only one "late" re-rupture in the surgical group [18].

A retrospective study of 111 patients reported no difference in return to work, patient satisfaction, sports performance, muscle strength, swelling, or re-rupture among operative or nonoperative patients [19]. In this study, pain on weight-bearing and cramps were seen mostly among patients who had received conservative care [19]. In a smaller study of 57 active duty military members [20], there was no statistically significant difference in incidence of tendon re-rupture between the two treatment groups (two in the nonsurgically treated group ($N = 30$) versus one in the surgically treated group ($N = 27$). In addition, there was no significant difference in occurrence of postoperative complications or deep venous thrombosis [20]. In a level I randomized, controlled clinical trial, there was no difference in outcome for patients treated nonoperatively or operatively if "controlled early motion" was implemented as part of the rehabilitation program [21]. Similar findings were reported among 200 patients in a 10-year period undergoing operative and nonoperative treatment for acute Achilles tendon rupture after using an identical rehabilitation program [22]. A more recent study on 210 conservatively treated patients showed 15 re-ruptures with a median time to re-rupture of 23 days after the end of treatment [23].

In summary, newer studies have shown overall similar outcome results in conservative care compared to surgery when early rehabilitation is used. Although, surgical repair may result in faster and better recovery of calf muscle strength [24], early rehabilitation remains an important feature when addressing an acute Achilles tendon rupture. Even if surgery is performed, early rehab has been shown to optimize outcomes [25, 26]. Early weight-bearing (initiated at 2 weeks) after surgical repair has been shown to improve function and strength when compared to 6 weeks of non-weight-bearing [25].

## What Do Systematic Reviews Reveal?

### *Rate of Re-rupture*

There are a number of systematic reviews focusing on re-rupture rate for Achilles tendon. The earliest review was reported in 2002 [27] with a meta-analysis of published studies from 1969 to 2000. Overall findings showed that there was less risk of re-rupture with surgical repair than nonoperative repair. Another study reviewing 12 trials also reported lower risk of re-rupture with surgical approach in comparison to nonoperative treatment [28]. Of interest, this study reported that among nonoperative patients, those who were treated with a functional brace did better than those who were treated with casting [28]. Amendola reported a statistically significant lower incidence of tendon re-rupture among surgical patients, 3.6% versus 8.8% [29].

Later, in 2010, a Cochrane database study of 12 trials with 844 patients reported a significantly lower risk of re-rupture in patients treated with surgical repair [30]. Other meta-analyses published in 2011 and 2012 also reported similar findings concluding that surgical repair was effective and a better choice [31–34]. As there has been more recent movement in implementing early rehabilitation in treatment of Achilles tendon ruptures, a 2015 published review of seven articles noted no significant difference in re-rupture rates between surgical and nonsurgical group [35].

Surgical treatment of the ruptured Achilles tendon inherits its own series of complications such as infection, adhesions, and skin sensation disturbances. It is suggested that if surgery is considered, percutaneous repair may provide a lower complication rate in comparison to open repair [28].

## *Return to Work*

Several meta-analysis studies [29, 31, 35] concluded return to work time to be shorter among the operative group. In these studies, surgical patients not only had higher patient satisfaction but were able to return to work earlier with improved functional outcome [35]. However, a retrospective study of 111 patients reported no difference in return to work or patient satisfaction among operative or nonoperative patients [19].

## *Return to Sports*

The current literature does not demonstrate significant differences in ability to return to pre-injury sports or ankle range of motion among the two groups [31, 32, 34].

## *Functional Outcome*

A systematic review by Holm et al. showed improved functional outcome in surgical patients [35]. However, in two separate meta-analyses, there was no difference noted regarding return to normal function in surgical versus conservative care [27, 31]. In three other meta-analyses, the authors could not make a definitive conclusion secondary to the small size of each trial [29, 30, 32] and differences in measurements and definition by each author [30]. Regardless, functional rehabilitation is proven to be the key to improved function. A literature search focusing on treatment complications and functional outcome revealed 10 studies demonstrating that functional rehabilitation with early range of motion (ROM) exercises resulted in good results with equivalent re-rupture rates for surgical and nonsurgical patients [36]. Therefore, the authors suggest that conservative care using functional rehabilitation should be considered as treatment of choice for Achilles tendon ruptures [36].

In a review of level II randomized, controlled studies, Wu et al. noted that the centers who offered functional rehabilitation had better outcomes with nonoperative treatment of Achilles tendon rupture [37]. The authors advocated use of conservative care in patients who have access to a functional rehabilitation program and suggest surgical treatment to be considered only in centers without an appropriate functional rehabilitation program [37].

### *Complications*

Surgery carries an absolute risk increase of 15.8% for complications not related to and other than re-rupture [36]. Risk of infection is reported to be higher in patients who were treated surgically [27, 29]. Interestingly, there were no differences in rate of deep venous thrombosis (DVT) or unwanted Achilles tendon lengthening in patients treated surgically or conservatively [29, 32, 34]. Sural nerve disturbances are rare but are mostly reported in patients who have undergone surgical repair of Achilles tendon [29].

## The Current Trend in Treatment

The incidence of Achilles tendon tear has been reported to have increased from 0.67/10,000 in 2005 to 1.08/10,000 in 2011 [38]. Along with an increase in incidence, the trend for nonoperative repair has also increased. In a 2014 study of 14,127 patients with acute Achilles tendon ruptures, more than 70% of the ruptures were treated nonoperatively [38]. A statistically significant trend toward nonsurgical treatment was also evidenced in a 2017 Canadian study [39]. In 2010, 21 out of 100 cases were considered for surgical repair. However, this number decreased to 6.4 cases per 100 undergoing surgical repair in 2014. Another study also reported an upward trend of nonoperative treatment as it accounted for 12% in 2011, 57% in 2012, and 84% in 2013 [20]. More recently, a level III retrospective study of a level I trauma center presented a decline in surgical treatment for Achilles tendon ruptures from 70% to 21% in a 6-year time period (2008–2014) [40]. Aujla et al. recommend early weight-bearing and an early ROM exercise protocol (individualized) in order to achieve an effective outcome in nonoperative treatment [41].

Although the literature remains unclear on the exact protocol for nonoperative care, it is well recognized that early ROM and weight-bearing are key to a successful result. However, female gender and increasing age may be associated with higher risk of a poor functional outcome in nonoperatively managed acute Achilles tendon rupture [41].

## Surgical Approach: Percutaneous or Open Repair?

Open surgical repair of an Achilles tendon rupture is associated with a higher risk of infection [30]. In a level III study of 270 consecutive cases [42], although there were no differences in re-rupture, sural neuritis, wound dehiscence, or infection rate, better outcomes were reported in patients treated percutaneously [42]. In this study, 98% of patients receiving percutaneous treatment ($N = 101$) were able to return to sports/activity within 5 months in comparison to 82% of patients receiving open repair ($N = 169$) [42]. In addition, there were no cases of DVT or re-rupture in either group [42].

In a level II prospective study of 82 patients, percutaneous repair was as safe as open treatment with the complication rate and return to work time being similar among the two groups [43]. The nature of the complications, however, was different as the percutaneous treatment group experienced three sural nerve entrapments, while the open procedure group experienced two superficial infections and one instance of skin necrosis. The AOFAS hind-foot score was similar in both groups, as was ROM [43].

## Repair of Chronic Achilles Tendon Rupture

The literature defines a chronic or neglected Achilles tendon tear as a tear that occurred at a minimum of 4 weeks prior to initiation of treatment [44, 45]. Symptomatic chronic or neglected Achilles tendon ruptures are assumed to be debilitating and more difficult to recover from [44–46]. Most surgeons agree that neglected ruptures should be repaired surgically in symptomatic patients. Direct repair is difficult, especially if the gap is more than 5 cm. End-to-end repair may be possible if the resultant gap is less than 2.5 cm.

A 2013 meta-analysis [46] could not determine the best treatment option for chronic Achilles tendon rupture as most of the identified studies were case series with a small sample size. The authors noted a need for randomized, controlled trials with "validated functional outcome measures" [46]. They concluded that if there are no contraindications, surgery is noted to be the recommended treatment for managing chronic ruptures [46].

Various surgical techniques are used in the repair of chronic Achilles tendon ruptures, including the use of local tendons versus allografts. Examples include

V-Y tendon plasty with or without fascia turn down [47], quadricep tendon autograft [48], semitendinosus tendon autograft [49], flexor hallucis longus (FHL) tendon [50], gracilis [51], and even use of peroneus brevis (PB) tendon [52]. In 17 patients who had V-Y tendon plasty with fascia turn down [47], the pre- and postoperative AOFAS ankle-hindfoot score improved from 64 to 95. There was no rerupture in the 17 patients; however, 2 patients experienced postoperative wound infections. In this study, the mean time from injury to surgical treatment was 7 months [47]. There was no difference in outcome reported when using FHL, PB, or semitendinosus for chronic Achilles tendon rupture ($N = 62$) [53]. In summary, although acute Achilles tendon ruptures are amenable to conservative treatment, surgical repair provides better options in cases of chronic or neglected Achilles tendon tears.

## References

1. Thompson T. A test for rupture of the tendo Achillis. Acta Orthop Scand. 1962;32:461–5.
2. Thompson T, Doherty J. Spontaneous rupture of tendon of Achilles: a new clinical diagnostic test. J Trauma. 1962;2:126–9.
3. Scott B, al Chalabi A. How the Simmonds-Thompson test works. J Bone Joint Surg Br. 1992;74:314–5.
4. Krackow KA, Thomas SC, Jone LC. Ligament-tendon fixation: analysis of a new stitch and comparison with standard techniques. Orthopedics. 1988;11:909–17.
5. Tallon C, Maffuli N, Ewen SW. Ruptured Achilles tendons are significantly more degenerated than tendinopathic tendons. Med Sci Sports Exerc. 2001;33:1983–90.
6. Hansen P, Kovanen V, Homich P, Krogsgaard M, Hansson P, Dahl M, Hald M, Aagaard P, Kjaer M, Magnusson SP. Micromechanical properties and collagen composition of ruptured human Achilles tendon. Am J Sports Med. 2013;4:437–43.
7. Magnusson SP, Qvortrup K, Larsen JO, Rosager S, Hanson P, Aagaard P, Krogsgaard M, Kjaer M. Collagen fibril size and crimp morphology in ruptured and intact Achilles tendons. Matrix Biol. 2002;21:369–77.
8. Jarvinen TA, Jarvinen TL, Kannus P, Jozsa L, Jarvinen M. Collagen fibers of the spontaneously rupture human tendons display decreased and crimp angle. J Orthop Res. 2004;22:1303–9.
9. Maffulli N, Waterston SW, Ewen SW. Ruptures Achilles tendons sow increased lectin stainability. Med Sci Sports Exerc. 2002;34:1057–64.
10. Saxena A, Bareither D. Magnetic resonance and cadaveric findings of the "watershed band" of the Achilles tendon. J Foot Ankle Surg. 2001;40:132–6.
11. Hess GW. Achilles tendon rupture: a review of etiology, population, anatomy, risk factors and injury prevention. Foot Ankle Spec. 2010;3:29–32.
12. Lantto I, Heikkinen J, Flinkkila T, Ohtonen P, Leppilahti J. Epidemiology of Achilles tendon ruptures: increasing incidence over a 33-year period. Scan J Med Sci Sports. 2015;25:133–8.
13. Seeger JD, West WA, Fife D, Noel GJ, Johnson LN, Walker AM. Achilles tendon rupture and its association with fluoroquinolone antibiotics and other potential risk factors in a managed care population. Pharmacoepidemiol Drug Saf. 2006;15:784–92.
14. Sode J, Obel N, Hallas J, Lassen A. Use of fluoroquinolone and risk of Achilles tendon rupture: a population-based cohort study. Eur J Clin Pharmacol. 2007;63:499–503.
15. Van der Linden PD, Sturkenboom MC, Herings RM, Leufkens HM, Rowlands S, Sticker BH. Increased risk of Achilles tendon rupture with quinolone antibacterial use, especially in elderly patients taking oral corticosteroids. Arch Intern Med. 2003;163:1801–7.

16. Mai HT, Alvarez AP, Freshman RD, Chun DS, Minhas SV, Patel AA, Nuber GW, Hsu WK. The NFL Orthopedic Surgery Outcomes Database (NO-SOD): the effect of common orthopedic procedures on football careers. Am J Sports Med. 2016;44:2255–62.
17. Minhas SV, Kester BS, Larkin KE, Hsu WK. The effect of an orthopaedic surgical procedure in the National Basketball Association. Am J Sports Med. 2016;44:1056–61.
18. Weber M, Niemann M, Lanz R, Muller T. Nonoperative treatment of acute rupture of the Achilles tendon: results of a new protocol and comparison with operative treatment. Am J Sports Med. 2003;31:685–91.
19. Miller D, Waterston S, Reaper J, Barrass V, Maffulli N. Conservative management, percutaneous or open repair of acute Achilles tendon rupture: a retrospective study. Scott Med J. 2005;50:160–5.
20. Renninger CH, Kuhn K, Fellars T, Youngblood S, Bellamy J. Operative and nonoperative management of Achilles tendon ruptures in active duty military population. Foot Ankle Int. 2016;37:269–73.
21. Twaddle BC, Poon P. Early motion for Achilles tendon ruptures: is surgery important? A randomized, prospective study. Am J Sports Med. 2007;35:2033–8.
22. Lim CS, Lees D, Gwynne-Jones DP. Functional outcome of acute Achilles tendon rupture with or without operative treatment using identical functional bracing protocol. Foot Ankle Int. 2017;38:1331–6.
23. Reito A, Logren HL, Ahonen K, Nurmi H, Paloneva J. Risk factors for failed nonoperative treatment and rerupture in acute Achilles tendon rupture. Foot Ankle Int. 2018;39(6):694–703. https://doi.org/10.1177/1071100717754042.
24. Lantto J, Heikkinen J, Flinkkila T, Ohtonen P, Siira P, Laine V, Lepilahti J. A prospective randomized trial comparing surgical and nonsurgical treatments of acute Achilles tendon ruptures. Am J Sports Med. 2016;44:2406–14.
25. Suchak AA, Bostick GP, Beaupre LA, Durand DC, Jomha NM. The influence of early weight-bearing compared with non-weight bearing after surgical repair of the Achilles tendon. J Bone Join Surg Am. 2008;90:1876–83.
26. McCormack R, Bovard J. Early functional rehabilitation or cast immobilization for the postoperative management of acute Achilles tendon rupture? A systematic review and meta-analysis of randomised controlled trials. Br J Sports Med. 2015;49:1329–35.
27. Bhandari M, Guyatt GH, Siddiqui F, Morrow F, Busse J, Leighton RK, Sprague S, Schemitsch EH. Treatment of acute Achilles tendon ruptures: a systematic overview and metaanalysis. Clin Orthop Relat Res. 2002;400:190–200.
28. Khan RJ, Fick D, Keogh A, Crawford J, Brammar T, Parker M. Treatment of acute Achilles tendon ruptures. A meta-analysis of randomized, controlled trials. J Bone Joint Surg Am. 2005;87:2202–10.
29. Amendola A. Outcomes of open surgery versus nonoperative management of acute Achilles tendon rupture. Clin J Sport Med. 2014;24:90–1. https://doi.org/10.1097/JSM.
30. Khan RJ, Carey Smith RL. Surgical interventions for treating acute Achilles tendon ruptures. Cochrane Database Syst Rev. 2010;(9):CD003674. https://doi.org/10.1002/14651858.
31. Zhao HM, Yu GR, Yang YF, Zhou JQ, Aubeeluck A. Outcomes and complications of operative versus non-operative treatment of acute Achilles tendon rupture: a meta-analysis. Chin Med J (Eng). 2011;124:4050–5.
32. Jiang N, Wang B, Chen A, Dong F, Yu B. Operative versus nonoperative treatment for acute Achilles tendon rupture: a meta-analysis based on current evidence. Int Orthop. 2012;36:765–73.
33. Wilkins R, Bisson LJ. Operative versus nonoperative management of acute Achilles tendon ruptures: a quantitative systematic review of randomized controlled trials. Am J Sports Med. 2012;40:2154–60.
34. Deng S, Sun Z, Zhang C, Chen G, Li J. Surgical treatment versus conservative management for acute Achilles tendon rupture: a systematic review and meta-analysis of randomized controlled trials. J Foot Ankle Surg. 2017;56:1236–43.

35. Holm C, Kjaer M, Eliasson P. Achilles tendon rupture-treatment and complication: a systematic review. Scand J Med Sci Sports. 2015;25:e1–10. https://doi.org/10.1111/sms.12209.
36. Soroceanu A, Sidhwa F, Aarabi S, Kaufman A, Glazebrook M. Surgical versus nonsurgical treatment of acute Achilles tendon rupture: a meta-analysis of randomized trials. J Bone Joint Surg Am. 2012;94:2136–43.
37. Wu Y, Lin L, Li H, Zhao Y, Liu L, Jia Z, Wang D, He Q, Ruan D. Is surgical intervention more effective than non-surgical treatment for acute Achilles tendon rupture? A systematic review of overlapping meta-analyses. Int J Surg. 2016;36(Pt A):305–11.
38. Erickson BJ, Cvetanoich GL, Nwachukwu BU, Villarroel LD, Lin JL, Bach BR Jr, McCormick FM. Trends in management of Achilles tendon ruptures in the United States Medicare population, 2005–2011. Orthop J Sports Med. 2014;2:2325967114549948.
39. Sheth U, Wasserstein D, Jenkinson R, Moineddin R, Kreder H, Jaglal S. Practice patterns in the care of acute Achilles tendon rupture: is there an association with level I evidence? Bone Joint J. 2017;99B(12):1629–36. https://doi.org/10.1302/0301-620x.99B12.
40. Haapasalo H, Peltoniemi U, Laine HJ, Kannus P, Mattila VM. Treatment of acute Achilles tendon rupture with a standardised protocol. Arch Orthop Trauma Surg. 2018;138(8):1089–96. https://doi.org/10.1007/s00402-018-2940-y.
41. Aujla R, Patel S, Jones A, Bhatia M. Predictors of functional outcome in non-operatively managed Achilles tendon ruptures. Foot Ankle Surg. 2018;24(4):336–41. https://doi.org/10.1016/j.fas.2017.03.007. Pii: S1268-7731(17)30062-0
42. Hsu AR, Jones CP, Cohen BE, Davis WH, Ellington JK, Anderson RB. Clinical outcomes and complications of percutaneous Achilles repair system versus open technique for acute Achilles tendon ruptures. Foot Ankle Int. 2015;36:1279–86.
43. Rozis M, Benetos J, Karampinas P, Polyzois V, Vlamis J, Pneumaticos S. Outcomes of percutaneous fixation of acute achilles tendon ruptures. Foot Ankle Int. 2018:10718757971. [Epub ahead of print].
44. Gross CE, Nunley JA. Treatment of neglected Achilles tendon ruptures with interpositional allograft. Foot Ankle Clin. 2017;22:735–43.
45. Maffulli N, Ajis A. Management of chronic ruptures of the Achilles tendon. J Bone Joint Surg Am. 2008;90:1348–60.
46. Hadi M, Young J, Cooper L, Costa M, Maffulli N. Surgical management of chronic ruptures of the Achilles tendon remains unclear: a systematic review of the management options. Br Med Bull. 2013;108:95–114.
47. Guelu B, Basat HC, Yildirim T, Bozduman O, Us AK. Long-term results of chronic Achilles tendon ruptures repaired with V-Y tendon plasty and fascia turndown. Foot Ankle Int. 2016;37:737–42.
48. Arriaza R, Gayoso R, Lopez-Videriero E, Aizpurua J, Agrasar C. Quadriceps autograft to treat Achilles chronic tears: a simple surgical technique. BMC Musculoskelet Disord. 2016;17:116. https://doi.org/10.1186.
49. Ellison P, Mason LW, Molloy A. Chronic Achilles tendon rupture reconstructed using hamstring tendon autograft. Foot (Edinb). 2016;26:41–4.
50. Rahm S, Spross C, Gerber F, Farshad M, Buck FM, Espinosa N. Operative treatment of chronic irreparable Achilles tendon ruptures with large flexor hallucis longus tendon transfers. Foot Ankle Int. 2013;34:1100–10.
51. Maffuli N, Spiezia F, Testa V, Capasso G, Longo UG, Denaro V. Free gracilis tendon graft for reconstruction of chronic tears of the Achilles tendon. J Bone Joint Surg Am. 2012;94:906–10.
52. Maffuli N, Spiezia F, Pintore E, Longo UG, Testa V, Capasso G, Denaro V. Peroneus brevis tendon transfer for reconstruction of chronic tears of the Achilles tendon: a long-term follow-up study. J Bone Joint Surg Am. 2012;94:901–5.
53. Maffulli N, Oliva F, Maffulli GD, Bunono AD, Gougoulias N. Surgical management of chronic Achilles tendon ruptures using less invasive techniques. Foot Ankle Surg. 2018;24:164–70.

# Chapter 10
# Charcot Neuroarthropathy

**Andrew J. Meyr and Kwasi Y. Kwaadu**

## Introduction

One sympathizes with French neurologist Jean-Martin Charcot, who of course is the namesake of the neuroarthropathic process on which this chapter is focused. He died in 1893, two years before the first X-ray was performed by Wilhelm Rontgen several hundred miles to the east in Germany. How, one wonders, was Dr. Charcot able to effectively evaluate and treat his patients suffering from this condition without the use of this imaging modality that plays such an important diagnostic and interventional role in contemporary medical practice? In the century which has passed since his initial description, the medical community has certainly advanced our knowledge boundaries related to this process, but, unfortunately, in many ways it was a limb-threatening and life-altering diagnosis in nineteenth-century France and remains one today.

The objective of this chapter is to provide a critical analysis of the medical literature with respect to factors associated with the pathogenesis, evaluation, and treatment of Charcot neuroarthropathy of the foot and ankle. This will be undertaken by posing and attempting to answer four presumably simple questions.

A. J. Meyr (✉) · K. Y. Kwaadu
Department of Surgery, Temple University School of Podiatric Medicine, Philadelphia, PA, USA
e-mail: ajmeyr@gmail.com; kwasi.kwaadu@temple.edu



D. E. Tower (ed.), *Evidence-Based Podiatry*,
https://doi.org/10.1007/978-3-030-50853-1_10

## Question 1: What Is the Value of Early Diagnosis in Charcot Neuroarthropathy?

A near universal tenet of the management of Charcot neuroarthropathy (CN) is the benefit of reaching an early diagnosis with the subsequent initiation of an appropriate protective treatment protocol. The thought process associated with this assertion makes intuitive sense. CN is generally considered to be a progressive condition roughly following the stages as outlined by Eichenholtz in 1966 [1]: inflammatory/developmental, coalescence, and reconstruction/remodeling. Given this progression, if the deformity reaches a stage of joint destruction and fragmentation, then substantial lower extremity deformity is the expected result. And, this resultant deformity is, at the very least, limiting when considering ambulatory function and, at worst, increases the likelihood of ulceration, infection, and amputation.

A clear level of agreement is found throughout the medical literature with respect to this recommendation for early recognition and immediate protective immobilization as a first-line intervention [2–15]. This immobilization is usually in the form of a total contact cast (TCC) but might also include various offloading devices including the Charcot Restraint Orthopedic Walker (CROW), for example. And, several authors have presented small sampled retrospective case series of the relative effectiveness of this technique. Pinzur and Schiff reported on 10 patients with an early diagnosis who were treated with a weight-bearing TCC changed biweekly [16]. All were able to be transitioned into shoes when deemed clinically stable, and although only generalized radiographic outcomes were reported, this transition to shoegear implies a lack of substantial deformity development. And, de Sousa found comparable positive clinical outcomes with a similar casting protocol in 33 of 34 feet with midfoot Charcot neuroarthropathy [17].

However, the inherent problem with this recommendation from a critical analysis of the medical literature standpoint is that there is no comparison and a relative lack of control for the intervention. Realistically, it would be of questionable ethical standards to design a comparative study where patients with diagnosed or suspected CN were recommended to weight-bear as tolerated in unsupportive shoegear. Therefore our collective information on the topic is relatively observational as in the studies above. Although this represents a relative criticism of the literature, it should be noted that a lack of high-powered clinical trials implies neither inaccuracy nor a lack of knowledge.

Probably the most appropriate comparison that might be invoked would be to retrospectively analyze groups where a relatively early vs. relatively late diagnosis was reached within a fairly standardized initial treatment protocol. In fact, this has been undertaken by two groups of investigators. Chantelau observed that 12 of 13 patients who had what he termed a late diagnosis/referral went on to joint fragmentation, while only 1 of 11 patients with an early diagnosis/referral did so [18]. Similarly, Wukich et al. retrospectively studied a group of 20 patients with CN who were initially misdiagnosed at two healthcare centers [19]. They found that those who did not progress to a destructive phase obtained appropriate referral after a mean of 4.1 weeks and experienced a complication rate of 14.3%, while those who did progress to joint destruction obtained appropriate referral after a mean of 8.7 weeks and experienced a complication rate of 66.7%. Both of these studies provide at least indirect evidence in support of deformity progression and the development of joint destruction with a delay in intervention, although the specific natural course of this process is still relatively unknown [20].

Another challenging aspect of the critical analysis of the medical literature related to this topic is our relative lack of definitive diagnostic criteria for CN. This makes the development of strict inclusion/exclusion criteria for interventional and comparative investigations difficult. It also likely indicates that some of the data on the topic is at risk for the inclusion of false-positive cases. In other words, if pathognomonic joint destruction does not develop following the initial clinical diagnosis, then these cases are generally considered to be a "success." But, it is at least possible that some of the cases as described above with a successful outcome were in fact other idiopathic inflammatory processes aside from neuroarthropathy. Early diagnosis is most often made clinically with the presence of a red, hot, swollen extremity, with associated sensory neuropathy, and often with some history of trauma. Although CN might be at the top of a differential diagnosis described in those clinical findings, it does not represent the entire list.

Attempts have been made to further objectify the diagnosis of CN with the use of skin temperature measurements [21–24], various advanced diagnostic imaging tools [25–31], and laboratory analyses [31–36]. This last point is perhaps the most interesting and could play the largest potential role in future investigations establishing diagnostic criteria. Studies of certain specific cytokines (i.e., RANKL, tumor necrosis factors, interleukins, etc.), as opposed to more generalized measures of inflammation (i.e., leukocyte count, C-reactive protein, erythrocyte sedimentation rate, etc.), thus far have primarily focused on the pathogenesis of the condition as it relates to bone metabolism but might at some point help contribute to early diagnosis as well.

Other interesting clinical questions that still remain to be answered with respect to the diagnosis of CN include whether all patients progress through all stages as described by Eichenholtz, the time frame of this progression, any variables associated with relatively faster/slower progressions, the radiographic natural course of joint destruction and deformity, and, again, an objective means of confidently reaching an early diagnosis.

## Question 2: What Is the Utility of Classification Systems for Charcot Neuroarthropathy?

Classification systems are generally considered to have intrinsic value in medicine if they meet two criteria. The first is if they are descriptive and facilitate communication between physicians. So, for example, two colleagues can confidently discuss the treatment of an ankle fracture based on a classification system without one or both of them actually seeing the radiographs of a specific fracture. Most classifications systems meet this condition of an inherently descriptive nature. A second criteria, however, is that the classification be prognostic and/or play a role in medical/surgical decision-making. Not as many classifications that are commonly encountered in the foot and ankle meet this second condition.

Perhaps the most widely utilized classification for CN was described by Eichenholtz in 1966 [1]. This proposed three separate and distinct but linear and progressive stages: developmental, coalescent, and reconstructive. It has also been subsequently amended to include a Stage 0 to describe expected findings after the initiation of the pathologic processes but before the presentation of clear clinical and radiographic findings [37–40]. As discussed in the previous section, however, a relative limitation of this classification is that the duration of each phase is variable and might potentially last on the order of weeks to months to years [1, 19, 37]. It is also the clinical experience of many physicians that there is a fair amount of "gray" between these stages that is more likely to represent a continuous spectrum than discrete categories. Another challenge is that there is no clear correlation between relatively subjective radiographic findings and the clinical appearance of the foot and/or functional outcomes. Despite these limitations, however, it has provided at least some foundational understanding for physicians leading to general guidelines as to the stage of the pathology and elucidating an expected course [2].

Most classifications systems for CN are more anatomic and describe the location of the involvement of the disease process. This includes those by Sanders and Frykberg, Brodsky, and Schon among others [2, 39, 41–43]. These essentially highlight basic epidemiologic findings of the likelihood of the location of the deformity. However, when viewed broadly, description of the specific pathoanatomy of midfoot remains relatively lacking considering that most deformities are primarily clustered around this area including the tarsometatarsal joints, naviculocuneiform joints, calcaneocuboid joint, and the talonavicular joint [39, 42–44]. Further, as there is still a great deal of variability that exists in the specific resultant deformity and clinical findings at each of these anatomic areas, these systems can only hope to provide basic information about treatment and expected outcomes. For example, Pinzur retrospectively studied a series of over 200 midfoot CN patients but observed differences in clinical outcomes if the resultant deformity was classified as valgus vs. varus vs. dislocated [45]. None of the above anatomic classification systems address deformity this specifically.

On a positive note, discussions about anatomy might help physicians generally understand the structural pathologic processes that lead to deformity. For example, the tarsometatarsal and naviculocuneiform joints are the most likely affected anatomic areas partly as a consequence of the cantilever bending forces caused by ground-reactive forces at the metatarsal heads, the deforming proximal pull of the Achilles tendon with resultant midfoot plantarflexion, and the associated inferiorly directed forces secondary to weight during gait [2]. Understanding this pathoanatomy should help increase the understanding behind treatment rationales, for example, the utility and importance of posterior muscle group lengthening. Further, the ankle and forefoot are affected with less frequency but are more likely to be associated with an acute and/or discrete trauma [2]. This knowledge might help with early recognition and diagnosis.

Another specific benefit of the anatomic classifications is with respect to the resultant inherent stability of the joint destruction. For example, midfoot CN is more often associated with valgus and sagittal collapse of the midfoot, forefoot abduction, preulcerative exostoses, and/or chronic neuropathic ulcerations over these exostoses. Once consolidated, these deformities are relatively more stable and might be more effectively managed with casting or other immobilizing devices. On the other hand, Charcot extending proximally beyond the naviculocuneiform joints to involve the talonavicular, subtalar, and ankle joints is generally associated with less stability but is also somewhat less likely to be associated with chronic ulceration and/or recurrence, particularly in the absence of associated frontal plane varus or valgus malalignment [46].

And finally, the specific anatomy of the disease process might provide some expectations with respect to wound healing and osseous consolidation. Sinacore reported that neuropathic wounds healed and that joint destruction consolidated faster in the forefoot compared to the midfoot, rearfoot, and ankle [47, 48].

## Question 3: What Is the Goal of Intervention for Charcot Neuroarthopathy?

- *3a: How does nonsurgical management help achieve this goal?*
- *3b: How does surgical management help achieve this goal?*

CN is a disease without a cure. In other words, once the abnormal pathophysiologic processes have initiated, then by definition there will be at least some permanent structural change to the extremity that cannot be reversed. And, even following the best possible surgical reconstruction, the resultant extremity should not be viewed as a return to "normal" in terms of anatomy and function. With this concession in mind, perhaps the broadest goal for intervention for CN might therefore be to limit structural damage and preserve function.

Structural damage and functional preservation are generally considered in terms of the presence or absence of a so-called "plantigrade" foot, and this should be considered both dynamically and statically. And, the dynamic function might further be best thought of in terms of a "stable" versus "unstable" extremity. Can it perform the most basic functions of stance and propulsion through a gait cycle? Certainly heel-to-toe propulsion with effective pronation/supination might be somewhat unrealistic, but can the foot at least accept body weight and allow for forward momentum? Even a shuffling, apropulsive gait with a rolling walker might meet this definition. Or is the deformity "unstable" where angular deformity and musculoskeletal imbalance make it unrealistic to perform these most basic functions?

Statically the structural damage is generally considered in terms of the risk for ulceration given the known pathway of ulceration-to-infection-to-amputation [2–15]. Is there a structural abnormality that is likely to lead to neuropathic ulceration? As midfoot CN is the most common anatomic location of involvement, this is also the area where plantar neuropathic ulcerations are most commonly seen. This is primarily on the plantar surfaces of the cuboid and medial cuneiform (or any medial column bone for that matter), although it is certainly possible at the forefoot, talus, calcaneus, tibia, or fibula in certain cases (Fig. 10.1).

Several investigators have attempted to objectify the risk of ulceration with static radiographic measurements. Bevan and Tomlinson found that the lateral talar-first metatarsal angle (or Meary's angle) and calcaneal-fifth metatarsal angles were sensitive parameters associated with ulceration in midfoot CN [49]. In fact, all patients with a plantar midfoot ulceration in their cohort had a Meary's angle more negative than −27 degrees. Wukich et al. described a strong association between the objective parameter of cuboid height (or lateral column height) on the lateral radiographic projection and plantar foot ulceration [50]. They observed a statistically significant difference in cuboid height in a retrospective series of midfoot CN patients with and without foot ulceration and reported that 40 (80%) of 50 patients with midfoot CN and a foot ulceration had a negative cuboid height. Hastings et al. further found that this cuboid height became progressively more negative in a group of diabetic patients with CN over a 2-year period [20], while Schon et al. quantified the lateral column height in groups of CN patients with differing midtarsus deformities [51]. However, Meyr and Sebag also investigated clinical outcomes with respect to cuboid height and did not observe robust measurements of positive predictive value, negative predictive value, sensitivity, or specificity for cuboid height with plantar midfoot ulceration [52]. One limitation to all of these studies examining the risk of ulceration is that they were performed from static radiographic measurements, as opposed to measuring the dynamic function of the foot.

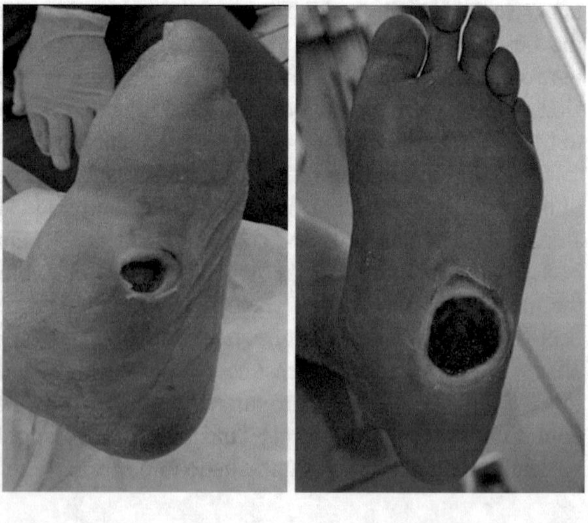

**Fig. 10.1** Classic clinical presentation of chronic plantar midfoot wounds in the setting of CN. CN of the lower extremity most commonly presents in the midfoot at or near the tarsometatarsal articulation. The resultant osseous deformity from joint destruction often results in neuropathic wound formation on the plantar-medial (left) or plantar-lateral (right) aspects of the midfoot

The differences in approach between the nonsurgical and surgical management of CN present an interesting dichotomy in the big picture of disease treatment. Although surgical intervention for CN has become more prevalent in recent decades, this is likely somewhat of a geographic phenomenon. In other words, it is not a service that is routinely offered in all areas of the world, and in fact it might even be reasonable to assume that the majority of patients who develop CN in the world might not have access to the possibility of a surgical intervention. This highlights the importance of maximizing nonoperative interventions in disease management.

## *3a: How Does Nonsurgical Management Help Achieve this Goal?*

The nonsurgical management of CN, almost by definition, should be considered proactive and reactionary to some degree in that it cannot realistically hope to alter structure. Instead the goal is essentially to preserve and protect a stable deformity before it becomes an unstable deformity at imminent risk of ulceration. This is most often thought of in terms of external support and protected immobilization.

### Protected Immobilization

There are many types of protective immobilization devices available, with characteristics and relative benefits that might be employed at different stages of the deformity. Historically, immobilization with casting has been recommended for the acute phase of this process as characterized by clinical inflammation (primarily warmth, erythema, and edema). It is thought that acute immobilization, most often in the form of a TCC, with or without ambulation, assists with reducing this inflammation and facilitating the progression into secondary stages of healing as defined by the Eichenholtz classification. Casting also likely provides effective activity modification, minimizing the overall cumulative pressure experienced by the foot.

The success of this intervention is primarily determined by decreasing levels of edema and warmth. Edema resolution can be monitored by subjective cast loosening, circumferential limb measurements, and water displacement models among other techniques [6, 16]. This can occur rapidly with effective cast application to the point that cast changes are recommended at most weekly and often more than once a week to avoid loosening which could otherwise further irritate the skin, leading to ulceration. Warmth can be objectified by means of external skin temperature analysis with serial measurements performed with an external probe at consistent anatomic sites [21–24]. The goal with this monitoring is to have the affected limb return to within approximately 2 degrees Celsius of the contralateral, non-affected extremity.

Rogers et al. described offloading as the most important management strategy during the acute phase and specifically recommended a TCC in order to achieve this [6]. This was initially replaced at 3 days and then subsequently checked weekly, to help reduce pistoning as the edema improved and the cast loosened. Although some have recommended a course of prolonged non-weight-bearing immobilization in the TCC, this is often not logistically possible or practical. Thus the traditional recommendation is for partial weight-bearing in the TCC, and this is likely to have similar efficacy without increased risk [9]. A few of the studies demonstrating the relative effectiveness of weight-bearing in a TCC have previously been described in this chapter [16, 17]. This technique has been reported to offload the forefoot and midfoot by as much as 80%, transferring the bulk of this pressure to the hindfoot and leg. As such, the weight-bearing TCC is not recommended for hindfoot deformities [10]. The cumulative duration of immobilization in a TCC and other immobilizing devices might extend up to 6 months depending on how quickly the patient progresses from the acute phase [9].

Once edema and warmth have resolved, this at least indirectly indicates that the patient is progressing into the next stage of the deformity [2]. And, following resolution of the acute phase, patients might be transitioned either into supportive diabetic footwear characterized by an extra-depth nature, wide toe box, and custom-molded Plastazote insole and rocker bottom sole or into a CROW with frequent monitoring.

### Bisphosphonates

Any discussion of the medical management of CN would not be complete without at least a reference to bisphosphonate therapy [53–58]. This represents the only current potential direct intervention into the disease process with an aim to decrease bone turnover associated with the acute phase. The thought process is simple: stabilize the underlying bone physiology as quickly as possible to decrease the likelihood that a joint destructive process with resultant deformity will ensue. However, the results of studies examining this intervention have been mixed and bring up the importance of analysis of outcomes measures as it relates to critical analysis of the medical literature. In other words, the use of bisphosphonates has been fairly clearly demonstrated to decrease skin temperatures, decrease inflammatory markers, and decrease bone turnover [53–56]. But this does not necessarily directly relate to what we established as our goals for intervention as limiting structural damage and preserving function. At least in theory, decreasing the time period of the acute inflammatory phase would decrease the risk of deformity presentation, but these are really two different outcomes with the potential for many confounding variables. And there is limited, if any, clear evidence that this therapy has an effect on clinical outcomes such as radiographic joint destruction/deformity, chronic neuropathic ulcer formation, or risk of amputation.

### *3b: How Does Surgical Management Help Achieve This Goal?*

At some point, particularly in the setting of substantial deformity, external offloading and support might not be enough to prevent chronic ulcer formation or relieve enough pressure to allow an ulceration to heal. Despite early recognition and appropriate immobilization, substantial deformity and instability can progress even with best efforts. It is in these situations that surgical management might be considered.

One consistent challenge when considering this topic with respect to the critical analysis of the medical literature is the lack of an objective indication for surgical intervention. Standardization of this is important if one is to draw comparisons across different studies. Sometimes the indication for surgery is relatively clear. This includes CN patients with infection, chronic nonhealing ulcers, pain, and instability [2, 9, 59]. This might be more challenging, however, in patients who are simply "at risk" for ulceration development. In one of the largest series of CN patients undergoing surgery to date, Pinzur and Schiff reported their indications to be a non-plantigrade foot with open wounds or osteomyelitis, a non-plantigrade foot with a postoperative goal to transition out of a brace and into a shoe, and/or the stabilization of an unstable deformity to decrease pain [45].

Another relative controversy exists with respect to the exact form of surgical intervention (i.e., exostectomy vs. reconstruction, internal vs. external fixation, plate constructs vs. intramedullary beaming procedures, the specific quantity and anatomic breadth of internal fixation, postoperative goals, etc.), but realistically these discussions are relatively undermined if a consistent surgical indication cannot be established. Further considerations to be aware of before undertaking a surgical plan of action include the individual level of experience with the procedures and potential complications [9], the acute vs. chronic stage of the deformity [60, 61], hemoglobin A1c values in the presence of diabetes mellitus [62], and the vascular status of the patient [63].

Surgical treatment options range from relatively simple procedures (such as an exostectomy at a source of increased pressure) to relatively intensive reconstructions (such as wedge resections and multiple joint arthrodeses with internal/external fixation). In the absence of associated instability or substantial deformity, a more basic surgical approach might be recommended to remove osseous prominences at a site of increased pressure with an exostectomy. Brodsky et al. were able to successfully treat 11 of 12 patients with midfoot CN with exostectomy, for example [63]. However, it is important to weigh the potential benefits of prominent bone removal against the risk of aggressive resection resulting in worsening instability with this technique. It is also unlikely to be effective in the long term in the setting of substantial deformity. For example, a Meary's angle more negative than −27 degrees has been associated with increased rate of wound recurrence when treated with only an exostectomy [49].

Operative reconstruction should be considered in patients with substantial deformity and instability, particularly progressive deformity in the sagittal plane and when the lateral column involvement becomes pronounced [50]. Contemporary trends in reconstruction advocate for advanced fixation techniques involving (1) arthrodesis extending far beyond the zone of injury in order to take advantage of fixation in uninvolved bone, (2) bone resection to shorten the underlying osseous architecture to facilitate reconstruction without increasing soft tissue tension, (3) utilization of the strongest fixation device that will be tolerated by the soft tissues, and (4) fixation devices placed in biomechanically optimal locations (such as the use of plantar plating and locked plating technology) [43, 59, 64]. These recommendations are relatively nonspecific when considering surgical intervention, and adherence to these principles might be achieved in a variety of ways. It might involve the use of internal fixation or external fixation or a combination of internal and external fixation, for example [43, 65–68]. It might also involve the use of extra-osseous plates or intramedullary axial beam constructs (Fig. 10.2). The former is more in accordance with traditional AO techniques, but the latter has received relatively recent attention as plating might be somewhat unpredictable in poorer quality bone [43, 68]. These axial beams can be delivered in retrograde fashion from the metatarsophalangeal joints into the talus through the medial column or in antegrade fashion from the talus into the metatarsals. It also involves the use of relatively smaller incisions, and they might also offer a mechanical advantage as they resist

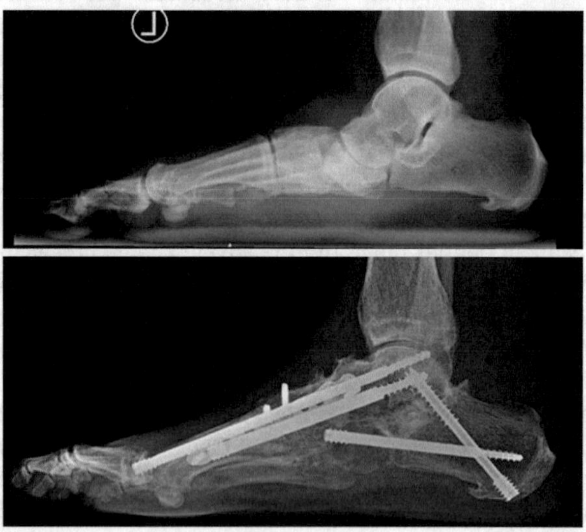

**Fig. 10.2** Example of surgical reconstruction constructs for midfoot CN. One of the most common reconstructive constructs for midfoot CN involves intramedullary axial fixation of the medial column. However, appropriate fixation constructs for this deformity might also include plate fixation with or without the use of external fixation. Although there are some general accepted principles of surgical reconstruction, surgeon preferences vary, and there is not a preponderance of data to support or refute one specific technique in comparison to another

cantilever bending forces and span completely across the zone of injury [43, 68, 69]. Although surgeon preferences vary, there is not a preponderance of data to support or refute one specific technique in comparison to another.

Following reconstruction, close follow-up several times a month is recommended until the soft tissue envelope heals as wound healing complications are frequent [46, 62]. And, patients should be monitored closely throughout the postoperative period as radiographic worsening of alignment over time has been reported even despite effective reconstruction. This finding is important and demonstrates that further deterioration might occur even after the active phase of CN has resolved [20]. Additionally, approximately 25% of patients will ultimately develop similar changes in the contralateral foot, further highlighting the importance of long term follow-up [2].

## Question 4: What Are Reasonable Expectations Following Intervention in Charcot Neuroarthropathy?

By way of conclusion, readers should appreciate that the value to any discussion about this condition comes if it results in a means to improve patient care. This might be particularly true in contemporary practice because of an increasing emphasis on outcome-based and value-based reimbursement strategies by healthcare institutions and insurance providers [70–74].

There are several general considerations to keep in mind when critically interpreting the literature relating to quality of life measures. One is to not overemphasize and instead look beyond the p-value of comparative results related to the change from pre- to post-intervention. It might be of more value to spend more time evaluating the absolute descriptive statistics of the cohort both before and after treatment. In other words, a critical reader should evaluate the demographic information related to the cohort and ask if this is a similar group of patients to what is experienced in their own practice. This doesn't necessarily represent a strength or a limitation of an individual study with respect to peer review and editing but is simply a question that should be asked by an individual critical reader. CN patients in downtown Philadelphia are likely to be somewhat different than CN patients in rural England, for example. This demographic data speaks to the applicability of results to some degree. The second is to look at the absolute numbers of the post-intervention outcome. A critical reader should not simply evaluate whether there is an improvement in the quality of life outcome but also whether the end result would constitute a "success" in the reader's individual practice. In other words, yes the quality of life might have improved compared to the pre-intervention measurement, but are you likely to be happy with this outcome as a provider and is your patient likely to be happy with this outcome in their daily life? Is this a patient with complaints that have been primarily resolved or one that still requires intensive care? A p-value is unable to answer these specific questions.

Several investigations have demonstrated that patients with CN have a relatively low quality of life at baseline compared to the general population. These groups have provided purely descriptive analyses of CN cohorts demonstrating low levels utilizing a variety of outcomes including the Short Musculoskeletal Function Assessment (SMFA), Short Form (SF)-36, AAOS outcomes instrument, and AOFAS score [75–77]. Others have performed a comparison between subsets of patients with varying comorbidities. Raspovic et al. completed two studies utilizing the SF-36 and Foot and Ankle Ability Measure (FAAM) [78, 79]. Patients with CN were found to have a lower quality of life than patients with diabetes without pedal problems, but no real differences were observed between those with CN and with and without foot ulcerations.

And, others still have looked at CN more broadly in terms of expectations. Wukich et al. found that patients with CN feared amputation even more than facing the possibility of dialysis, the possibility of infection, and even death [80]. Amputation represents a valid and major concern in these patients. Saltzman observed a 31% major amputation rate in a cohort of CN patients treated nonsurgically who suffered from a recurrent ulceration [81]. Further, in a retrospective review of over 1,000 patients with CN, Sohn et al. found a 28.3% 5-year mortality rate with 63% of patients experiencing a foot ulceration [82]. And Pakarinen et al. also found a relatively high mortality rate (29%) at a mean follow-up of 8 years [83].

In terms of more comparative investigations, one study was identified by Kroin et al. who found improved SMFA scores following reconstructive surgery for midfoot CN [84]. Interestingly however, the authors did not report the absolute values for the outcome scores, only the change from preoperative values.

Other studies have performed slightly more advanced comparisons with respect to outcomes. Pinzur et al. retrospectively reviewed over 200 patients during a 12-year period undergoing reconstructive surgery for midfoot CN and determined that 77.6% had a favorable outcome defined as no wounds or major amputation [45]. However, they also found that patients who initially had a valgus deformity had a higher rate of favorable outcome (87.0%) compared to those with a varus (56.3%) or dislocated (70.3%) deformity initially. And Eschler et al. studied complications following Charcot reconstructions in relation to the PEDIS (perfusion, extension, depth, infection, sensation) score and suggested a threshold score of 7 as being somewhat predictive of complication [85]. In fact, patients with a PEDIS score greater than 7 experienced about twice as many complications as patients with a PEDIS score less than 7.

The preceding represents a reasonable collection of quality of life data indicating that Charcot is associated with a relatively poor long term prognosis. Although intervention seems to consistently improve quality of life, a "normal" result is probably an unrealistic outcome. Patients should appreciate that their extremity is unlikely to ever return to baseline and should have realistic expectations for both outcome and function. Potential future avenues for investigation on this topic include long term morbidity and mortality data following diagnosis, realistic expectations of conservative and surgical intervention, and risk factors for complication following surgical intervention.

## References


1. Eichenholtz SN, editor. Charcot joints. Springfield: Charles C. Thomas; 1966. p. 7–8.
2. Brodsky J. The diabetic foot. In: Coughlin MJ, Mann RA, Saltzman CL, editors. Surgery of the foot and ankle. 8th ed. Philadelphia: Mosby Elsevier; 2007. p. 1281–368.
3. Frykberg RG. Charcot foot: an update on pathogenesis and management. In: Boulton AJM, Connor H, Cavanagh PR, editors. The foot in diabetes. 3rd ed. Chichester: Wiley; 2000. p. 235–60.
4. Sanders LE, Frykberg RG, Rogers LC. The diabetic Charcot foot: recognition, evaluation, and management. In: Armstrong DG, Lavery LA, editors. Clinical care of the diabetic foot. 2nd ed. Alexandria: American Diabetes Association; 2010. p. 79–96.
5. Zgonis TM, Stapleton JJ, Roukis TS. Charcot foot and ankle deformity. In: Southerland JT, Boberg JS, Downey MS, Am N, Rabjohn LV, editors. McGlamry's comprehensive textbook of foot and ankle surgery. 4th ed. Philadelphia: Lippincott, Williams & Wilkins; 2013. p. 1008–21.
6. Rogers LC, Frykberg RG, Armstrong DG, Boulton AJ, Edmonds M, Van GH, Hartemann A, Game F, Jeffcoate W, Jirkovska A, Jude E, Morbach S, Morrison WB, Pinsur M, Pitocco D, Sanders L, Wukich DK, Uccioli L. The Charcot foot in diabetes. Diabetes Care. 2011;34(9):2123–9.
7. La Fontaine J, Lavery L, Jude E. Current concepts of Charcot foot in diabetic patients. Foot (Edinb). 2016;26:7–14.
8. Strotman PK, Reif TH, Pinzur MS. Charcot arthropathy of the foot and ankle. Foot Ankle Int. 2016;37(11):1255–63.
9. Frykberg RG, Zgonis T, Armstrong DG, Driver VR, Giurini JM, Kravitz SR, Landsman AS, Lavery LA, Moore JC, Schuberth JM, Wukich DK, Andersen C, Vanore JV. Diabetic foot disorders. A clinical practice guideline (2006 revision). J Foot Ankle Surg. 2006;45(5 Suppl):S1–66.
10. Varma AK. Charcot neuroarthropathy of the foot and ankle: a review. J Foot Ankle Surg. 2014;52(6):740–9.
11. Blume PA, Sumpio B, Schmidt B, Donegan R. Charcot neuroarthropathy of the foot and ankle: diagnosis and management strategies. Clin Podiatr Med Surg. 2014;31(1):151–72.
12. Wukich DK, Sung W. Charcot arthropathy of the foot and ankle: modern concepts and management review. J Diabetes Complicat. 2009;23(6):409–26.
13. Hyer CF, Pinzur MS, Ellington JK, Davis WH, Jones CP. Charcot arthropathy: operative and nonoperative management. Foot Ankle Spec. 2014;7(4):286–90.
14. Labovitz JM, Shapiro JM, Satterfield VK, Smith NT. Excess cost and healthcare resources associated with delayed diagnosis of Charcot foot. J Foot Ankle Surg. 2018;57(5):952–6.
15. Schade VL, Andersen CA. A literature-based guide to the conservative and surgical management of the acute Charcot foot and ankle. Diabet Foot Ankle. 2015;6:26627.
16. Pinzur MS, Lio T, Posner M. Treatment of Eichenholtz stage 1 foot arthropathy with a weightbearing total contact cast. Foot Ankle Int. 2006;27(5):324–9.
17. de Souza LJ. Charcot arthropathy and immobilization in a weight-bearing total contact cast. J Bone Joint Surg Am. 2008;90(4):754–9.
18. Chantelau E. The perils of procrastination: effects of early vs. delayed detection and treatment of incipient Charcot fracture. Diabet Med. 2005;22(12):1707–12.
19. Wukich D, Sung W, Wipf AM, Armstrong D. The consequences of complacency: managing the effects of unrecognized Charcot feet. Diabet Med. 2011;28:195–8.
20. Hastings MK, Johnson JE, Strube MJ, Hildebolt CF, Bohnert KL, Prior FW, Sinacore DR. Progression of foot deformity in Charcot neuropathic osteoarthropathy. J Bone Joint Surg Am. 2013;95(13):1206–13.
21. Armstrong DG, Lavery LA, Liswood PJ, Todd WF, Tredwell JA. Infrared dermal thermometry for the high-risk diabetic foot. Phys Ther. 1997;77(2):176–7.

22. Moura-Neto A, Fernandes TD, Zantut-Wittman DE, Trevisan RO, Sakaki MH, Santos AL, Nery M, Parsisi MC. Charcot foot: skin temperature as a good clinical parameter for predicting disease outcome. Diabetes Res Clin Pract. 2012;96(2):e11–4.
23. van Netten JJ, Prijs M, van Baal JG, Liu C, van der Heijden F, Bus SA. Diagnostic value for skin temperature assessment to detect diabetes-related foot complications. Diabetes Technol Ther. 2014;16(11):714–21.
24. Sousa P, Felizardo V, Oliveira D, Couto R, Garcia NM. A review of thermal methods and technologies for diabetic foot assessment. Expert Rev Med Devices. 2015;12(4):439–48.
25. Chantelau E, Richter A, Schmidt-Grigoriadis P, Scherbaum WA. The diabetic Charcot foot: MRI discloses bone stress injury as trigger mechanism of neuroarthropathy. Exp Clin Endocrinol Diabetes. 2006;114(3):118–23.
26. Peterson N, Widnall J, Evans P, Jackson G, Platt S. Diagnostic imaging of diabetic foot disorders. Foot Ankle Int. 2017;38(1):86–95.
27. Rogers LC, Bevilacqua NJ. Imaging of the Charcot foot. Clin Podiatr Med Surg. 2008;25(2):263–74.
28. Short DJ, Zgonis T. Medical imaging in differentiating the diabetic Charcot foot from osteomyelitis. Clin Podiatr Med Surg. 2017;34(1):914.
29. Schlossbauer T, Mioc T, Sommerey S, Kessler SB, Reiser SB, Pfeifer KJ. Magnetic resonance imaging in early stage Charcot arthropathy: correlation of imaging findings and clinical symptoms. Eur J Med Res. 2008;13(9):409–14.
30. Pickwell KM, van Kroonenburgh MJ, Weijers RE, van Hirtum PV, Huijberts MS, Schaper NC. F-18 FDG PET/CT scanning in Charcot disease: a brief report. Clin Nucl Med. 2011;36(1):8–10.
31. Commean PK, Smith KE, Hildebolt CF, Bohnert KL, Sinacore DR, Prior FW. A candidate imaging marker for early detection of Charcot neuroarthropathy. J Clin Densitom. 2017;21:485.
32. Mabilleau G, Petrova N, Edmonds ME, Sabokbar A. Number of circulating CD14-positive cells and the serum levels of TNF-alpha are raised in acute Charcot foot. Diabetes Care. 2011;34(3):33.
33. Petrova NL, Dew TK, Musto RL, Sherwood RA, Bates M, Moniz CF, Edmonds ME. Inflammatory and bone turnover markers in a cross-sectional and prospective study of acute Charcot osteoarthropathy. Diabet Med. 2015;32(2):267–73.
34. Jansen RB, Christensen TM, Bulow J, Rordam L, Jorgensen NR, Svendsen OL. Markers of local inflammation and bone resorption in the acute diabetic Charcot foot. J Diabetes Res. 2018;208:5647981.
35. Jansen RB, Christensen TM, Bulow J, Rordam L, Jorgensen NR, Svendsen OL. Bone mineral density and markers of bone turnover and inflammation in diabetes patients with or without a Charcot foot: an 8.5-year prospective case-control study. J Diabetes Complicat. 2018;32(2):164–70.
36. Gough A, Abraha H, Li F, Purewal TS, Foster AV, Watkins PJ, Moniz C, Edmonds ME. Measurement of markers of osteoclast and osteoblast activity in patients with acute and chronic diabetic Charcot neuroarthropathy. Diabet Med. 1997;14(7):527–31.
37. Yu GV, Hudson JR. Evaluation and treatment of stage 0 Charcot's neuroarthropathy of the foot and ankle. J Am Podiatr Med Assoc. 2002;92(4):210–20.
38. Shibata T, Tada K, Hashizume C. The results of arthrodesis of the ankle for leprotic neuroarthropathy. J Bone Joint Surg Am. 1990;72(5):749–56.
39. Sella EJ, Barrette C. Staging of Charcot neuroarthropathy along the medial column of the foot in the diabetic patient. J Foot Ankle Surg. 1999;38(1):34–40.
40. Holmes C, Schmidt B, Munson M, Wrobel JS. Charcot stage 0: a review and considerations for making the correct diagnosis early. Clin Diabetes Endocrinol. 2015;18(1):18.
41. Rogers LC, Frykberg RG. The Charcot foot. Med Clin North Am. 2013;97(5):847–56.
42. Schon LC, Easley ME, Weinfeld SB. Charcot neuroarthropathy of the foot and ankle. Clin Orthop Relat Res. 1998;349:116–31.

43. Sammarco VJ. Superconstructs in the treatment of Charcot foot deformity: plantar plating, locked plating and axial screw fixation. Foot Ankle Clin. 2009;14(3):393–407.
44. Harris JF, Brand PW. Patterns of disintegration of the tarsus in the anaesthetic foot. J Bone Joint Surg Br. 1996;48(1):4–16.
45. Pinzur MS, Schiff AP. Deformity and clinical outcomes following operative of Charcot foot: a new classification with implications for treatment. Foot Ankle Int. 2018;39(3):265–70.
46. Wukich DK, Sadoskas D, Vaudreuil NJ, Fourman M. Comparison of diabetic Charcot patients with and without foot wounds. Foot Ankle Int. 2017;38(2):140–8.
47. Sinacore DR. Healing times of diabetic ulcers in the presence of fixed deformities of the foot using total contact casting. Foot Ankle Int. 1998;19(9):613–8.
48. Sinacore DR. Acute Charcot arthropathy in patients with diabetes mellitus: healing times by foot location. J Diabetes Complicat. 1998;12(5):287–93.
49. Bevan WP, Tomlinson MP. Radiographic measures as a predictor of ulcer formation in diabetic charcot midfoot. Foot Ankle Int. 2008;29(6):568–73.
50. Wukich DK, Raspovic KM, Hobizal KB, Rosario B. Radiographic analysis of diabetic midfoot charcot neuroarthropathy with and without midfoot ulceration. Foot Ankle Int. 2014;35(11):1108–15.
51. Schon LC, Weinfeld SB, Horton GA, Resch S. Radiographic and clinical classification of acquired midtarsus deformities. Foot Ankle Int. 1998;19(6):394–404.
52. Meyr AJ, Sebag JA. Relationship of cuboid height to plantar ulceration and other radiographic parameters in midfoot Charcot neuroarthropathy. J Foot Ankle Surg. 2017;56(4):748–55.
53. Game FL, Catlow R, Jones GR, Edmonds ME, Jude EB, Rayman G, Jeffcoate WJ. Audit of acute Charcot's disease in the UK: the CDUK study. Diabetologia. 2012;55(1):32–5.
54. Richard JL, Almasri M, Schuldiner S. Treatment of acute Charcot foot with bisphosphonates: a systematic review of the literature. Diabetologia. 2012;55(5):1258–64.
55. Jude EB, Selby PL, Burgess J, Lilleystone P, Mawer EB, Page SR, Donohue M, Foster AV, Edmonds ME, Boulton AJ. Bisphosphonates in the treatment of Charcot neuroarthrpathy: a double-blind randomized controlled trial. Diabetologia. 2001;44(11):2032–7.
56. Parkarinen TK, Laine HJ, Maenpaa H, Kahonen M, Mattila P, Lahtela J. Effect of immobilization, off-loading and zoledronic acid on bone mineral density in patients with acute Charcot neuroarthropathy: a prospective randomized trial. Foot Ankle Surg. 2013;19(2):121–4.
57. Petrova NL, Edmonds ME. Medical management of Charcot arthropathy. Diabetes Obes Metab. 2013;15(3):193–7.
58. Smith C, Kumar S, Causby R. The effectiveness of non-surgical interventions in the treatment of Charcot foot. JBI Libr Syst Rev. 2007;5(10):558–76.
59. Schneekloth BJ, Lowery NJ, Wukich DK. Charcot neuroarthropathy in patients with diabetes: an updated systematic review of surgical management. J Foot Ankle Surg. 2016;55(3):586–90.
60. Burns PR, Wukich DK. Surgical reconstruction of the Charcot rearfoot and ankle. Clin Podiatr Med Surg. 2008;25(1):95–120.
61. Simon SR, Tejwani SG, Wilson DL, Santner TJ, Denniston NL. Arthrodesis as an early alternative to nonoperative management of Charcot arthropathy of the diabetic foot. J Bone Joint Surg Am. 2000;82-A(7):939–50.
62. Wukich DK, Crim BE, Frykberg RG, Rosario BL. Neuropathy and poorly controlled diabetes increase the rate of surgical site infection after foot and ankle surgery. J Bone Joint Surg Am. 2014;96(10):832–9.
63. Brodsky JW, Rouse AM. Exostectomy for symptomatic bony prominences in diabetic Charcot feet. Clin Orthop Relat Res. 1993;296:21–6.
64. Marks RM, Parks BG, Schon LC. Midfoot fusion technique for neuroarthropathic feet: biomechanical analysis and rationale. Foot Ankle Int. 1998;19(8):507–10.
65. Dayton P, Feilmeier M, Thompson M, Whitehouse P, Reimer RA. Comparison of complications for internal and external fixation for Charcot reconstruction: a systematic review. J Foot Ankle Surg. 2015;54(6):1072–5.

66. Zgonis T, Roukis TS, Lamm BM. Charcot foot and ankle reconstruction: current thinking and surgical approaches. Clin Podiatr Med Surg. 2007;24(3):505–17.
67. Lamm BM, Gottlieb HD, Paley D. A two-stage percutaneous approach to Charcot diabetic foot reconstruction. J Foot Ankle Surg. 2010;49(6):517–22.
68. Lamm BM, Siddiqui NA, Nair AK, LaPorta G. Intramedullary foot fixation for midfoot Charcot neuroarthropathy. J Foot Ankle Surg. 2012;51(4):531–6.
69. Kann JN, Parks BG, Schon LC. Biomechanical evaluation of two different screw positions for fusion of the calcaneocuboid joint. Foot Ankle Int. 1999;20:33–6.
70. Bosco JA 3rd, Sachdev R, Shapiro LA, Stein SM, Zuckerman JD. Measuring quality in orthopaedic surgery: the use of metrics in quality management. Instr Course Lect. 2014;63:473–85.
71. Katz G, Ong C, Hutzler L, Zuckerman JD, Bosco JA 3rd. Applying quality principles to orthopaedic surgery. Instr Course Lect. 2014;63:465–72.
72. Snyder CF, Aaronson NK. Use of patient-reported outcomes in clinical practice. Lancet. 2009;374(9687):369–70.
73. Walijee JF, Nellans K. Quality assessment in hand surgery. Hand Clin. 2014;30(3):259–68.
74. Andrawis JP, Chenok KE, Bozic KJ. Health policy implications of outcomes measurement in orthopaedics. Clin Orthop Relat Res. 2013;471(11):3475–81.
75. Kroin E, Schiff A, Pinzur MS, Davis ES, Chaharbakhshi E, DiSilvio FA Jr. Functional impairment of patients undergoing surgical correction for Charcot foot Arthropathy. Foot Ankle Int. 2017;38(7):705–9.
76. Pinzur MS, Evans A. Health-related quality of life in patients with Charcot foot. Am J Orthop (Belle Mead NJ). 2003;32(10):492–6.
77. Sochocki MP, Verity S, Atherton PJ, Huntington JL, Sloan JA, Embil JM, Trepman E. Health related quality of life in patients with Charcot arthropathy of the foot and ankle. Foot Ankle Surg. 2008;14(1):11–5.
78. Raspovic KM, Wukich DK. Self-reported quality of life in patients with diabetes: a comparison of patients with and without Charcot neuroarthropathy. Foot Ankle Int. 2014;35(3):195–200.
79. Raspovic KM, Hobizal KB, Rosario BL, Wukich DK. Midfoot Charcot neuroarthropathy in patients with diabetes: the impact of foot ulceration on self-reported quality of life. Foot Ankle Spec. 2015;8(4):255–9.
80. Wukich DK, Raspovic KM, Suder NC. Patients with diabetic foot disease fear major lower-extremity amputation more than death. Foot Ankle Spec. 2018;11(1):17–21.
81. Saltzman CL, Hagy ML, Zimmerman B, Estin M, Cooper R. How effective is intensive non-operative initial treatment of patients with diabetes and Charcot arthropathy of the feet? Clin Orthop Relat Res. 2005;435:185–90.
82. Sohn MW, Lee TA, Stuck RM, Frykberg RG, Budiman-Mak E. Mortality risk of Charcot arthropathy compared with that of diabetic foot ulcer and diabetes alone. Diabetes Care. 2009;32(5):816–21.
83. Pakarinen TK, Laine HJ, Maenpaa H, Mattila P, Lahtela J. Long-term outcome and quality of life in patients with Charcot foot. Foot Ankle Surg. 2009;15(4):187–91.
84. Kroin E, Chaharbakhshi EO, Schiff A, Pinzur MS. Improvement in quality of life following operative correction of midtarsal Charcot foot deformity. Foot Ankle Int. 2018;39(7):808–11.
85. Eschler A, Gradl G, Wussow A, Mittlmeier T. Prediction of complications in a high-risk cohort of patients undergoing corrective arthrodesis of late stage Charcot deformity based on the PEDIS score. BMC Musculoskeletal Disord. 2015;16:349.

# Chapter 11
# Congenital Talipes Equinovarus

Daniel J. Hatch

One of the more common deformities of the foot and ankle present at birth is congenital talipes equinovarus (CTEV) or clubfoot. Clubfoot is a three-dimensional deformity that has an incidence of 1/1,000 in the Caucasian population [1]. There is a higher incidence in South African blacks and Polynesians (6/1,000) [2]. Males are more frequently affected than females at a ratio of three to one. Forty percent of cases are bilateral [3]. When untreated, clubfoot can be very disabling resulting in pain, severe deformity, inability to wear shoes, and inability to ambulate (Fig. 11.1).

## Definition

CTEV is comprised of four components: equinus, varus, adductus, and cavus [4] (Fig. 11.2). Equinus is the foot in a plantarflexed position compared to the lower leg. Varus is in reference to the position of the calcaneus. Adduction is the relationship of the forefoot to the rearfoot. Cavus is the overall increase in height of the arch of the foot. There are four basic classifications of clubfoot: congenital (idiopathic), teratologic, syndromic, and positional [5]. Idiopathic is the most common and can present at birth as an isolated defect. It may be first diagnosed in utero by ultrasound at 15–16 weeks gestation [6]. Sometimes this can be identified as early as 12 weeks gestation [7]. Aurell et al. evaluated the ultrasound anatomy of 30 untreated clubfeet in 22 children in their neonatal clubfoot study [8]. The authors found close proximity of the navicular and medial malleolus along with capsular thickening medially. Teratologic clubfoot types are associated with neuromuscular disease processes such as spina

D. J. Hatch (✉)
Clinical Instructor: Scholl College of Podiatric Medicine, North Chicago, IL, USA

Director of Surgery: North Colorado Podiatric Surgical Residency, Greeley, CO, USA

Private Practice: Foot and Ankle Center of the Rockies, Denver, CO, USA
e-mail: dhatch@facrockies.com



D. E. Tower (ed.), *Evidence-Based Podiatry*,
https://doi.org/10.1007/978-3-030-50853-1_11

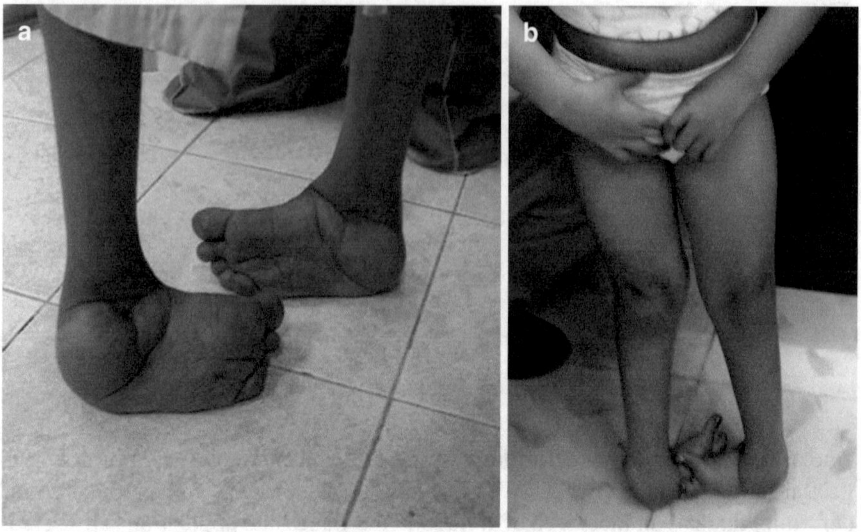

**Fig. 11.1** Neglected clubfoot

**Fig. 11.2** Idiopathic clubfoot

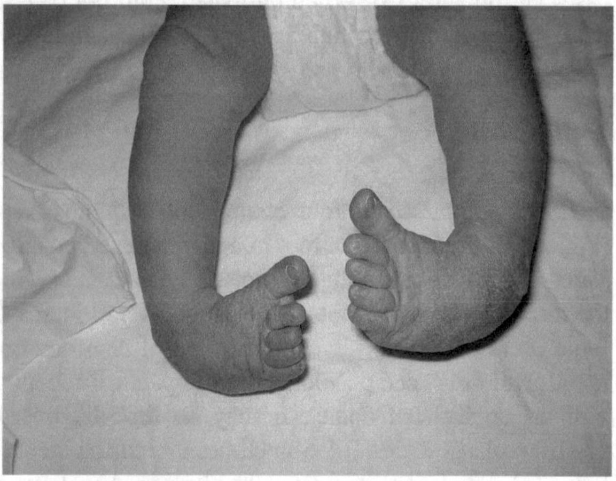

bifida and myelomeningocele. Syndromic clubfoot is associated with genetic abnormalities and other disease processes of which clubfoot commonly occurs. Examples of this type would include arthrogryposis, Larsen syndrome, and moebius syndrome [2, 9, 10]. Positional (sometimes called postural) clubfoot is a relatively normal foot that was held in an abnormal position in utero. This type is more easily corrected and usually does not require treatment with an Achilles tenotomy or extensive bracing.

## Etiology

The etiology of idiopathic clubfoot is multifactorial and involves several common theories. Idiopathic clubfoot results from in utero rather than embryonic conditions. The more frequently cited factors involved in the development of clubfoot include in utero positioning, environmental factors, neuromuscular with increased collagen synthesis, and genetic origin. Some less frequently reported causes include intrauterine developmental arrest [11], a defect in the germ plasm of the talus [12, 13], hypoplastic dorsalis pedis artery [14], and neurological defects affecting muscles of the lower extremity [15].

In utero malpositioning was identified by Hippocrates [16] and supported by Browne [17, 18]. Additionally, it has been reported that there is a greater incidence of clubfoot after amniocentesis [19]. Farrell et al. found that amniocentesis at 12 weeks correlated with a statistically significant 1.3% increased chance of clubfoot [20]. The authors found this timing correlated with a maximal amount of foot and ankle growth. It is believed that the loss of amniotic fluid contributes to the "crowding" of the uterine cavity [20].

Environmental factors are rare and would include drug exposures [21] and smoking [4, 22].

Ippolito and Ponseti's histological study of five clubfeet and three normal feet in aborted fetuses found shortening and thickening of the talonavicular and spring ligaments suggesting a possible etiology of clubfoot to be a "retracting fibrosis" [23]. The authors also found that the distal leg muscles showed a decrease in size and number of muscle fibers. Other studies have supported the theory of increase in fetal myosin and ensuing fibrosis [15, 24–26].

There is a high genetic influence in clubfoot [2, 27–32]. Idelberger in 1939 found a concordance of clubfoot in 32.5% of monozygotic twins and only 2.9% of dizygotic twins [33]. Wynne-Davies found that if one child in a family had clubfoot, then the second child's chance of clubfoot would be 1/35 [2]. In 2008, Gurnett et al. reported on a genetic variance of the gene PITX1 that was found to be associated with clubfoot deformity [34]. Additional gene factors have been identified including TBX4, RBM10, HOXA, and HOXD [22, 35]. Idiopathic clubfoot is an isolated condition without other musculoskeletal findings and accounts for the majority (80%) of congenital clubfoot. The idiopathic deformity is present with a polygenic threshold influence [22, 35, 36]. The genetic influence may not only determine the incidence of clubfoot, but it may also influence the severity and type of deformity.

## Pathoanatomy

In 1803, Antonio Scarpa described the abnormal anatomy of congenital clubfoot recognizing that there was medial displacement of the navicular, cuboid, and calcaneus with respect to the talus [37]. Several studies have been performed on fetuses of varying ages [4, 38]. When unilaterally present, the clubbed foot is smaller both in length and girth and the calf muscles are retracted and less developed compared to the contralateral side. The head and neck of the talus are deviated medially and plantarly, while the body of the talus is rotated laterally [12, 39, 40]. The navicular is subluxed medially and may at times even closely juxtapose the medial malleolus [4]. Ponseti would utilize his thumb as a method of measurement to document the distance between the navicular tuberosity and the medial malleolus as an indicator of treatment progression (Ponseti IV, Personal Communication, 2003). The

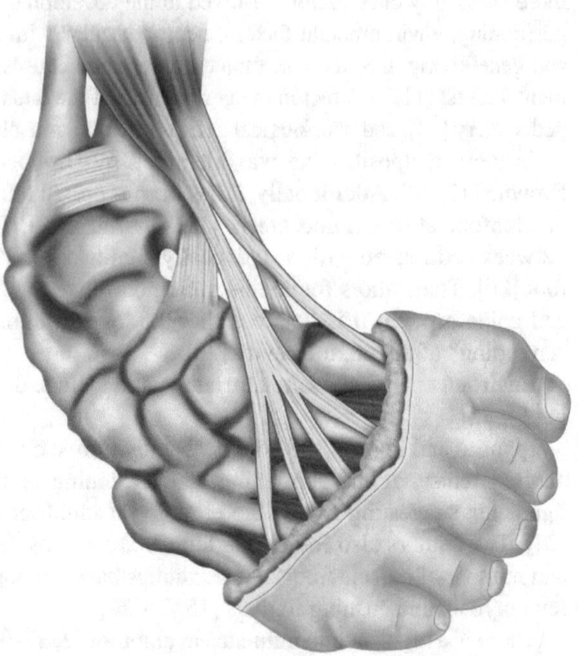

**Fig. 11.3** Medially displaced tendons

calcaneus is plantarflexed and inverted with tight medial ligaments and tendons. This gives the appearance of an "empty heel" where the calcaneal tuberosity is elevated. The extensor tendons are medially displaced due to the position of the foot in relation to the leg [4] (Fig. 11.3). The posterior muscle groups are tight and contracted with proximal migration of the posterior muscle bellies.

While Ponseti was not an advocate of radiographs in the infant due to lack of ossification and reliable measurements, it is noted that on the AP radiograph that Kite's angle is decreased, occasionally to zero along with increased forefoot adduction. On the lateral projection, the talus and calcaneus are in equinus.

## Kinesiology

The understanding of clubfoot mechanics date back to Farabeauf [41] and were further expanded by Huson [42, 43]. Farabeauf, a French anatomist, detailed his thoughts on foot mechanics in his "Precis de manual operative" first published in 1872. Huson wrote his doctoral dissertation in 1961 on "A Functional and Anatomical study of the Tarsus" and noted that the tarsal joints rotate about a moving axis rather than around a fixed hinge [42]. Ponseti attributes Huson with his understanding of foot mechanics that provided him the understanding to treat clubfoot successfully [4] (Ponseti IV, Personal Communication, 2003). Motion of the calcaneus is not simply inversion and eversion in the frontal plane. Farabeauf likened the motion to the keel of a ship in which it would pitch, roll, and yaw. The calcaneus' motion is in all three planes with the interosseous talocalcaneal ligament serving as the axis point. It is an interesting anatomic observation that this ligament lies within the same axis as the subtalar joint which has been described as being approximately 42 ° from the transverse plane and 16 ° from the sagittal plane [44–46]. The main tenant of Ponseti's conservative treatment for clubfoot incorporates this overall understanding of subtalar joint mechanics. In order for the body of the calcaneus to evert, the anterior process of the calcaneus must first abduct [47] (Fig. 11.4). Abduction of the anterior process of the calcaneus is accomplished by abducting the forefoot as a single unit about the rearfoot by applying counter-pressure against the lateral aspect of the talar head. This tri-plane maneuver initiated by the transverse plane abduction allows the heel to freely move under the talus into a more everted position with the anterior process of the calcaneus in a more abducted and dorsiflexed position.

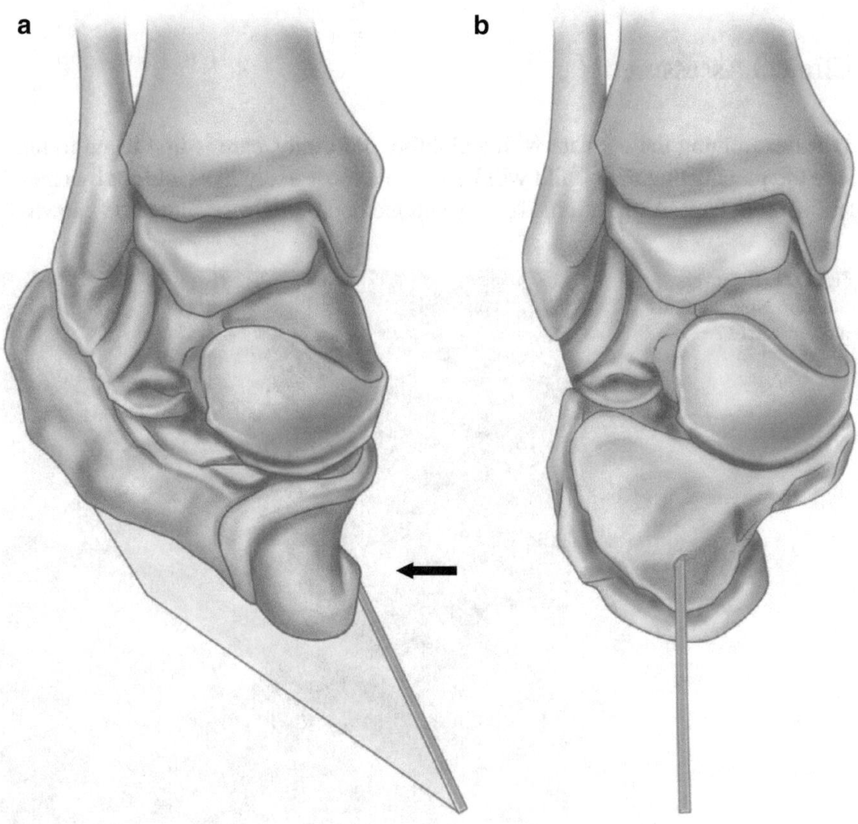


**Fig. 11.4** Abduction of the calcaneal beak initiates eversion of the heel. (**a**) In clubfoot, the anterior beak of the calcaneus is positioned under the head of the talus. (**b**) Abduction of the beak in relation to the talar head will allow correction of the heel varus

## Terminology

Clubfeet can be placed into five categories based upon treatment status including untreated, neglected, recurrent, resistant, and complex or atypical [5, 48]. Untreated clubfoot is defined as a child under 2 years of age who has not been previously treated, whereas a neglected clubfoot occurs in a child over 2 years of age who has not been previously treated. A recurrent clubfoot, or relapse, presents in a child previously treated who has re-developed equinus and varus position of the heel. Recurrence of clubfoot deformity is most often due to lack of adherence to the treatment protocols and bracing (Fig. 11.5). A resistant clubfoot is more difficult to treat conservatively and usually involves an underlying neuromuscular disorder such as spina bifida. The complex or atypical clubfoot is a unique and challenging entity that is treated in a different fashion compared to typical idiopathic types. The complex clubfoot has a pronounced calcaneal equinus, a central crease in the arch, and a short first metatarsal due to forefoot equinus (Fig. 11.6).

## Clinical Assessment

When examining the neonate with a clubfoot deformity, care is first taken to reassure the parents that their child will be fine and most likely has clubfoot by chance and without fault. A gestational history and method of delivery should be known. A

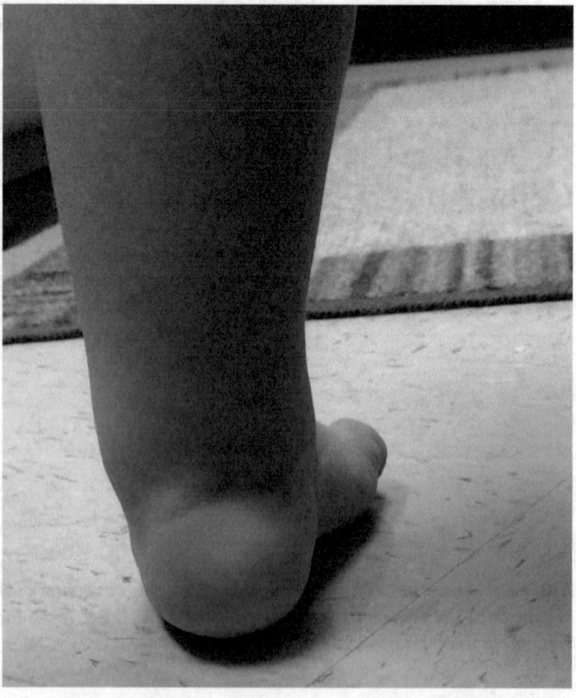

**Fig. 11.5** Recurrent clubfoot. Note: equinus and varus heel

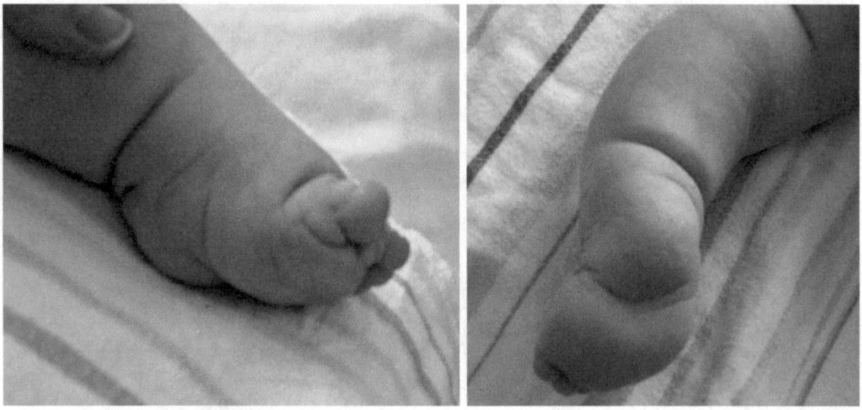

**Fig. 11.6.** Complex clubfoot. Note: equinus, plantar crease and overall increased girth of foot and ankle along with short hallux

neuromuscular examination should be performed along with examination of the child's lower back (indentations/hair growth) and hips for signs of dislocation. Once the overall assessment is performed, attention is then directed to the lower legs and feet. Care is taken to identify any creases posteriorly or in the arch that would indicate severe contractures. Additionally, the rigidity of the deformity is assessed by evaluating the reducibility of the equinus and forefoot adductovarus. While there have been various classification schemes, the two more frequently cited are the Dimeglio and the Pirani systems. At times these schemas are even used concurrently [49]. Dimeglio et al. proposed a 20-point scoring system based upon four reduction of deformity attributes: equinus, heel varus, forefoot adduction about the hindfoot, and forefoot derotation about the talus. Each of the attributes are given up to four points for minimum reducibility with an additional point added for each of the following: presence of a posterior crease, presence of a medial crease, presence of cavus deformity and muscle condition [50] (Fig. 11.7, Table 11.1). Dimeglio's classification emphasizes reducibility of the contracted deformity in the sagittal, frontal, and horizontal planes. Pirani et al. developed a 6-point scale giving one point for the presence of each of the following clinical signs: posterior crease, presence of an empty heel, rigid equinus, curvature of lateral border of the foot, medial crease, and prominent lateral aspect of the talar head. The posterior crease sign implies a posterior contracture of the ankle joint. The emptiness of the heel refers to the inability to palpate the tuberosity of the calcaneus due to rigid equinus of the heel. The medial crease implies a more medial contracture of the foot (Fig. 11.8).

Each clinical sign is graded on a point scale with 0 = normal, 0.5 = mild, and 1.0 = severe [51, 52] (Table 11.2, Fig. 11.9). Pirani's classification emphasizes foot morphology as it correlates with severity of deformity; however, he added transverse plane reduction of the forefoot about the lateral talar head (prominent lateral aspect of the talar head) and rigidity of the equinus deformity. Attempts are being made to utilize these classifications as predictors of treatment types and success [53, 54].

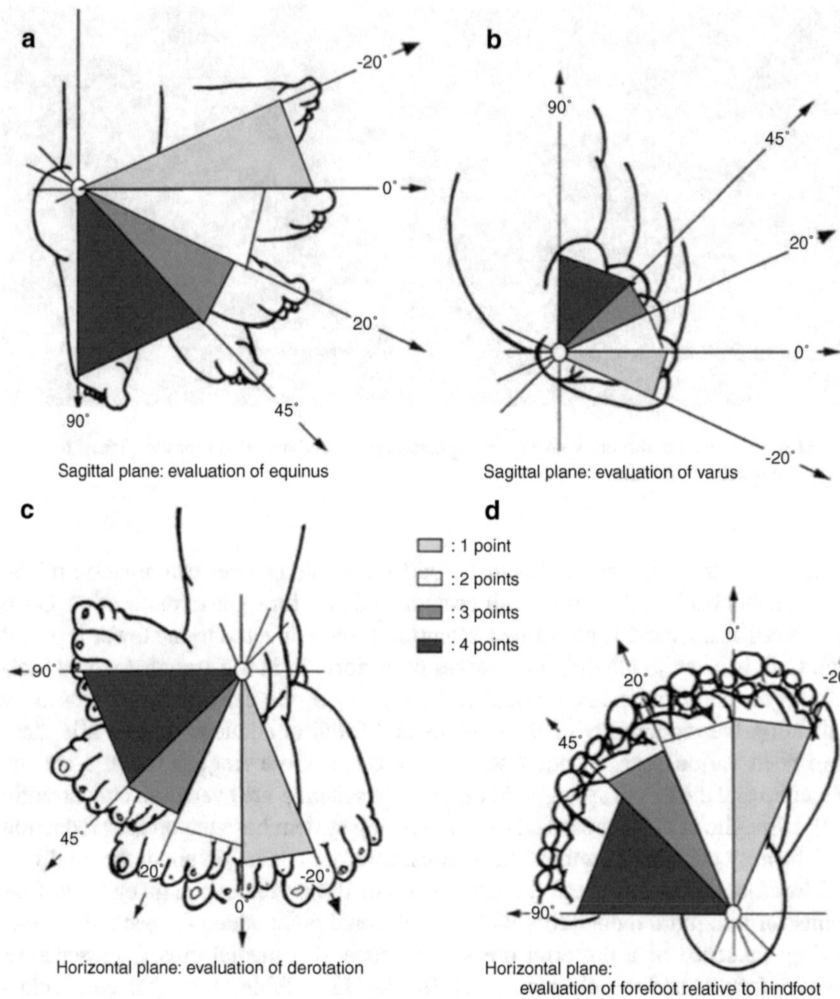


**Fig. 11.7** Dimeglio's classification of clubfoot

## Treatment History and Options

Plaster casts were first applied for the treatment of clubfoot in 1838 by Guerin [43]. Early treatment of clubfoot was attempted by forceful manipulations using the Thomas wrench [43]. In 1908, Robert Jones reported favorable results if treatment was initiated early [55]. He would first manipulate and cast the deformity followed by wedge resection of the tarsus, only if needed. Kite published his method in 1930 [56]. He claimed a 95% success rate and, subsequently, his treatment was popular in the orthopedic world for many years [56, 57]. Unfortunately, Kite's method could not be reproduced with outcomes comparable to his study. The treatment was a long

**Table 11.1** Dimeglio scoring system. (see Fig 11.7 for visual representation of deformities and scoring)

Points are based upon the degree of contracted deformity:
90°–45° = 4 points
45°–20° = 3 points
20°–0° = 2 points
0°–(-20°) = 1 point
<–20° = 0 points

| Deformity | Points | Maximum point Deformity/position |
|---|---|---|
| Equinus | 0–4 | 4 points = 90° plantarflexed |
| Heel varus | 0–4 | 4 points = 90° inverted |
| Forefoot derotation | 0–4 | 4 points = 90° rigid internal rotation |
| Forefoot adduction | 0–4 | 4 points = 90° adduction |
| Posterior crease | 1 point | Present |
| Medial crease | 1 point | Present |
| Cavus | 1 point | Present |
| Muscle condition | 1 point | |
| Total points | Range from 0 to 20; min = 0; max = 20 | |

process addressing each clubfoot component individually. Kite would first treat the forefoot adduction by abducting the forefoot against counter-pressure at the cuboid. Heel varus was then corrected followed lastly by improving the ankle equinus. Repair of the heel varus was difficult, and Kite's method was met with frequent failures that resulted in a high incidence of surgical intervention. Recent literature has compared Kite's method to Ponseti's with more favorable outcomes in the Ponseti treatment method [58–60].

There has been a paradigm shift in the surgical treatment of clubfoot since the early 1900s. This is due to an improved understanding of foot mechanics and the success of the Ponseti casting technique. Presently, surgical repair should be reserved for the most difficult deformities related to neglected, syndromic, and teratologic conditions. Initially, surgical repair was performed due to lack of improvement with conservative options. From a historical perspective, surgical treatment started in the early 1900s by Codivilla with his medial approach [61, 62]. While there have been a variety of methods proposed in the surgical treatment of clubfoot, there appear to be several surgical approaches that are considered classic surgical treatments. These include the methods of Turco, Carroll, and Crawford. These various incisional approaches attempted to alleviate contracted structures and tighten the soft tissue laxity. Turco proposed a posterior to medial incision to isolate the contracted tissues [63, 64] (Fig. 11.10). Norris Carroll advocated a two incision approach in 1990 [65]. This involved a medial incision and a posterior incision. He further explained his technique in an article in 1993 [66] (Fig. 11.11). Crawford popularized the "Cincinnati" incision for clubfoot, advocating improved exposure and surgical scar [67] (Fig. 11.12). All these approaches had the goal of a

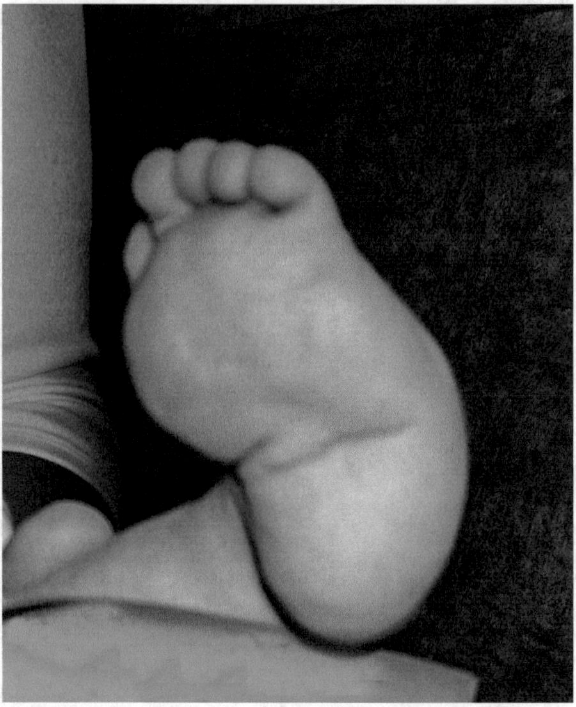

**Fig. 11.8** Medial crease. A sign of medial contractures

**Table 11.2** Pirani scoring system

| Hindfoot contracture | Points/ Rating |
|---|---|
| (a) Posterior crease (PC) | 0, 0.5, 1 |
| (b) "Empty heel" (EH) | 0, 1 |
| (c) Rigidity of equinus (RE) | 0, 0.5, 1 |
| Midfoot contracture | |
| (a) Curvature of lateral border of foot (CLB) | 0, 0.5, 1 |
| (b) Medial arch crease (MC) | 0, 0.5, 1 |
| (c) Reduction of lateral talar head (LHT) | 0, 0.5, 1 |
| Total Points | Range from 0–6; min = 0; max = 6 |
| | 0 = more normal; 6 = more problematic/rigid |

plantigrade foot and being able to wear shoes. In their 2016 study, Mahapatra and Abraham found the Cincinnati approach to have less wound complications and better functional result than the Turco method [68]. Subsequent soft tissue procedures have been described for realignment of the foot; however, problems with scarring, stiffness, and arthrosis have occurred [69–71]. These factors along with the surgical complications of over- and under-correction have led most surgeons to reserve surgical repair for the most resistant, recalcitrant deformities. In fact, Zionts compared

**Fig. 11.9** Pirani's schematic classification examples

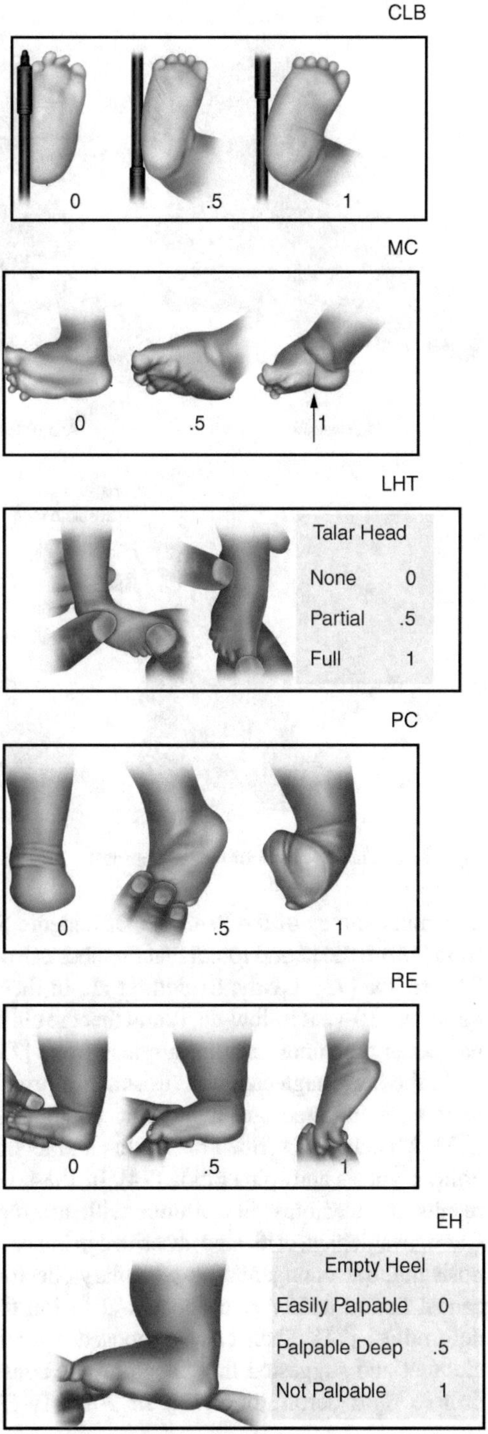

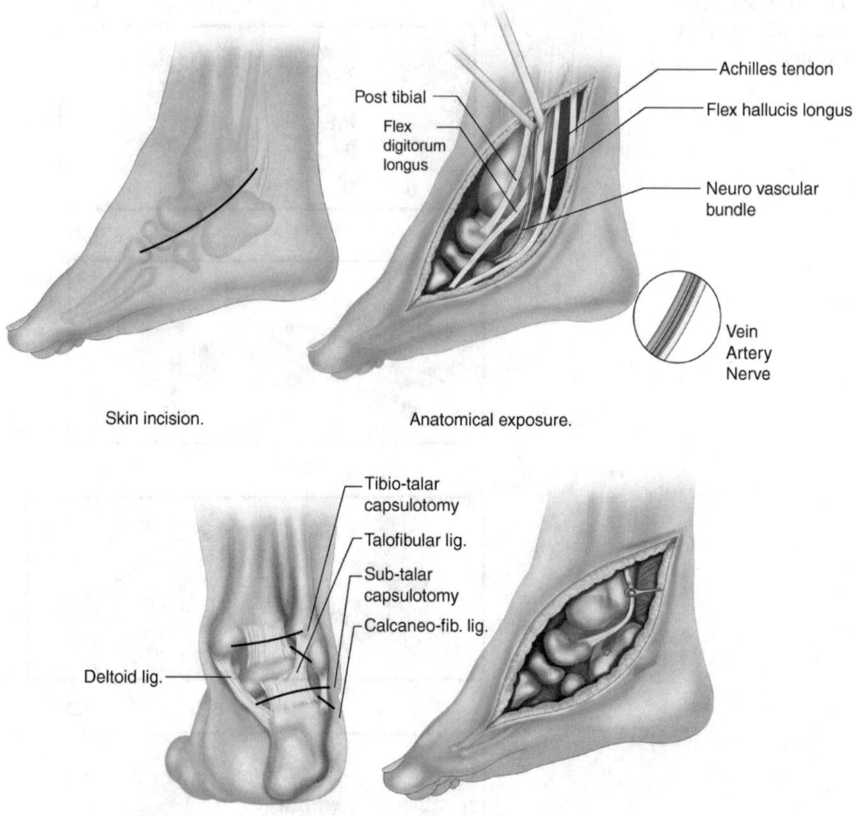


**Fig. 11.10** Turco's posterior medial approach

a member survey of the Pediatric Orthopedic Society of North America (POSNA) from 2001 to 2012 and found that member use of extensive surgical release fell from 54% to 7% [72]. Lastly, Švehlík et al., in their long term prospective trial with a minimum 10-year follow-up, found that the children treated with the Ponseti method had better outcomes than the surgical group [73].

In the most neglected and resistant deformities, including rigid conditions seen in more syndromic and teratologic conditions, talectomy may be employed. In 1971, Menelaus described his results and technique of talectomy for patients with arthrogryposis and spina bifida [74]. In 1984, Green et al. discussed their favorable results of talectomy in children with arthrogryposis multiplex congenita [75]. Chotigavanichaya et al. also described primary talectomy in patients with arthrogryposis multiplex congenita [76]. Primary talectomy can be combined with tibial calcaneal fusion and/or calcaneocuboid fusion to help prevent future recurrence of deformities [77]. Shah et al. proposed a treatment algorithm for non-idiopathic clubfeet and suggested that talectomy be considered for the neurogenic and syndromic rigid deformities [78]. In 2015, El-Sherbini et al. reported satisfactory

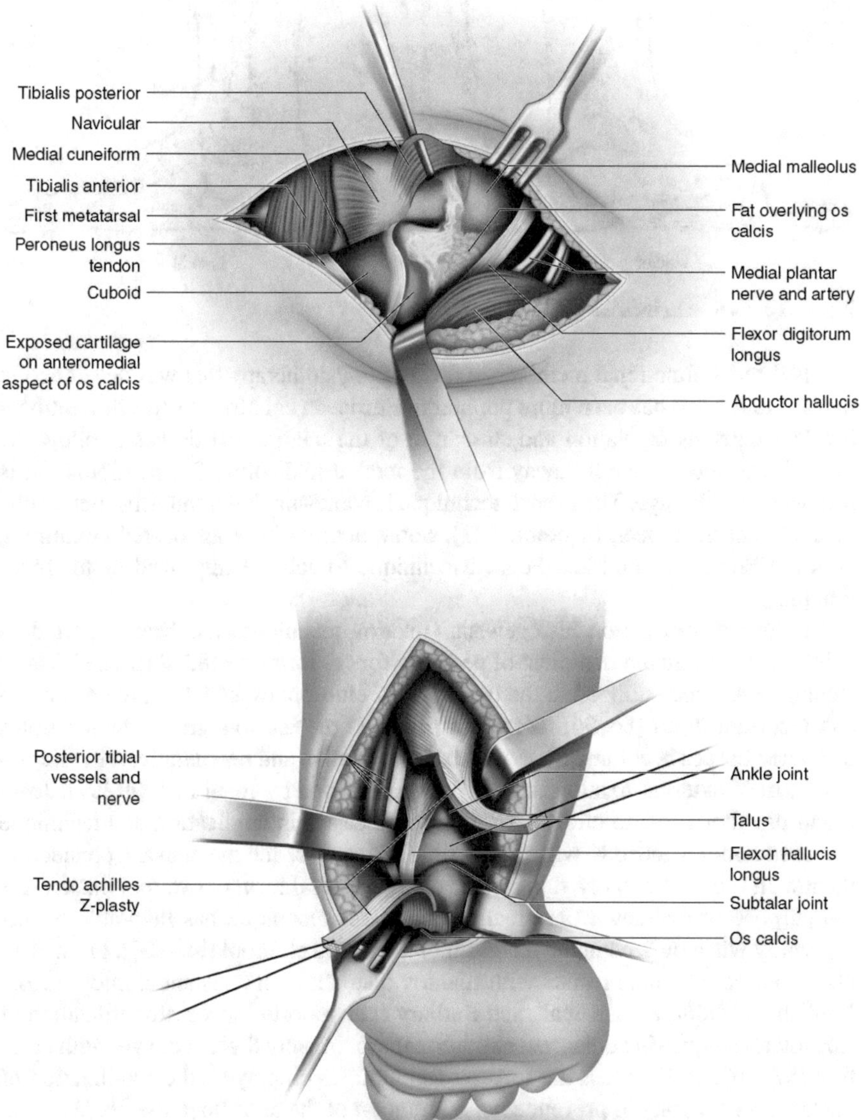


**Fig. 11.11** Carroll's medial and posterior approach

results of talectomy in 19 feet with severe rigid equinovarus deformities with a minimum 6.4 year follow-up [79]. Talectomy can be successful for the rigid equinovarus deformity as long as there is complete excision of the talus and the tibial calcaneal axis is optimized by correct alignment.

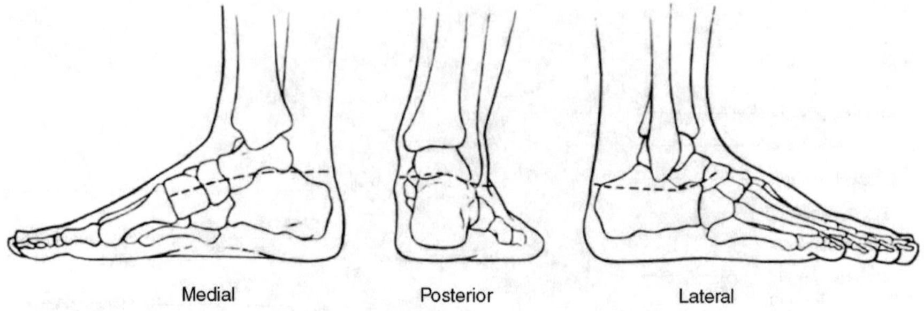


**Fig. 11.12** Cincinatti incision

The French functional method is a form of physiotherapy that was developed in the late 1970s and has been more popular in European countries [80]. The treatment involves daily manipulation and stretching of the medial soft tissues to allow the navicular to move laterally away from the medial malleolus. The manipulation is followed by splintage. The French technique is somewhat labor intensive but results of treatment have been favorable [81]. Some authors have advocated combining both the French method and Ponseti technique to achieve improved motor function [82].

The use of distraction histogenesis (Ilizarov technique) has been reported as being successful in the treatment of pediatric foot deformities [83–85]. The Ilizarov technique has been utilized in the treatment of clubfoot especially in the neglected and recurrent types [86–96]. Ilizarov's principle of "tension stress" demonstrates distracted tissues becoming more metabolically active and regenerative. An alternative form of external fixation for CTEV was reported by Joshi in 1999 [97]. Joshi found his alternative to circular fixation to be easier in application and technique and used non-tensioned K-wires in the tibia, calcaneus, and metatarsals, connecting them with rods. Essentially, this created a mono-lateral form of external fixation for the purpose of distraction and realignment. This technique has favorable results especially when utilized in the recurrent or neglected clubfoot [98–100]. Prem et al. also reported favorable results with Ilizarov distraction in resistant clubfoot [101]. Bradish and Noor, Franke et al., and Barbary et al. reported successful utilization of Ilizarov techniques in adolescent children (approximately 8 years of age) with clubfoot [87, 102, 103]. When the Ilizarov technique is employed, the stabilization of the talus is necessary to prevent external rotation of the talus upon the fibula during correction. Stabilization of the talus is also important in order to allow the mechanics of the subtalar joint to facilitate abduction of the anterior process of the calcaneus and subsequent eversion of the heel. This author has successfully employed the use of circular external fixation with both constrained and unconstrained constructs for the treatment of neglected, recurrent, syndromic, and teratologic clubfoot in older children where initial casting was unsuccessful (Fig. 11.13). This particular external fixation construct allowed the rotation of the forefoot about the fixed talar pivot point. The use of external distraction histogenesis is an alternative to acute surgical correction techniques as advocated by Dwyer, Evans, and Japas. When

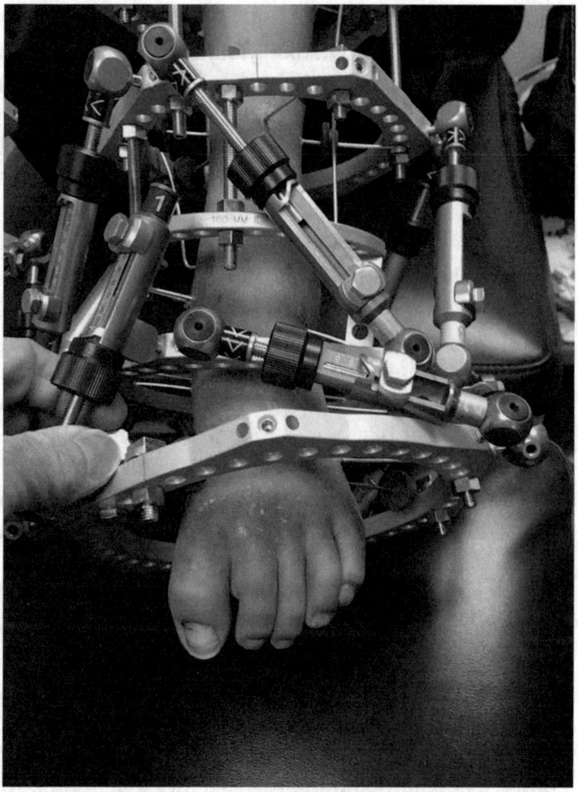

**Fig. 11.13** Example of multiplanar frame treatment in neglected 12 y/o male

these latter methods are performed to offer correction in skeletally immature adolescents, further shortening of the foot, arthrosis, and premature closure of physeal plates are possible outcomes.

In 2000, Delgado reported the ability to avoid surgery with the use of botox injections [104]. The use of botulinum toxin has also been reported favorably by Alvarez [105]. This author has used botox in the contracted muscle groups in cases of syndromic and teratologic clubfoot to facilitate manipulation and casting. While this helped facilitate some conditions with castings, those with more rigid contractures went on to be treated with circular external distraction histogenesis.

Ignacio Ponseti (6/3/1914-10/18/2009) started his technique of conservative treatment for clubfoot in the 1950s after realizing that surgery left a very scarred and stiff, non-functional foot that often required additional surgeries. He based his concepts on the understanding of foot mechanics initially described by the French anatomist Farabeuf and later by Huson in his dissertation [4, 43]. The main premise of treatment is that the anterior process of the calcaneus must first abduct before heel eversion can occur. This is accomplished by abducting the forefoot with counterpressure being applied at the lateral aspect of the talar head. Even though Ponseti developed this technique in the 1950s, it didn't become popular until the 1990s with the advent of the internet [106]. Frustrated parents would compare clubfoot treatment results on the internet yielding a renewed interest in Ponseti's technique. Presently, the Ponseti technique is considered the "gold standard" in the treatment of idiopathic clubfoot. There are numerous articles in the current literature that support this technique as the first treatment option for idiopathic clubfoot [107–116]. Ponseti and Smoley reported on their series of 67 patients with 94 clubfeet in 1963 [47]. They had 5–12 years of follow up and reported 71% good results. In 1980, Laaveg and Ponseti reported on 104 feet in 70 patients yielding good results in 88.7% of the cases [117]. In 1992, Ponseti stated that he had an 89% success rate but a recurrence rate of 50% [118]. At that time, Ponseti was recommending splinting for only 2 years after his treatment. Later studies would recommend a longer period of splinting (4–5 years) in an attempt to resist the aggressive collagen synthesis up until this age. Recurrence rates would then decrease with improved adherence to the treatment plan and duration of splinting [109]. In 1995, Cooper and Dietz reported on a 30-year follow-up of patients treated with the Ponseti technique [119]. They studied 45 patients with 71 clubfeet and found that 78% had good to excellent results. In 2002, Herzenberg reported his control group of standard serial casting (Kite's method) had 32/34 posterior medial surgical release (PMR), and those treated with Ponseti technique had only 1/34 PMR [120]. In 2006, Dobbs et al. reported on 34 patients who underwent an extensive soft tissue release with a mean follow-up of 30 years. Their results illustrated the poor foot function and decreased quality of life in patients undergoing surgical treatment for the correction of clubfoot [1]. In 2006, at the Pediatric Orthopedic Symposium of North America, Lovell et al. reported a 50-year follow-up on patients treated for idiopathic clubfoot with Ponseti technique exhibiting satisfactory long term results and function [121]. Since 2006 there have been many articles in the literature that support the Ponseti technique as the primary method in treating idiopathic clubfoot [60, 71, 114, 122]. In a 2014 Cochrane review of 14 trials with 607 participants, Gray et al. found lower post-treatment Pirani scores in the Ponseti group versus Kite group [60]. Patients in the Kite group also required more extensive surgery after initial treatment. Additionally, the Ponseti technique is also being utilized in neglected clubfeet in older children [123–127]. With the understanding of foot mechanics and Ponseti's principles, this conservative manipulation technique is being successfully utilized in previously resistant cases such as arthrogryposis [128, 129], in older age groups with neglected clubfoot [123, 126, 127, 130], and even in a "reverse Ponseti" technique for the treatment of rocker-bottom flatfoot and vertical talus [131].

## Treatment Protocols: Ponseti

Ideally, the conservative treatment for clubfoot should begin as soon as possible after birth and is best within the first week when the condition is more amenable to manipulation and casting. However, some authors have advocated treatment after the first 30 days of birth to 3 months in order to let the mother and child acclimate to home surroundings [53, 132]. Microscopically, the collagen fibers have a wavy appearance known as crimp. It is the stretching of the collagen and subsequent reappearance of crimp after several days that allows the casting technique to be successful [52]. Additionally, Pirani et al. reported on MRI studies demonstrating that joint adaptation and realignment has occurred after casting [133]. A CT study by Ippolito also confirms realignment [134]. In Ponseti's conservative manipulation treatment protocol, the foot deformities of cavus, adduction, and varus are all treated simultaneously, and the equinus is treated last. The initial cast focuses on the cavus deformity by supinating the forefoot while abducting against counter-pressure on the lateral aspect of the talar head (Fig. 11.14). Ponseti identified a common error attempting to get the foot down by pronation. Pronation of the foot is an absolute contraindication that increases the deformity. The forefoot is in varus and any attempt to pronate the forefoot will increase the amount of cavus. Subsequent manipulations and casting are continued until the abduction of the foot relative to the leg is approximately 70 degrees. These 70 degrees are a result of motion about the subtalar joint, midtarsal joint, and foot compared to the leg. The average number of treatments to reach this stage is three to six (Figs. 11.15 and 11.16). However, each child is different, and manipulations are not stressed or forced to achieve that

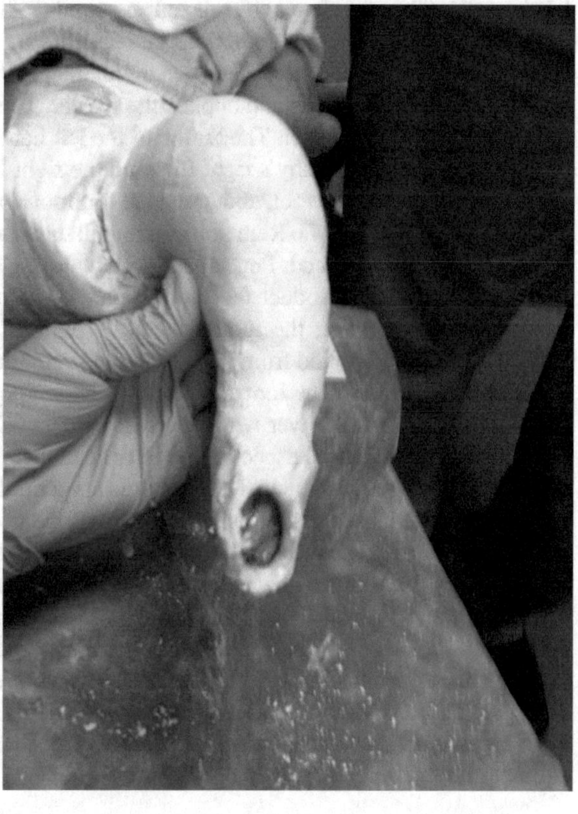

**Fig. 11.14** First cast

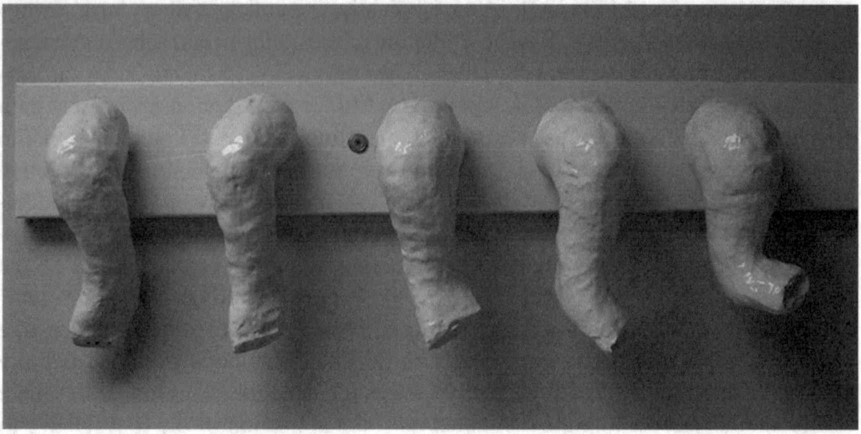

**Fig. 11.15** Casting series. (Photo by author from Dr Ponseti's clinic showing typical casting series)

goal. It sometimes takes more treatment utilizing a gentle stretch to resistance. Gentle manipulations and casting with plaster (Gypsona®) are performed each visit. It is important for the infant to be relaxed and comfortable. Preferably, it is advisable to feed the child during manipulations and casting. It is also desirable to have two people involved in the casting. One person maintains the foot in its corrected position, while the other molds and applies the plaster. The manipulations involve performing Ponseti's maneuver. The thumb of the left hand is against the lateral aspect of the talar head of the baby's right foot and the right hand with full contact along the plantar surface of the foot, abducting the forefoot against the counter-pressure of the left thumb (Fig. 11.17). Remember, manipulations and casting are performed to resistance and never forced. Ponseti advocated casting above the knee, to the groin in order to be able to abduct the foot around the talus relative to the lower leg. Additionally, in treating the infant, the long leg cast helps to prevent slippage. Webril® padding is applied from the toes to the knee. Plaster is then applied over the padding while molding the foot and posterior heel. The foot is held in its new position with Ponseti's maneuver while the cast hardens. Care is taken to avoid excessive pressure at the lateral aspect of the talar head that may result in a pressure sore once the plaster has hardened. The plaster is snug on the lower leg, and it must be very well molded, especially around the back of the heel/Achilles tendon. Padding is then applied over the proximal portion of the cast to the groin with the knee bent at 90 degrees. The plaster above the knee may be applied with more gentle tension. The toe of the cast is open to visualize vascular status of the digits (Fig. 11.18). An average of six casts are applied with the final ones focusing on the ankle equinus component of the deformity. If resistance is met in correcting the equinus, the decision for a tenotomy of the Achilles tendon is considered. The tenotomy is performed in an average of 85–90% of cases and is a safe procedure for those with the knowledge of the anatomy [135]. It can easily be done in a clinic setting with local

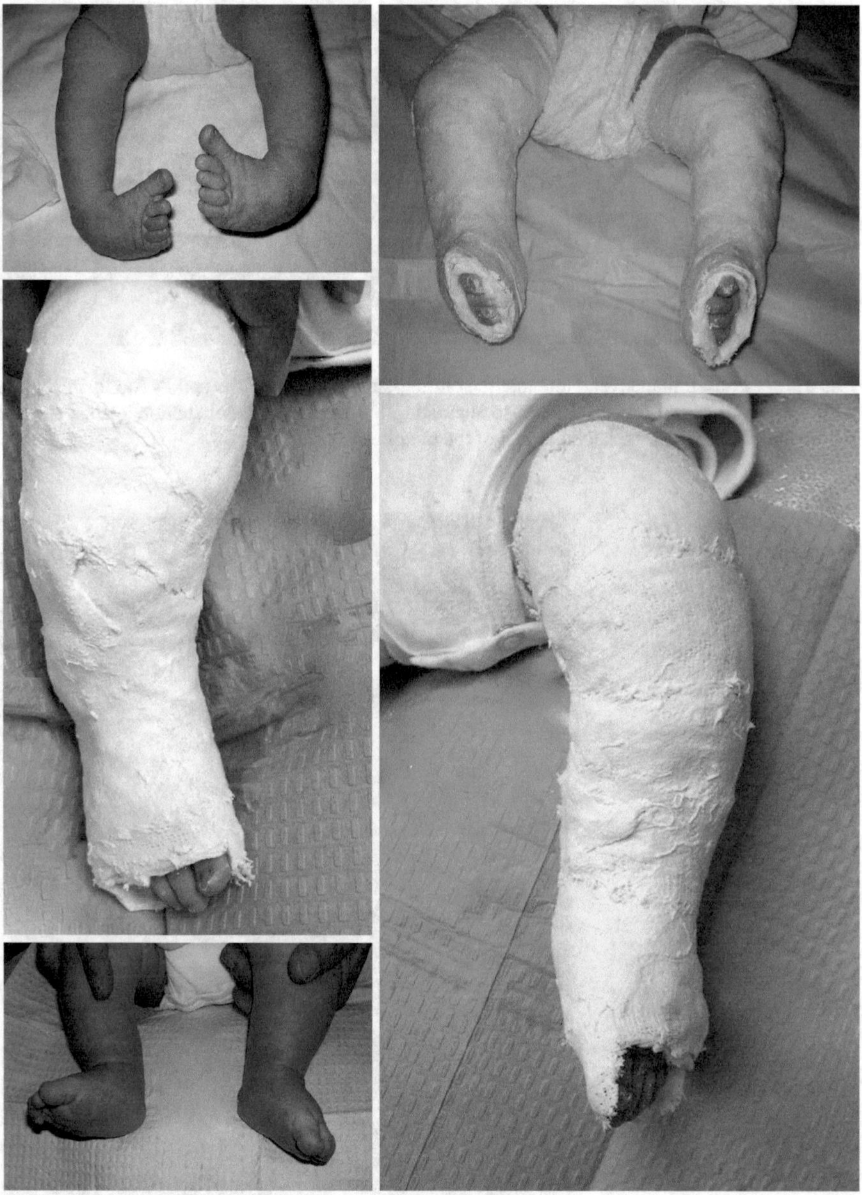

**Fig. 11.16** Typical sequence from initial presentation, 1st cast, 3rd cast and to final presentation

anesthetic, thus avoiding a general anesthetic at this age. Grigoriou et al. found that an Achilles tenotomy was as useful as an Achilles tenotomy and posterior capsular release in clubfoot treatment [136]. Therefore these authors did not recommend a posterior capsular release. Before the procedure, a topical anesthetic cream is

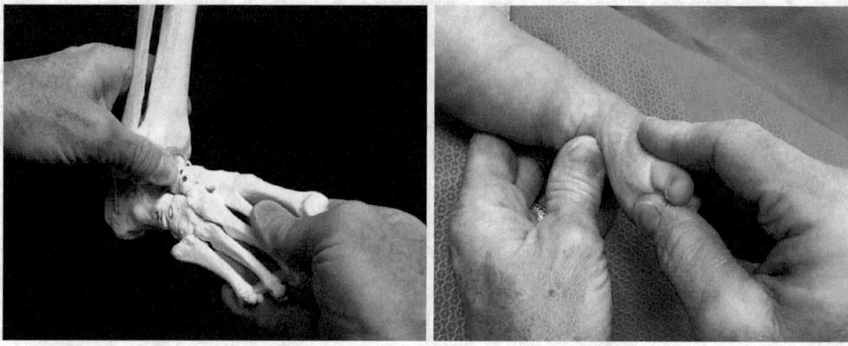

**Fig. 11.17** Ponseti maneuver. Note that the entire plantar surface of the child's foot is in contact with the length of my fingers. I am also supinating the forefoot with abduction against the left thumb pressing against the lateral aspect of the talar head

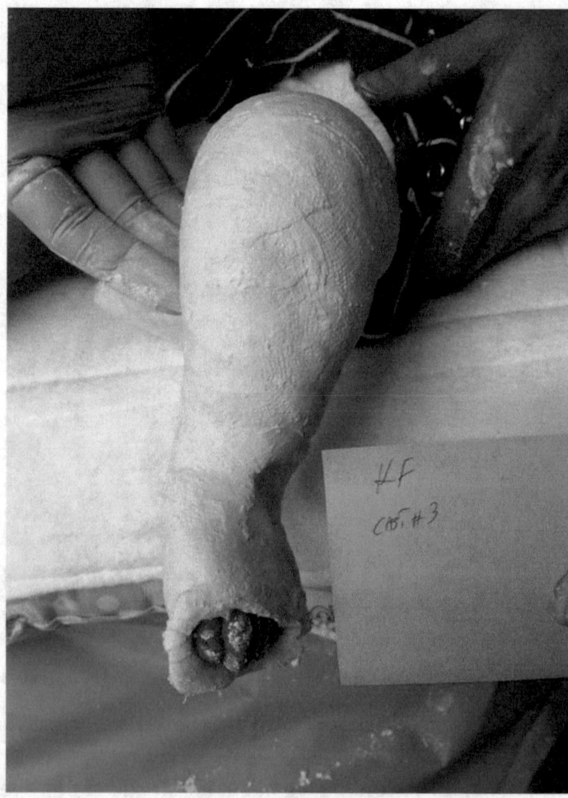

**Fig. 11.18** Typical cast appearance

applied for several hours under occlusion. After a surgical prep, a small subcutaneous wheal of 1% lidocaine plain is created over the Achilles tendon approximately 1 cm above the superior aspect of the os calcis. Care is taken to avoid using too much fluid to obscure palpation of the Achilles tendon. Holding the foot in dorsiflexion to create tension on the Achilles tendon, a small stab incision is made with a beaver blade (ex. #67) adjacent to the lateral aspect of the tendon. Palpation of the tendon is performed, and it is transected in its entirety such that a noticeable release is felt and heard. After the tenotomy is performed, one final cast is applied for 3 weeks. The tendon heals quite readily in this time frame, and ultrasound studies have shown that healing is complete in this time frame [137]. The cast is then removed and straight lasted shoes on an abduction bar (splint) with the amount of abduction set at approximately 70 degrees for the involved foot/feet is applied (Fig. 11.19). Initially, this splint is kept on for 3 months for 23 hours per day. Thereafter, the use of the splint is maintained on for naps and sleeping averaging approximately 16 hours per day. Periodic evaluations, every 4 months, are made to assess adherence to treatment plan and monitor growth and any chance of recurrence [138]. Later in his career, Ponseti advocated splinting while sleeping until the age of five to help reduce the chance of recurrence. Ponseti believed the rapid rate of collagen synthesis beginning at birth contributed to recurrence of the deformity and started to taper down at the age of 5 [4].

Other adjunctive treatment options have been utilized with casting techniques and include the use of the French functional method (discussed earlier), especially after completion of the Ponseti casts and the use of botulinum toxin as reported by Alvarez.

## Recurrence/Relapse

A relapse in the treatment of clubfoot is a partial recurrence of the original deformity, usually as a result of premature cessation of treatment [139]. A relapse is mostly exhibited by equinus and supination of the foot (Fig. 11.5). Periodic

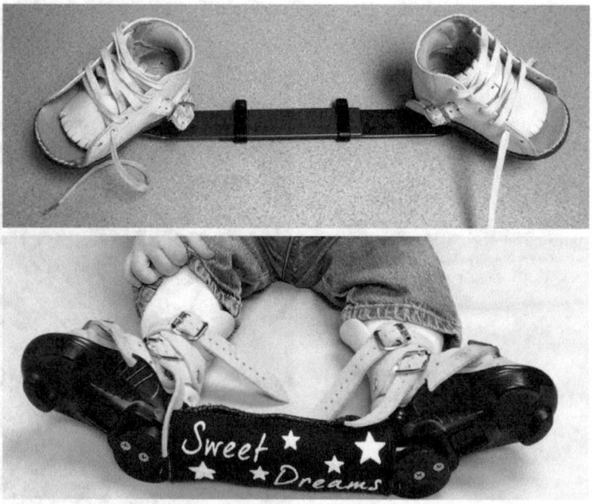


**Fig. 11.19** Splinting types

monitoring of the patient after initial treatment (every 3–4 months) is recommended to check for any signs of relapse and proper fit of the shoes and splint. Relapses are infrequent after the age of five, in part due to the maturity of the collagen fibers. However, it may occur even to the age of 11 as reported by Morcuende [140].

Treatment of a relapsed clubfoot begins with repeat serial casting followed by bracing. If the equinus component isn't corrected to 10° dorsiflexion after four to five casts in a child less than 4 years of age, then a repeat tenotomy may be necessary [141]. After development of the primary ossification center of the lateral cuneiform and in children over the age of three, a tibialis anterior tendon transfer may be performed if there is dynamic supination of the foot [142, 143]. The treatment of a recurrent clubfoot by the tibialis anterior tendon transfer is supported by various authors [144–146]. Corrective casting is employed initially, in part, to improve the alignment of the foot in order to achieve a better functional transfer of the tibialis anterior [143]. This technique has been described by Dr. Vincent Mosca in the Global Health monograph edited by Dr. Lynn Staheli [52]. The tibialis anterior tendon transfer procedure is performed by a two incision approach: one is over the insertion of the tendon and the other over the lateral cuneiform. Incision placement is aided by the use of fluoroscopy. The tendon is carefully freed from its attachment medially and tagged with 2-0 absorbable suture and then passed subcutaneously to the lateral incision keeping the

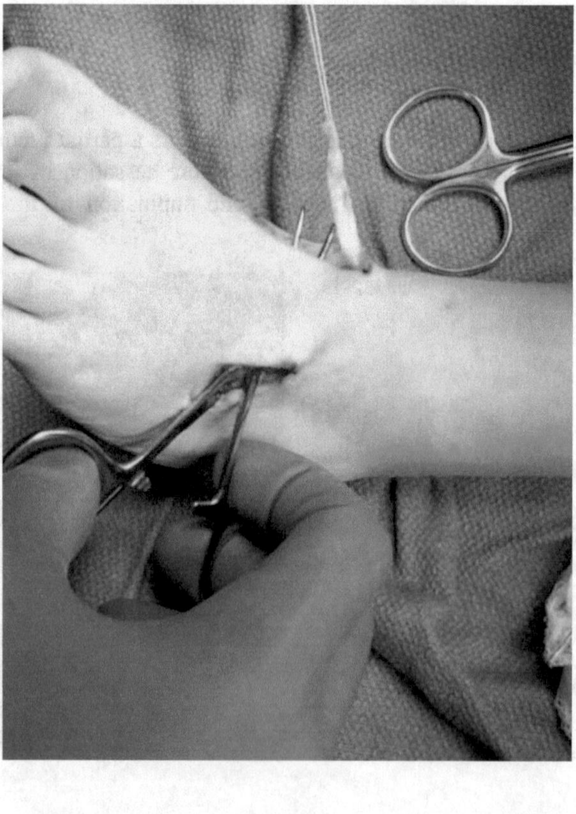

**Fig. 11.20** Intra-operative photo of tibialis anterior tendon transfer

superior retinaculum intact (Fig. 11.20). A drill hole is made in the lateral cuneiform and the tendon is passed through the hole under tension while the foot is held in dorsiflexion by using Keith needles. The needles and tendon are passed through the bottom of the foot and tied over rolled gauze and sterile buttons. An above knee cast is applied for 6 weeks to facilitate tenodesis. Usually bracing is not needed afterward.

## Complications

While the Ponseti method is a safe and reliable method for treating idiopathic clubfoot, complications may arise during treatment. The majority of complications are due to casting errors and include overcorrection, rocker bottom flatfoot deformity, lateral displacement of the fibula, flattening of the talar dome, and complex/atypical clubfoot [147].

Overcorrection is usually isolated to abduction of the forefoot at Lisfranc's joint. This usually evolves after applying counter-pressure along the lateral column of the foot (cuboid) as opposed to the lateral aspect of the talar head. A rocker-bottom flatfoot deformity (Fig. 11.21) is achieved by early dorsiflexion of the foot relative to the leg before adequate eversion of the heel is achieved. It is also accomplished by dorsiflexing the forefoot alone rather than the entire foot relative to the leg. The example in Fig. 11.21a was treated successfully by a "reverse Ponseti" technique to help realign the talonavicular joint as indicated by Fig. 11.21b.

Lateral displacement of the fibula occurs when the talus externally rotates within the ankle mortise and usually occurs when the heel is still locked in a varus position. Counter-pressure against the lateral aspect of the talar head is important in preventing this complication. A flat talar dome may be seen on a lateral projection radiograph and is usually due to excessive external rotation of the foot to the lower leg.

The atypical clubfoot is an entity that may include clubfoot associated with other conditions that may make it more difficult to treat. These include syndromic, teratologic, and neurogenic conditions. A unique, atypical clubfoot that occurs during the

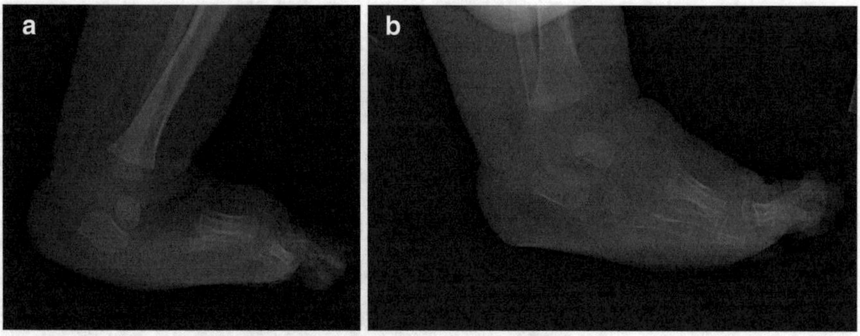


**Fig. 11.21** Example of rocker bottom foot. (**a**) Pre treatment. (**b**) Post treatment (reverse Ponseti)

casting process in otherwise normal children is called complex or resistant clubfoot [148]. This foot type is usually represented by an increase in girth and has a pronounced equinus component to it both at the ankle and the forefoot. This results in a plantarflexed first ray giving the hallux a shorter appearance. The complex clubfoot is stiffer and also presents with a central crease in the arch (Fig. 11.6). The metatarsals are plantarflexed in addition to the heel. Any attempt at reducing heel varus in the usual fashion will lead to hyperabduction of the metatarsals. There are various theories regarding the etiology of atypical clubfoot ranging from error in treatment to a sympathetic mediated response during treatment (Fig. 11.22). While complex regional pain syndromes have been reported in pediatric patients, this has not been well documented in infants [149]. The complex clubfoot is a condition that occurs during treatment of clubfoot and not at the onset. An initial sign of concern

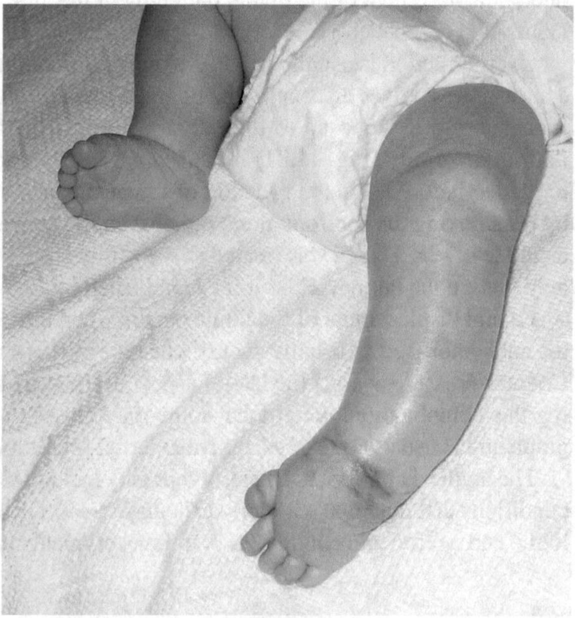

**Fig. 11.22** Complex clubfoot appearance. Note increased girth, hyperemia and taught skin along with short appearing hallux

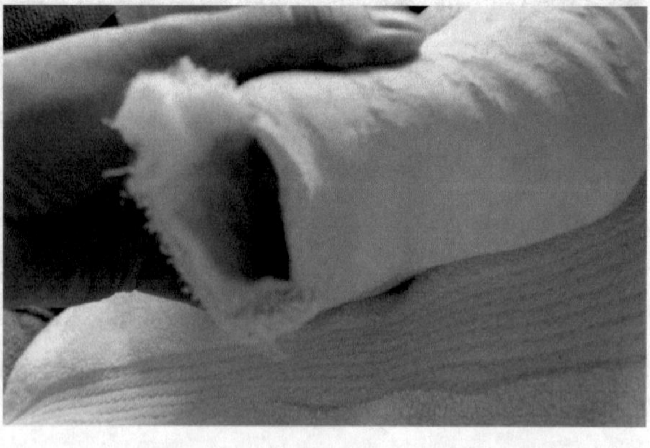

**Fig. 11.23** Toes appear retracted in cast

to the practitioner is when the toes appear to be retracting within the cast, indicating that the foot has taken on a more equinus position (Fig. 11.23). The treatment for complex clubfoot is modified to address the unique nature of the deformity. After applying standard Ponseti technique and getting the foot to approximately 30 degrees of external rotation, attention is directed to address the equinus component. The clinician's thumbs are pressed along the first and fifth metatarsals, while the index fingers are on the head of the talus. The cavus and equinus components are addressed simultaneously. A tenotomy of the Achilles tendon in these cases is most always necessary.

## Summary

While the Ponseti technique is presently considered the "gold standard" for the treatment of idiopathic clubfoot, there are still some conditions that may be resistant to this method and may require surgical intervention. Most recently, Wright stated "The Ponseti protocol has completely changed the treatment of clubfoot with results so obviously superior to extensive surgical release that a randomized controlled trial would not be appropriate" [71]. Ponseti stated in his book on *Congenital Clubfoot: Fundamentals of Treatment*: "a well conducted orthopedic treatment based upon a sound understanding of the functional anatomy of the foot and on the biologic response of young connective tissue and bone to the changes in direction of mechanical stimuli, can gradually reduce or almost eliminate these deformities in most clubfeet."

## References

1. Dobbs MB, Nunley R, Schoenecker PL. Long-term follow up of patients with clubfeet treated with extensive soft tissue release. JBJS. 2006;88-A:986–96.
2. Wynne DR. Family study and the cause of clubfoot. J Bone Joint Surg. 1964;46:445–63.
3. Cartlidge I. Observations on the epidemiology of club foot in Polynesian and Caucasian populations. J Med Genet. 1984;21:290–2.
4. Ponseti IV. Congenital clubfoot: fundamentals of treatment. USA: Oxford University Press; 1996.
5. Ponseti I, Staheli LT. Clubfoot: ponseti management. Seattle: Global-HELP; 2005.
6. Burgan HE, Furness ME, Foster BK. Prenatal ultrasound diagnosis of clubfoot. J Pediatr Orthop. 1999;19:11–3.
7. Keret D, Ezra E, Lokiec F, Hayek S, Segev E, Wientroub S. Efficacy of prenatal ultrasonography in confirmed club foot. J Bone Joint Surg Br. 2002;84:1015–9.
8. Aurell Y, Johansson A, Hansson G, Jonsson K. Ultrasound anatomy in the neonatal clubfoot. Eur Radiol. 2002;12:2509–17.
9. Silvani S, DeValentine SJ, Karlin JM, SBL. Moebius syndrome and TEV. JAPA. 1981;71:604–6.
10. Purushothamdas S, Rayan F, Gayner A. Correction of neglected clubfoot deformity in children with Moebius syndrome. J Pediatr Orthop B. 2009;18:73–5.
11. Böhm M. The embryologic origin of club-foot. J Bone Joint Surg Am. 1929;11:229–59.

12. Irani RN, Sherman MS. The pathological anatomy of club foot. J Bone Joint Surg Am. 1963;45:45–52.
13. Tachdjian MO. The child's foot. Philadelphia: Saunders; 1985.
14. Greider TD, Siff SJ, Gerson P, Donovan MM. Arteriography in club foot. J Bone Joint Surg Am. 1982;64:837–40.
15. Isaacs H, Handelsman JE, Badenhorst M, Pickering A. The muscles in club foot--a histological histochemical and electron microscopic study. J Bone Joint Surg Br. 1977;59-B:465–72.
16. Adams F. The genuine works of Hippocrates. Baltimore: Williams & Wilkins; 1939.
17. Browne D. Congenital deformities of mechanical origin. Br Med J. 1936;1:1182.
18. Dunn PM. Sir Denis Browne (1892-1967) and congenital deformities of mechanical origin. Arch Dis Child Fetal Neonatal Ed. 2005;90:F88–91.
19. Tabor A, Alfirevic Z. Update on procedure-related risks for prenatal diagnosis techniques. Fetal Diagn Ther. 2010;27:1–7.
20. Farrell SA, Summers AM, Dallaire L, Singer J, Johnson J-AM, Wilson RD. Club foot, an adverse outcome of early amniocentesis: disruption or deformation? J Med Genet. 1999;36:843–6.
21. Yazdy MM, Mitchell AA, Louik C, Werler MM. Use of selective serotonin-reuptake inhibitors during pregnancy and the risk of clubfoot. Epidemiology. 2014;25:859–65.
22. Bacino CA, Hecht JT. Etiopathogenesis of equinovarus foot malformations. Eur J Med Genet. 2014;57:473–9.
23. Ippolito E, Ponseti IV. Congenital club foot in the human fetus. A histological study. J Bone Joint Surg Am. 1980;62:8–22.
24. Ponseti IV, Campos J. Observations on pathogenesis and treatment of congenital clubfoot. Clin Orthop Relat Res. 1972;84:50–60.
25. Fukuhara K, Schollmeier GUH. The pathogenesis of clubfoot. JBJS Br. 1994;76:450–7.
26. Sano H, Uhthoff HK, Jarvis JG, Mansingh A, Wenckebach GF. Pathogenesis of soft-tissue contracture in club foot. J Bone Joint Surg Br. 1998;80:641–4.
27. Klein D. Genetics of clubfoot. J Genet Hum. 1964;13:385–6.
28. Cowell HR, Wein BK. Current concepts review: genetic aspects of club foot. J Bone Joint Surg. 1980;62-A:1381–4.
29. Chapman C, Stott NS, Port RV, Nicol RO. Genetics of club foot in Maori and Pacific people. J Med Genet. 2000;37:680–3.
30. Wang JH, Palmer RM, Chung CS. The role of major gene in clubfoot. Am J Hum Genet. 1988;42:772–6.
31. Dietz F. The genetics of idiopathic clubfoot. Clin Orthop Relat Res. 2002:39–48.
32. Dobbs MB. Clubfoot: etiology and treatment: editorial comment. Clin Orthop Relat Res. 2009;467:1119–20.
33. Idelberger K. Die ergebnisse der zwillingsforschung beim angeborenen klumpfuss. Verh Dtsch Orthop Ges. 1939;33:272.
34. Gurnett CA, Alaee F, Kruse LM, Desruisseau DM, Hecht JT, Wise CA, Bowcock AM, Dobbs MB. Asymmetric lower-limb malformations in individuals with homeobox PITX1 gene mutation. Am J Hum Genet. 2008;83:616–22.
35. Dobbs MB, Gurnett CA. Update on clubfoot: etiology and treatment. Clin Orthop Relat Res. 2009;467:1146–53.
36. Wynne-Davies R, Littlejohn A, Gormley J. Aetiology and interrelationship of some common skeletal deformities. (Talipes equinovarus and calcaneovalgus, metatarsus varus, congenital dislocation of the hip, and infantile idiopathic scoliosis). J Med Genet. 1982;19:321–8.
37. Scarpa A. In: di Scarpa A, editor. Memoria chirurgica sui piedi torti congeniti dei fanciulli e sulla maniera di correggere questa deformita. Pavia: G. Comini; 1803.
38. Ippolito E. Update on pathologic anatomy of clubfoot. J Pediatr Orthop B. 1995;4:17–24.
39. Carroll NC. Pathoanatomy of congenital clubfoot. In: Symposium on pediatric clubfoot; 1978. p. 225–32.

40. Herzenberg JE, Carroll NC, Christofersen MR, Lee EH, White S, Munroe R. Clubfoot analysis with three-dimensional computer modeling. J Pediatr Orthop. 1988;8:257.
41. Farabeuf LH. In: Farabeuf LH, editor. Precis de Manuel Operatoire par. 4th ed. Paris: Masson; 1893.
42. Huson A. Een Ontleedkundig-functioneel Onderzoek Van de Voetwortel: (An anatomic and functional study of the tarsus). Leiden: Leiden University; 1961.
43. Dobbs MB, Morcuende JA, Gurnett CA, Ponseti IV. Treatment of idiopathic clubfoot: an historical review. Iowa Orthop J. 2000;20:59–64.
44. Manter JT. Movements of the subtalar and transverse tarsal joints. Anat Rec. 1941;80:397–410.
45. Hicks JH. The mechanics of the foot I. The joints. J Anat. 1953;87:345–57.
46. Sarrafian SK. Biomechanics of the subtalar joint complex. Clin Orthop Relat Res. 1993;290:17–26.
47. Ponseti IV, Smoley EN. Congenital club foot: the results of treatment. J Bone Joint Surg. 1963;45:261–344.
48. Irani RN, Sherman MS. The pathological anatomy of idiopathic clubfoot. Clin Orthop Relat Res. 1972;84:14–20.
49. Cosma D, Vasilescu DE. A clinical evaluation of the Pirani and Dimeglio idiopathic clubfoot classifications. J Foot Ankle Surg. 2015;54:582–5.
50. Diméglio A, Bensahel H, Souchet P, Mazeau P, Bonnet F. Classification of clubfoot. J Pediatr Orthop B. 1995;4:129–36.
51. Pirani S, Hodges D, Sekeramayi F. A reliable & valid method of assessing the amount of deformity in the congenital clubfoot deformity. J Bone Joint Surg Br. 2008;90-B:53.
52. Staheli L. Clubfoot: ponseti management. Seattle: Global HELP Organization; 2009.
53. Zionts LE. What's new in idiopathic clubfoot? J Pediatr Orthop. 2015;35:547–50.
54. Lampasi M, Abati CN, Stilli S, Trisolino G. Use of the Pirani score in monitoring progression of correction and in guiding indications for tenotomy in the Ponseti method: are we coming to the same decisions? J Orthop Surg. 2017;25:2309499017713916.
55. Jones R. Discussion on the treatment of club-foot. Br Med J. 1909;2:1065–71.
56. Kite JH. Non-operative treatment of congenital clubfeet: a review of one hundred cases*. South Med J. 1930;23:337–44.
57. Kite JH. Principles involved in the treatment of congenital club-foot. 1939. Clin Orthop Relat Res. 1972;84:4–8.
58. Sud A, Tiwari A, Sharma D, Kapoor S. Ponseti's vs. Kite's method in the treatment of clubfoot--a prospective randomised study. Int Orthop. 2008;32:409–13.
59. Rijal R, Shrestha B, Singh G, Singh M, Nepal P, Khanal G, Rai P. Comparison of Ponseti and Kite's method of treatment for idiopathic clubfoot. Indian J Orthop. 2010;44:202.
60. Gray K, Pacey V, Gibbons P, Little D, Frost C, Burns J. Interventions for congenital talipes equinovarus (clubfoot). Cochrane Database Syst Rev. 2012;(4):CD008602.
61. Codivilla A. Sulla Cura del piede equino varo congenito. Arch Ortop. 1906;23:245–56.
62. Sanzarello I, Nanni M, Faldini C. The clubfoot over the centuries. J Pediatr Orthop B. 2017;26:143–51.
63. Turco VJ. Surgical correction of the resistant club foot. One-stage posteromedial release with internal fixation: a preliminary report. J Bone Joint Surg Am. 1971;53:477–97.
64. Turco VJ. Resistant congenital clubfoot-one stage posteriomedial release with internal fixation. J Bone Joint Surg. 1979;61:805–14.
65. Carroll NC, Gross RH. Operative management of clubfoot. Orthopedics. 1990;13:1285–96.
66. Carroll NC. Surgical technique for talipes equinovarus. Oper Tech Orthop. 1993;3:115–20.
67. Crawford AH, Marxen JL, Osterfeld DL. The Cincinnati incision: a comprehensive approach for surgical procedures of the foot and ankle in childhood. J Bone Joint Surg Am. 1982;64:1355–8.
68. Mahapatra S, Abraham VT. A comparative analysis of the two most common surgical exposures for clubfoot. Int Surg J. 2016;3:1283–6.

69. van Gelder JH, van AGP R, Visser JD, PGM M, Van Gelder JH, et al. Long-term results of the posteromedial release in the treatment of idiopathic clubfoot. J Pediatr Orthop. 2010;30:700–4.
70. Alkar F, Louahem D, Bonnet F, Patte K, Delpont M, Cottalorda J. Long-term results after extensive soft tissue release in very severe congenital clubfeet. J Pediatr Orthop. 2017;37:500–3.
71. Wright JG. Commentary on articles by Kelly A. Jeans, MS, et al.: "Functional outcomes following treatment for clubfoot. ten-year follow-up," and Bibek Banskota, MRCS, MS, et al.: "Outcomes of the ponseti method for untreated clubfeet in nepalese patients seen between the ages of one and five years and followed for at least 10 years". J Bone Joint Surg Am. 2018;100:e149.
72. Zionts LE, Sangiorgio SN, Ebramzadeh E, Morcuende JA. The current management of idiopathic clubfoot revisited: results of a survey of the POSNA membership. J Pediatr Orthop. 2012;32:515.
73. Švehlík M, Floh U, Steinwender G, Sperl M, Novak M, Kraus T. Ponseti method is superior to surgical treatment in clubfoot – long-term, randomized, prospective trial. Gait Posture. 2017;58:346–51.
74. Menelaus MB. Talectomy for equinovarus deformity in arthrogryposis and spina bifida. J Bone Joint Surg Br. 1971;53:468–73.
75. Green AD, Fixsen JA, Lloyd-Roberts GC. Talectomy for arthrogryposis multiplex congenita. J Bone Joint Surg Br. 1984;66-B:697–9.
76. Chotigavanichaya C, Ariyawatkul T, Eamsobhana P, Kaewpornsawan K. Results of primary talectomy for clubfoot in infants and toddlers with arthrogryposis multiplex congenita. J Med Assoc Thail. 2015;98:S38–41.
77. Nicomedez FPI, Li YH, Leong JCY. Tibiocalcaneal fusion after talectomy in arthrogrypotic patients. J Pediatr Orthop. 2003;23:654–7.
78. Shah IP, Crawford AH, Tamai J, Parikh SN. Management of non-idiopathic clubfeet. Int J Paediatr Orthop. 2016;2:27–32.
79. El-Sherbini MH, Omran AA. Midterm follow-up of talectomy for severe rigid equinovarus feet. J Foot Ankle Surg. 2015;54:1093–8.
80. Faulks S, Richards BS. Clubfoot treatment: ponseti and French functional methods are equally effective. Clin Orthop Relat Res. 2009;467:1278–82.
81. Dimeglio A, Canavese F. The French functional physical therapy method for the treatment of congenital clubfoot. J Pediatr Orthop B. 2012;21:28–39.
82. Zapata KA, Karol LA, Jeans KA, Jo C-H. Gross motor function at 10 years of age in children with clubfoot following the French physical therapy method and the Ponseti technique. J Pediatr Orthop. 2018;38:e519–23.
83. Paley D, Foot N, Correction D. Principles of foot deformity correction: Ilizarov technique. In: Gould JS, editor. Operative foot surgery. Philadelphia: WB Saunders; 1994. p. 476–514.
84. Reinker KA, Carpenter CT. Ilizarov applications in the pediatric foot. J Pediatr Orthop. 1997;17:796–802.
85. Lamm BM, Standard SL, Galley IJ, Herzenberg JE, Paley D. External fixation for the foot and ankle in children. Clin Podiatr Med Surg. 2006;23:137–66.
86. Grill F, Franke J. The Ilizarov distractor for the correction of relapsed or neglected clubfoot. J Bone Joint Surg Br. 1987;69:593–7.
87. Franke J, Grill F, Hein G, Simon M. Correction of clubfoot relapse using Ilizarov's apparatus in children 8-15 years old. Arch Orthop Trauma Surg. 1990;110:33–7.
88. de la Huerta F. Correction of the neglected clubfoot by the Ilizarov method. Clin Orthop Relat Res. 1994:89–93.
89. Wallender H, Hansson G, Tjernström B. Correction of persistent clubfoot deformities with the Ilizarov external fixator. Acta Orthop Scand. 1996;67:283–7.

90. Choi IH, Yang MS, Chung CY, Cho TJ, Sohn YJ. The treatment of recurrent arthrogrypotic club foot in children by the Ilizarov method. A preliminary report. J Bone Joint Surg Br. 2001;83:731–7.
91. Hosny GA. Correction of foot deformities by the Ilizarov method without corrective osteotomies or soft tissue release. J Pediatr Orthop B. 2002;11:121–8.
92. Utukuri MM, Ramachandran M, Hartley J, Hill RA. Patient-based outcomes after Ilizarov surgery in resistant clubfeet. J Pediatr Orthop B. 2006;15:278–84.
93. Burns JK, Sullivan R. Correction of severe residual clubfoot deformity in adolescents with the Ilizarov technique. Foot Ankle Clin. 2004;9:571–82.
94. Ferreira RC, Costa MT, Frizzo GG, Santin RAL. Correction of severe recurrent clubfoot using a simplified setting of the Ilizarov device. Foot Ankle Int. 2007;28:557–68.
95. Peterson HA. The Ilizarov method for the treatment of resistant clubfoot: is it an effective solution? Yearbook Orthop. 2007;2007:52–3.
96. Kocaoğlu M, Eralp L, Atalar AC, Bilen FE. Correction of complex foot deformities using the Ilizarov external fixator. J Foot Ankle Surg. 2002;41:30–9.
97. Joshi BB, Laud NS, Warrier S, Kanaji BG. Treatment of CTEV by Joshi's external stabilization system (JESS). Textbook of orthopaedics and trauma. 1st ed. New Delhi: Jaypee Brothers Medical Publishers; 1999.
98. Suresh S, Ahmed A, Sharma VK. Role of Joshi's external stabilisation system fixator in the management of idiopathic clubfoot. J Orthop Surg. 2003;11:194–201.
99. MarthyaH A, Marthya A. Short term results of Correction of CTEV with JESS distractor. J Orthop. 2004;1:e3.
100. Manjappa CN. Joshi's external stablization system (JESS) application for correction of resistant club-foot. Internet J Orthop Surg. 2010;18:1. https://doi.org/10.5580/1408.
101. Prem H, Zenios M, Farrell R, Day JB. Soft tissue Ilizarov correction of congenital talipes equinovarus--5 to 10 years postsurgery. J Pediatr Orthop. 2007;27:220–4.
102. Bradish CF, Noor S. The Ilizarov method in the management of relapsed club feet. J Bone Joint Surg Br. 2000;82:387–91.
103. El Barbary H, Abdel Ghani H, Hegazy M. Correction of relapsed or neglected clubfoot using a simple Ilizarov frame. Int Orthop. 2004;28:183–6.
104. Delgado MR, Wilson H, Johnston C, Richards S, Karol L. A preliminary report of the use of botulinum toxin type A in infants with clubfoot: four case studies. J Pediatr Orthop. 2000;20:533–8.
105. Alvarez CM, De Vera MA, Chhina H, Williams L, Durlacher K, Kaga S. The use of botulinum type a toxin in the treatment of idiopathic clubfoot: 5-year follow-up. J Pediatr Orthop. 2009;29:570–5.
106. Morcuende JA, Egbert M, Ponseti IV. The effect of the internet in the treatment of congenital idiopathic clubfoot. Iowa Orthop J. 2003;23:83–6.
107. Doherty R. Long term follow up. BMJ. 1999;318:233.
108. Colburn M, Williams M. Evaluation of the treatment of idiopathic clubfoot by using the Ponseti method. J Foot Ankle Surg. 2003;42:259–67.
109. Morcuende JA, Dolan LA, Dietz FR, Ponseti IV. Radical reduction in the rate of extensive corrective surgery for clubfoot using the Ponseti method. Pediatrics. 2004;113:376–80.
110. Zwick EB, Kraus T, Maizen C, Steinwender G, Linhart WE. Comparison of Ponseti versus surgical treatment for idiopathic clubfoot: a short-term preliminary report. Clin Orthop Relat Res. 2009;467:2668–76.
111. Clarke NMP, Uglow MG, Valentine KM. Comparison of Ponseti versus surgical treatment in congenital talipes equinovarus. J Foot Ankle Surg. 2011;50:529–34.
112. Zionts LE, Zhao G, Hitchcock K, Maewal J, Ebramzadeh E. Has the rate of extensive surgery to treat idiopathic clubfoot declined in the United States? J Bone Joint Surg Am. 2010;92:882. https://doi.org/10.2106/JBJS.I.00819.

113. Halanski MA, Davison JE, Huang J-C, Walker CG, Walsh SJ, Crawford HA. Ponseti method compared with surgical treatment of clubfoot: a prospective comparison. J Bone Joint Surg Am. 2010;92:270–8.
114. Lykissas MG, Crawford AH, Eismann EA, Tamai J. Ponseti method compared with soft-tissue release for the management of clubfoot: a meta-analysis study. World J Orthop. 2013;4:144–53.
115. Mayne AIW, Bidwai AS, Beirne P, Garg NK, Bruce CE. The effect of a dedicated Ponseti service on the outcome of idiopathic clubfoot treatment. Bone Joint J. 2014;96:1424–6.
116. Ganesan B, Luximon A, Al-Jumaily A, Balasankar SK, Naik GR. Ponseti method in the management of clubfoot under 2 years of age: a systematic review. PLoS One. 2017;12:e0178299.
117. Laaveg SJ, Ponseti IV. Long-term results of treatment of congenital club foot. J Bone Joint Surg Am. 1980;62:23–31.
118. Ponseti IV. Treatment of congenital club foot. J Bone Joint Surg Am. 1992;74:448–54.
119. Cooper DM, Dietz FR. Treatment of idiopathic clubfoot. A thirty-year follow-up note. J Bone Joint Surg Am. 1995;77:1477–89.
120. Herzenberg JE, Radler C, Bor N. Ponseti versus traditional methods of casting for idiopathic clubfoot. J Pediatr Orthop. 2002;22:517–21.
121. Lovell ME, Oji DE, Dolan LA, Ponseti IV. Others health and function of patients with treated idiopathic clubfeet: 50 year follow-up study. In: Annual Meeting of the Pediatric Orthopedic Society of North America. San Diego.
122. Jowett CR, Morcuende JA, Ramachandran M. Management of congenital talipes equinovarus using the Ponseti method: a systematic review. J Bone Joint Surg Br. 2011;93B:1160–4.
123. Banskota B, Banskota AK, Regmi R, Rajbhandary T, Shrestha OP, Spiegel DA. The Ponseti method in the treatment of children with idiopathic clubfoot presenting between five and ten years of age. Bone Joint J. 2013;95(B):1721–5.
124. Aroojis A, Pirani S, Banskota B, Banskota AK, SDA. Clubfoot etiology, pathoanatomy, basic Ponseti technique, and Ponseti in older patients. In: Global orthopedics. New York: Springer; 2014. p. 357–68.
125. Faizan M, Jilani LZ, Abbas M, Zahid M, Asif N. Management of idiopathic clubfoot by Ponseti technique in children presenting after one year of age. J Foot Ankle Surg. 2015;54:967–72.
126. Digge V, Desai J, Das S. Expanded age indication for Ponseti method for correction of congenital idiopathic talipes equinovarus: a systematic review. J Foot Ankle Surg. 2018;57:155–8.
127. van Praag VM, Lysenko M, Harvey B, Yankanah R, Wright JG. Casting is effective for recurrence following Ponseti treatment of clubfoot. J Bone Joint Surg Am. 2018;100:1001–8.
128. Morcuende JA, Dobbs MB, Frick SL. Results of the Ponseti method in patients with clubfoot associated with arthrogryposis. Iowa Orthop J. 2008;28:22–6.
129. Kowalczyk B, Felus J. Ponseti casting and achilles release versus classic casting and soft tissue releases for the initial treatment of arthrogrypotic clubfeet. Foot Ankle Int. 2015;36:1072–7.
130. Lourenço AF, Morcuende JA. Correction of neglected idiopathic club foot by the Ponseti method. J Bone Joint Surg Br. 2007;89:378–81.
131. Dobbs MB, Purcell DB, Nunley R, Morcuende JA. Early results of a new method of treatment for idiopathic congenital vertical talus. J Bone Joint Surg Am. 2006;88:1192–200.
132. Liu Y-B, Li S-J, Zhao L, Yu B, Zhao D-H. Timing for Ponseti clubfoot management: does the age matter? 90 children (131 feet) with a mean follow-up of 5 years. Acta Orthop. 2018;89:662–7.
133. Pirani S, Zeznik L, Hodges D. Magnetic resonance imaging study of the congenital clubfoot treated with the Ponseti method. J Pediatr Orthop. 2001;21:729.
134. Ippolito E, Fraracci L, Farsetti P, Di Mario M, Caterini R. The influence of treatment on the pathology of club foot. CT study at maturity. J Bone Joint Surg Br. 2004;86:574–80.
135. Dobbs MB, Gordon JE, Walton T, Schoenecker PL. Bleeding complications following percutaneous tendoachilles tenotomy in the treatment of clubfoot deformity. J Pediatr Orthop. 2004;24:353.

136. Grigoriou E, Abol Oyoun N, Kushare I, Baldwin KD, Horn BD, Davidson RS. Comparative results of percutaneous Achilles tenotomy to combined open Achilles tenotomy with posterior capsulotomy in the correction of equinus deformity in congenital talipes equinovarus. Int Orthop. 2015;39:721–5.
137. Niki H, Nakajima H, Hirano T, Okada H, Beppu M. Ultrasonographic observation of the healing process in the gap after a Ponseti-type Achilles tenotomy for idiopathic congenital clubfoot at two-year follow-up. J Orthop Sci. 2013;18:70–5.
138. Shabtai L, Segev E, Yavor A, Wientroub S, Hemo Y. Prolonged use of foot abduction brace reduces the rate of surgery in Ponseti-treated idiopathic club feet. J Child Orthop. 2015;9:177–82.
139. Dobbs MB, Rudzki JR, Purcell DB, Walton T, Porter KR, Gurnett CaBeck RW. Factors predictive of outcome after use of the Ponseti method for the treatment of idiopathic clubfeet. JBJS. 2004;86-A:22–7.
140. McKay SD, Dolan LA, Morcuende JA. Treatment results of late-relapsing idiopathic clubfoot previously treated with the Ponseti method. J Pediatr Orthop. 2012;32:406–11.
141. Dietz FR. Treatment of a recurrent clubfoot deformity after initial correction with the Ponseti technique. Instr Course Lect. 2006;55:625–9.
142. Alonso J, Davis N, Harris R. Surgical relevance of delayed ossification of lateral cuneiform in children with clubfoot. J Bone Joint Surg Br. 2009;91-B:56–7.
143. Holt JB, Oji DE, Yack HJ, Morcuende JA. Long-term results of tibialis anterior tendon transfer for relapsed idiopathic clubfoot treated with the Ponseti method. J Bone Joint Surg. 2015;97:47–55.
144. Garceau GJ, Manning KR. Transposition of the anterior tibial tendon in the treatment of recurrent congenital club-foot. J Bone Joint Surg Am. 1947;29:1044–8.
145. Kuo KN, Hennigan SP, Hastings ME. Anterior tibial tendon transfer in residual dynamic clubfoot deformity. J Pediatr Orthop. 2001;21:35–41.
146. Holt JB, Oji DE, Yack HJ, Morcuende JA. Long-term results of tibialis anterior tendon transfer for relapsed idiopathic clubfoot treated with the Ponseti method: a follow-up of thirty-seven to fifty-five years. J Bone Joint Surg Am. 2015;97:47–55.
147. Ponseti IV. Common errors in the treatment of congenital clubfoot. Int Orthop. 1997;21:137–41.
148. Ponseti IV, Zhivkov M, Davis N, Sinclair M, Dobbs MB, Morcuende JA. Treatment of the complex idiopathic clubfoot. Clin Orthop Relat Res. 2006;451:171–6.
149. Low AK, Ward K, Wines AP. Pediatric complex regional pain syndrome. J Pediatr Orthop. 2007;27:567–72.

# Chapter 12
# Chronic Wound Management

**Jeffrey D. Lehrman**

Chronic ulcers of the lower extremity are among the most devastating pathologies treated by podiatrists. Chronic ulcers carry with them high morbidity and mortality, along with a high rate of failure to heal. For example, 49% of all diabetic foot ulcers may fail to heal despite traditional good ulcer care [1], and 50% of venous leg ulcers have been present for at least 9 months before first presentation to a doctor [2]. Chronic ulcers present not only a dire situation but also an emergent one as evidenced by the fact that diabetic foot ulcers whose percentage area reduction is not at least 53% after 4 weeks of traditional treatment only go on to heal by the 12-week mark 9% of the time [3]. These foreboding statistics are among the many that support the need for advanced treatment options and evidence-based decisions when caring for chronic ulcers. Whereas a "wound" is something acute and normally secondary to trauma or surgery, this chapter focuses only on the care of chronic wounds, those "wounds" that have been present for at least 4 weeks and have not improved as would be expected in an uncompromised, healthy host. A wound that is chronic may also be referred to as an "ulcer."

## Comorbidities

Before making treatment decisions regarding the ulcer itself, it is important to first take a step back and evaluate comorbid conditions that may have contributed to the development of the ulcer and/or its chronicity. This can be daunting when considering data from the US Wound Registry indicates that patients seen in outpatient wound centers have an average of eight comorbid conditions [4]. However, a

J. D. Lehrman (✉)
A Step Ahead Foot & Ankle Center, Fort Collins, CO, USA
e-mail: JeffLehrman@LehrmanConsulting.com



D. E. Tower (ed.), *Evidence-Based Podiatry*,
https://doi.org/10.1007/978-3-030-50853-1_12

thorough history taken in a methodical fashion should allow for the detection of all potentially complicating factors. Table 12.1 lists some potential comorbidities that may complicate chronic ulcers. Upon detection, it is important that any of these comorbid conditions be addressed and managed as best as possible. This may require referral to another specialist. Ignoring a contributing systemic condition may render any local care futile.

## Ulcer Evaluation

Consistent evaluation and documentation of ulcer characteristics is an essential component of chronic ulcer management. This allows for consistency between different providers, tracking of progress, and is also important for risk management. Table 12.2 contains a list of ulcer characteristics which should be noted and documented.

**Table 12.1** Potential comorbidities that may complicate chronic ulcers

| |
|---|
| Malnutrition |
| Immobility |
| Obesity |
| Cardiopulmonary disease |
| Poor glycemic control in patients with diabetes |
| Peripheral arterial disease |
| Venous insufficiency |
| Immunodeficiency |
| Advanced age |
| Neuropathic conditions |
| Metabolic disorders |
| Hematologic disorders |
| Neoplastic conditions |
| Infection (both local and systemic) |
| Tobacco use |
| Psychosocial issues |

**Table 12.2** Notable ulcer characteristics

| |
|---|
| Location of ulcer |
| Ulcer length, width, and depth |
| Quantity, color, and type of drainage |
| Color, texture, and condition of ulcer bed and surrounding tissue |
| Absence/presence of necrotic tissue |
| Vascularity |
| Temperature surrounding the ulcer |
| Presence or absence of undermining/tunneling and, if present, orientation and extent |

## Infection Management

Contamination, colonization, and infection are all states with which ulcer care providers should be familiar. Contamination indicates the presence of non-replicating organisms in the ulcer bed. All chronic ulcers are contaminated [5]. It is for this reason that superficial culture swabs cannot be relied upon to determine if an ulcer is infected, nor should they be used to identify causative organisms in the presence of infection [6]. Colonization indicates the presence of replicating organisms that are not causing tissue damage. This usually represents skin flora. Infection sets in when these replicating organisms begin to cause tissue damage. It is best to culture an ulcer only when infection is suspected [7]. This helps to avoid false positives and overutilization of antimicrobials. When culture is warranted, it is best to be performed, when possible, as a deep tissue culture under sterile conditions. When infection is confirmed, antimicrobial therapy should be targeted based on culture and sensitivity reports.

## Offloading

The evaluation of the ulcer should include evaluation for the need to offload. This includes a gait analysis and checking for any underlying bony prominences. For podiatrists, plantar foot ulcers can be especially stubborn when not properly offloaded. There are so many offloading options. In a book that focuses on evidence-based decisions, the literature surrounding the use of some of these options is especially interesting. The rigid, flat-bottom postsurgical shoe is intended to accommodate bulky postsurgical dressings and was never intended to serve as an offloading device. There is no statistically significant data to suggest that a rigid, flat-bottom postsurgical shoe offloads the plantar foot more than a regular shoe. The same is true for the offloading abilities of forefoot and rearfoot wedge shoes. True offloading is best achieved with a total contact cast. Total contact casting heals up to 90% of nonischemic diabetic foot ulcers [8]. Not only is total contact casting extraordinarily impactful in healing diabetic foot ulcers; the time to healing is fast at an average of just 34 days [7]. Removable cast boots have proven to offload just as effectively as total contact casts [9]. The problem is removable cast boots are flawed because they can be removed by patients, which can take place 72% of the time [10]. However, when used correctly, irremovable cast boots offload just as effectively as total contact casts with equal rates of ulcer healing [8]. While remaining cost-conscious about treatment decisions, it is important to note the incredible efficacy of offloading alone compared to the inferior efficacy of much more expensive treatment options.

## Debridement

Debridement is indicated for most chronic ulcers. Any necrotic and/or nonviable tissue should be removed from the ulcer bed as well as its margins and periphery, and this is normally best accomplished via debridement. Necrotic and/or nonviable tissue can serve as a medium for infection. It is a barrier to healing, contributes to the formation of matrix metalloproteinases, and increases the bioburden of the ulcer bed.

There are multiple forms of debridement. Biosurgical debridement refers to maggot or larval therapy. This is a selective form of debridement as the maggot species that are used only feed on nonviable tissue and will not disrupt healthy tissue. By means of proteolytic enzymes, maggots liquefy and ingest necrotic tissue. Enzymatic debridement refers to the use of exogenous enzyme(s) to cleave the strands of collagen that anchor necrotic tissue to the bed of the ulcer. Whereas enzymatic debridement relies on exogenous enzymes, autolytic debridement enlists the body's own endogenous enzymes. This is typically a slow form of debridement for those with chronic ulcers as it relies upon natural processes and the proteolytic enzymes produced endogenously. The use of dressings that help to maintain moisture can facilitate autolytic debridement. These include hydrogels, hydrocolloids, and honey. Chemical debridement usually refers to the use of silver nitrate to address hypergranulation tissue. Mechanical debridement most often refers to a wet-to-dry or moist-to-dry dressing. These two types of mechanical debridement are considered substandard and should not be used [11]. Other forms of mechanical debridement include irrigation, pulse lavage, whirlpool, and scrubbing. Low-frequency ultrasound-assisted debridement may be employed in the form of noncontact or contact ultrasound. Finally, sharp debridement may be performed with scissors, forceps, lasers, hydrosurgical options, curettes, and/or scalpels. The frequency with which sharp debridements are performed should be based on literature, and this is a situation where the standard of care does not always match the gold standard. Recent literature [12] tells us that chronic ulcers demonstrate better healing with more frequent debridements. This is likely due to the fact that biofilm returns quickly after sharp debridement, beginning to reform within 24 hours [13] and re-establishing itself within 3 days [14]. Not only should sharp debridement be performed frequently, there are multiple studies that suggest ulcer progression is improved when sharp debridement is combined with enzymatic debridement rather than choosing one or the other [15–17].

There may be situations where debridement is not indicated. One example is an ulcer with a dry, intact eschar that does not exhibit any sign of underlying infection [18]. In most cases, these dry eschars are best left intact. Enzymatic debridement may not be appropriate in infected ulcers, and sharp debridement should not be performed if malignancy is suspected or, in most cases, if there is underlying arterial disease which has not been addressed.

## Topical Agents

In addition to the enzymatic debriders referenced above, other topical agents exist. There are different types of topical growth factor therapies, including both autogenous and platelet-derived. Autologous platelet-rich plasma mimics the natural healing process [19]. Topical platelet-derived growth factor is also available commercially and has demonstrated both increased and faster rates of healing in diabetic foot ulcers compared to placebo [20]. Other topical agents are available, mostly in the form of antimicrobials. Silver has traditionally enjoyed a high rate of utilization, but, recently, clinically relevant silver resistance has been identified [21]. This realization should play a role in conscientious dressing selections that not only protect the patient being treated but also protect the community.

## Dressings

Too often what we decide to dress an ulcer with is based on convenience or cost, whereas this decision should be guided by good quality data. Among many dressings, options include alginates, foam, hydrocolloids, hydrogels, silver, and collagen. Interestingly, more expensive dressings may offer no advantage over less expensive dressings [22]. Of the many dressing options available, hydrocolloid matrix was shown in a systematic review to have the highest probability to offer the best chance of healing diabetic foot ulcers [22].

## Negative-Pressure Wound Therapy

Negative-pressure wound therapy (NPWT) delivers subatmospheric pressure to the ulcer bed. It also offers vacuum-assisted drainage which should facilitate the removal of microorganisms, debris, and other unwanted components of the ulcer bed that can delay healing. NPWT should also contribute to the removal of interstitial fluid, which should, in turn, contribute to a decrease in edema. With a decrease in edema, capillary exchange should be increased, which should allow for improved perfusion and delivery of oxygen and growth factors needed for healing. NPWT is available in both disposable and non-disposable forms with each offering their own advantages and disadvantages. While the knowledge of the effectiveness of NPWT seems to be well-known, the decision regarding pressure settings is another area where standard of care is not always consistent with best practices. One decision that needs to be made for most NPWT types is the pressure mode, with the options being continuous, intermittent, and variable. Studies show a higher degree of granulation under intermittent and variable pressure than under continuous pressure [23].

While the typical pressure range is between 50 and 150 mmHg, we now know [24] that higher pressures should be used when there is more exudate and when a bridge dressing is used.

## Grafts

Graft options for chronic ulcers include both autologous grafts and skin substitutes. While autologous grafts are normally preferred over any other option as far as effectiveness, they may not always be available or the best option. This is when skin substitute options may be considered. There are many different types of skin substitute products, and they include xenografts, synthetic bilayers, allogenic epidermal substitutes, allogenic dermal substitutes, composite allografts, allograft placental tissue, allograft human skin cells, and autologous cultured skin. There are many different options when it comes to product selection. When making this selection, each of these different product types have their own literature to consider. However, it is critical to note that in a Cochrane review of 17 studies regarding the use of skin grafts and tissue replacement products for diabetic foot ulcers, no evidence was found that allows for the recommendation of one type of skin graft or tissue replacement product over another [25]. This same Cochrane paper concluded that while skin grafts and tissue replacements increase the healing rate of foot ulcers, evidence of using anything less compromises the chances no certainty of cost-effectiveness [25].

## Compression

Evidence-based treatment of venous leg disease and venous leg ulcers mandates the use of compression when indicated [26]. However, just employing any type of compression may not be sufficient. It must be graduated, consistent compression at an adequate level. The initial pressure required to collapse a vessel is 30–40 mmHg [27]. Therefore, therapeutic compression should achieve at least this degree of pressure. Too often prescription or purchase of inadequate compression options leads to undesirable results.

In many cases, healing venous leg ulcers is easier than preventing their recurrence. With such a high rate of recurrence, evidence-based decision-making is a must. Adequate below-knee graduated compression stockings or hosiery that patients can tolerate and use as indicated are likely to prevent recurrence of venous leg ulcers [28]. The key terms and phrases in the previous sentence include "adequate," "patients can tolerate," and "use as indicated." It is incumbent on the prescriber to find a compression option that provides an adequate degree of compression that the patient can actually tolerate. Using compression with a lower degree of pressure in an effort to trade effectiveness for convenience often results in poor outcomes. Class III compression provides 25–35 mmHg, and using anything less compromises the chances of actually preventing recurrence.

## Hyperbaric Medicine

Hyperbaric medicine involves exposing a patient to hyperbaric oxygen, 100% oxygen at a pressure that is greater than normal. Although controversial in some circles, the evidence-based outlook on the use of hyperbaric medicine for chronic ulcers can be simply stated: healing processes of chronic ulcers have been shown to accelerate under the influence of hyperbaric oxygen [29].

## References

1. Papanas N, et al. Benefit-risk assessment of becaplermin in the treatment of diabetic foot ulcers. Drug Saf. 2010;33:455–61.
2. Hess C. Lower extremity wound checklist. Adv Skin Wound Care. 2009;22(9):144.
3. Sheehan P, et al. Percent change in wound area of diabetic foot ulcers over a 4-week period is a robust predictor of complete healing in a 12-week prospective trial. Diabetes Care. 2003;26(6):1879–82.
4. Horn SD, et al. Development of a wound healing index for patients with chronic wounds. Wound Repair Regen. 2013;21(6):823–32.
5. Frank C, et al. Lower extermity wounds: a problem-based approach. Can Fam Physician. 2005;51(10):1352–9.
6. Kallstrom G. Are quantitative bacterial wound cultures useful? J Clin Microbiol. 2014;52(8):2753–6.
7. Frantz RA. Identifying infection in chronic wounds. Nursing. 2005. 2005;35(7):73.
8. Nabuurs-Franssen MH. Total contact casting of the diabetic foot in daily practice: a prospective follow-up study. Diabetes Care. 2005 Feb;28(2):243–7.
9. Fibreglass total contact casting, removable cast walkers, and irremovable cast walkers to treat diabetic neuropathic foot ulcers: a health technology assessment. Health Quality. Ont Health Technol Assess Ser. 2017;17(12):1–124.
10. Armstrong DG, et al. Activity patterns of patients with diabetic foot ulceration. Diabetes Care. 2003;26(9):2595–7.
11. Association for the Advancement of Wound Care. Guideline of pressure ulcer guidelines; Association for the Advancement of Wound Care; McLean, VA. 2010. p. 9.
12. Wilcox JR, et al. Frequency of debridements and time to heal: a retrospective cohort study of 312 744 wounds. JAMA Dermatol. 2013;149(9):1050–8.
13. Carpenter S, et al. Bilayered skin-substitute technology for the treatment of diabetic foot ulcers: current insights. Wounds. 2016;28(6 Suppl):S1–S20.
14. Wolcott RD, et al. Biofilm maturity studies indicate sharp debridement opens a time- dependent therapeutic window. J Wound Care. 2010;19(8):320–8.
15. Motley TA, et al. Clinical outcomes associated with serial sharp debridement of diabetic foot ulcers with and without clostridial collagenase ointment. Wounds. 2014;26:57–64.

16. Jiminez JC, et al. Enzymatic debridement of chronic nonischemic diabetic foot ulcers: results of a randomized, controlled trial. Wounds. 2017;29:133–9.
17. Tallis A, et al. Clinical and economic assessment of diabetic foot ulcer debridement with collagenase: results of a randomized controlled study. Clin Ther. 2013;35:1805–20.
18. Lauerman MH, Scalea TM, Eglseder WA, Pensy R, Stein DM, Henry S. Efficacy of wound coverage techniques in extremity necrotizing soft tissue infections. Am Surg. 2018;84(11):1790–5.
19. Lacci KM, et al. Platelet-rich plasma: support for its use in wound healing. Yale J Biol Med. 2010;83(1):1–9.
20. Wieman TJ, et al. Efficacy and safety of a topical gel formulation of recombinant human platelet-derived growth factor-BB (becaplermin) in patients with chronic neuropathic diabetic ulcers. A phase III randomized placebo-controlled double-blind study. Diabetes Care. 1998;21:822–7.
21. Finley P. J. Unprecedented silver resistance in clinically isolated enterobacteriaceae: major implications for burn and wound management. Antimicrob Agents Chemother. 2015;59(8):4734–41.
22. Dumville JC, et al. Systematic review and mixed treatment comparison: dressings to heal diabetic foot ulcers. Diabetologia. 2012;55(7):1902–10.
23. Malmsjö M, et al. The effects of variable, intermittent, and continuous negative pressure wound therapy, using foam or gauze, on wound contraction, granulation tissue formation, and ingrowth into the wound filler. Eplasty. 2012;12:e5.
24. Borgquist O, et al. The influence of low and high pressure levels during negative-pressure wound therapy on wound contraction and fluid evacuation. Plast Reconstr Surg. 2011;127(2):551–9.
25. Santema TB, et al. Skin grafting and tissue replacement for treating foot ulcers in people with diabetes. Cochrane Database Syst Rev. 2016;(2):CD011255.
26. Dogra S, et al. Summary of recommendations for leg ulcers. Indian Dermatol Online J. 2014;5(3):400–7.
27. Hegarty M. The clinical effectiveness of negative pressure wound therapy: a systematic review. Today's Wound Clin. 2010;5:490.
28. Nelson EA, et al. Compression for preventing recurrence of venous ulcers. Cochrane Database Syst Rev. 2000;(4):CD002303.
29. Opasanon S, et al. Clinical effectiveness of hyperbaric oxygen therapy in complex wounds. J Am Coll Clin Wound Spec. 2014;6(1–2):9–13.

# Chapter 13
# Total Ankle Arthroplasty

**Jeremy J. Cook, Emily A. Cook, Philip Basile, Bryon McKenna, Elena Manning, and Samantha Miner**

## Evaluation of the Literature

In 2018, Noordin and Malik published a citation analysis of the 50 most cited articles on total ankle arthroplasty [1]. They found 2,445 relevant articles published between 1979 and 2013. The top five most cited articles were published between 1998 and 2007. These 5 most cited articles contributed over 1,100 of the 5,608 citations for the top 50 articles. More importantly, 74% of the studies were level 4, while the remaining 18% were equal parts level 3 and level 5. The most cited article was a systematic review of second-generation ankle replacements [1, 2]. Evidence-based medicine requires constant attentiveness, and the fact that the most cited article as of 2018 was a 2007 review article that discussed outcomes, a generation removed from contemporaries is untenable. The aim of this chapter is to present recent literature published in peer-reviewed journals to provide the best possible updated evidence-based medicine on topics concerning total ankle replacements. In order to complete this aim, an extensive systematic review was performed on PubMed, Embase, Web of Science, and Cochrane using medical subject headings (MeSH): "ankle," "replacement," "arthroplasty," and "prosthesis." We included all papers published in the English language between 2013 and 2018 in peer-reviewed journals. This search resulted in 2,543 papers. After excluding papers that were not in the English language, published prior to 2013, published in non-peer-reviewed journals, case reports, and basic science papers, the result was 126 articles. The abstracts for these 126 articles were reviewed; the pertinent articles for each section of this chapter were then included in the review. Papers published prior to 2013 that were relevant to the discussions were referenced.

J. J. Cook (✉) · E. A. Cook (✉) · P. Basile · B. McKenna · E. Manning · S. Miner
Department of Surgery, Mount Auburn Hospital, Cambridge, MA, USA
e-mail: jeremycook@post.harvard.edu; emilycook@post.harvard.edu



D. E. Tower (ed.), *Evidence-Based Podiatry*,
https://doi.org/10.1007/978-3-030-50853-1_13

## Current Concepts in Total Ankle Replacements

### *Patient Selection*

When considering total ankle replacements, the first and most critical step is proper patient selection. A total ankle replacement performed on the correct patient is imperative. Age, functional level, BMI, presence of comorbidities, tobacco use, deformity, and severity of adjacent joint arthritis are all important considerations [3].

Steck et al. published a chart of indications, relative contraindications, and absolute contraindications for total ankle arthroplasty in 2009. Historically, the best patient candidate for a total ankle implant would be a nonobese, nonsmoker, greater than 55 years old, without immunosuppression and with adequate neurovascular status. The patient would have low physical demand with good bone stock and have an ankle in neutral alignment with a competent deltoid ligament and minimal to no adjacent joint arthritis [3, 4]. Steck and colleagues also delineated relative contraindications in 2009 which included patients less than 55 years old, smoking, immunosuppression, diabetes, obesity, osteoporosis, poor bone stock, avascular necrosis of talus (only if the necrotic portion of the talus remains after the bone cuts), bone loss from prior severe trauma, ankle deformity (varus, valgus, procurvatum, recurvatum), and workman compensation cases. Absolute contraindications included patients with high physical demands (i.e., runners), poor vascularity, significant all cause neuropathy, neuromuscular deficits and or paralysis, non-reconstructable deformity or incompetent deltoid ligament, infection, severe soft tissue compromise (prior multiple incisions, flaps), avascular necrosis involving the entire talar body, and patient noncompliance [4].

Technological advances in implant design, like polyethylene inserts of varying thicknesses, development of implants with enhanced component stability, and virtual resurfacing of the talus, have made proper patient selection the more critical element. Essentially, technology and technique have progressed enough that patient factors are the greater limitation to successful outcomes. These implant design advances have allowed foot and ankle surgeons to expand candidate populations, while indications and contraindications for total ankle replacement continue to evolve.

#### Age

The unique challenge of end-stage ankle arthritis is that the majority are due to post-traumatic etiology (65–80%), as contrasted to the hip and knee [5, 6]. Since these patients on average are much younger, long-term implant survivorship is a significant concern. Therefore, age is an important consideration for ankle replacement candidacy. For many years the majority of surgeons would not implant a TAA in patients younger than 65 years of age. The primary concern was that the likelihood of revision was elevated. This was attributed to the extended life expectancy in younger patients as well as increased activity resulting in increased wear and tear on the implant. Although well-grounded logically, there was little evidence to support this age cutoff in the literature. More recent literature indicates that the patient's age has become less of a deterrent and experienced surgeons are performing total ankle arthroplasty in younger individuals with great success with new implant designs. Spirt et al. evaluated complications and revisions after TAA and reported that the 5-year implant survival rate for patients 54 years of age or younger was 74%, compared to 89% for patients 55 years of age and older. They also found that patients 54 years of age and younger had a 1.45 times higher risk for reoperation and 2.64 times increased risk for implant failure. This data is based on older implant designs [7].

Recently, Demetracopoulos et al. performed a level 2 prospective comparative study to evaluate the effects of age on outcomes in TAA [8]. In this study, the authors included 395 consecutive TAA patients who underwent primary TAA from June 2007 to July 2011 from multiple centers. Patients were divided into three groups, <55 years of age ($N = 81$), 55–70 years of age ($N = 221$), and >70 years of age ($N = 93$). Patient-reported outcome scores, American Orthopaedic Foot & Ankle Society (AOFAS) function score, Visual Analog Scale (VAS), and weight-bearing radiographs were used to assess the patients preoperatively and at their annual postoperative visit. After a mean follow-up of 3.5 years, there were no differences between any of the three age groups in changes in VAS, physical performance outcomes, wound complications, or need for reoperation and revisions. In fact, the only statistically significant difference between the age groups was patients <55 years of age had greater improvement in postoperative Short-Form 36 (SF-36) ($P = 0.026$) and AOFAS function scores ($P < 0.001$) compared to patients >70 years of age. Although very encouraging, this study is limited by a mean short-term follow-up of 3.5 years. Reviewing our own meta-analysis with publications from 2013 to 2018, the median age for studies were dichotomized into younger than and older than 62.65 years of age for comparison. The survivorship was 90.3% in studies below the median and 95.5% in studies above the median age. This relationship was not statistically significant, $P = 0.362$ [9]. Mean survivorship was better in the more recent studies than those reported in Sprit's manuscript regardless of age. Clearly more research is needed to evaluate the longevity of the newer generation implants in younger patients as the indication for total ankle replacements continues to broaden.

## Immunosuppression

A common etiology of end-stage ankle arthritis is inflammatory arthropathy such as rheumatoid arthritis. The principal treatment modality for the arthropathies is immunosuppression, which has been associated with poor surgical outcomes and more frequent complications [10–14].

Pedersen et al. published a multi-center cohort study comparing clinical outcomes of TAA in patients with rheumatoid arthritis (RA) and noninflammatory arthritis. One hundred patients met selection criteria and were included in the analysis. Fifty RA patients were then matched with 50 noninflammatory arthritis patients. The two groups were matched based on implant system, BMI, and length of follow-up, with the average follow-up being a mean of 63.8 months within the RA group and 65.6 months within the noninflammatory group. The RA group had a slightly younger population with a mean age of 58.5 compared to 61.2 years of age for the control group. The RA group had eight major complications in six patients, while nine major complications occurred in nine patients in the noninflammatory arthritis group. Although the revision rate was not statistically different between groups, a major difference was the average time to revision. In the RA group, revision surgery occurred after a mean of 43 months (range 12–70 months). The time to revision was much longer in the noninflammatory patients, 78 months (range 51–120 months). The authors did cite that patients with RA did have worse overall pain and disability scores preoperatively that were statistically equivalent to the control group postoperatively. After 5 years, both groups had similar postoperative outcomes [15].

Raikin et al. reported an increased risk of major wound complications associated with underlying inflammatory arthritis with an odds ratio of 14.03, requiring additional operation [16]. Althoff compared the risk of periprosthetic joint infections in 6,977 patients and found that inflammatory arthritis was an independent risk factor that increased the odds of infections (OR 2.38; $P < 0.0001$) [17]. Ultimately, patients with inflammatory arthritis can have a significant improvement in pain and function after TAA, but appropriate surgical precautions must be taken to minimize complications. An important consideration is that the time to revision seems to be much shorter in RA patients [15].

## Diabetes

Another immunocompromised class of patients frequently encountered by foot and ankle surgeons is the diabetic patient. It is considered well established that patients with diabetes have an elevated risk of complications and worse outcomes compared to nondiabetics following foot and ankle surgery [18–20]. The extent that this disease impacts ankle joint replacement has had far less discussion. A large national database study evaluated risks for complications following 169,406 total joint arthroplasties. Diabetes was noted to be one of the greatest risk factors for readmission and complications [21].

A 2015 study investigated the impact of diabetes in 2,973 patients undergoing TAA. Diabetics had an overall complication rate of 7.8%, while nondiabetics had a rate of 4.7%. Their multivariate analysis determined that diabetes carried a complication rate that was four times higher than nondiabetics (RR = 4.1, $P = 0.02$). Moreover, diabetes was independently associated with increased risk of blood transfusion (RR = 9.8, $P = 0.03$), longer length of stay (difference = 0.41 days, $P < 0.001$), and more frequent non-home discharge (RR = 1.88, $P < 0.001$) [22].

Also in 2015, Gross et al. assessed the effects of diabetes on complications after total ankle replacements. This retrospective cohort included 50 patients diagnosed with diabetes and 55 patients in the nondiabetic patient population. Results found that approximately 20% of all diabetic patients required reoperation and revision or developed implant failure which was equivalent to the nondiabetics. This study suffers from significant limitations but does support that diabetes is not an absolute contraindication for TAA [23].

In 2010, Raikin et al. performed a level 2 prognostic study evaluating the risk factors for incision healing complications following TAA in 106 patients. Diabetes was associated with a significant increased risk for wound healing complications. Although a past medical history significant for diabetes was associated with a higher risk of wound complications, these complications responded well to local wound care. It is worth noting that only patients with well-controlled diabetes were included and that patients with peripheral neuropathy, neuroarthropathy, and compromised circulation were excluded [16].

Although specific guidelines for glycemic control have not been determined for ankle replacement procedures, there is good data available for the risk of infection following joint replacements. In Cancienne and co-workers' 2017 study of 7,736 diabetic patients treated with total hip arthroplasty, patients with an HbA1c level of 7.5 mg/dL or greater had more than double the odds of deep infection compared to patients below that threshold (odds ratio, 2.6; 95% CI, 1.9–3.4; $P < 0.0001$) [24].

With regard to patients with diabetes, TAA is not absolutely contraindicated. Diabetic patients are more vulnerable to complications and tend to have longer hospital stays and are less likely to be discharged home. Wound complications and infection are more likely. Optimizing glycemic control prior to surgery and during the postoperative course is crucial to avoiding catastrophic complications. Although no study has ever explored the negative consequences of using a TAA implant in neuropathic patients, all manufactures' literature list neuropathy, Charcot joint, avascular necrosis, and infection as surgical technique complications. In 2003, Parvizi showed a high reoperation rate in 40 Charcot knees undergoing joint replacement [25]. A 2011 case study by Yasin and colleagues confirmed that Charcot joints remain more vulnerable to implant failure and instability than in non-Charcot patients [26]. The most recent knee arthroplasty literature in 2018 found that 10-year survivorship was 70% due to higher rates of complications in patients with Charcot [27]. Chalmers and colleagues followed 12 total hip arthroplasties in patients with Charcot for a mean of 5 years. The complication rate was 58% overall, and 33% required a reoperation within 5 years [28].

## Obesity

Another risk factor independent from diabetes but frequently found in tandem is obesity. The most common cutoff for obesity in the literature is a BMI greater than 30 kg/m$^2$ per the definition of the World Health Organization (WHO). The American obesity epidemic has been worsening for decades with no end in sight. As a result of this ubiquitous health issue, the likelihood is high that at least some of these patients will be candidates for TAA. There has been significant debate regarding performing TAA on obese patients. Controversy engulfs this topic since recent literature suggests differences in outcomes and complication rates among obese and nonobese patients [29].

There is extensive literature evaluating effects of obesity on the outcomes of total hip and knee replacements. This literature has shown that obese patients are at increased risk for revision surgery after total knee and total hip replacements [30, 31]. In the foot and ankle literature, however, there are contradictory studies regarding the association of obesity and an increased risk for revision concerning total ankle replacements.

In one study, Werner et al. retrospectively compared complication rates in nonobese and obese patients undergoing ankle arthrodesis and total ankle arthroplasty in 23,029 patients (5,361 with TAA and 17,668 with ankle arthrodesis). In the TAA cohort, they found that obese patients had a higher risk for complications within 90 days of surgery as compared to nonobese patients. These included a wide array of pathologies, such as major, minor, local, systemic, venous thromboembolic, infectious, and medical complications. They also found that obese patients who underwent TAA had a higher rate of revision than the nonobese group. Interestingly, the complication rate and revision rate was similarly increased in obese patients in the ankle arthrodesis cohort [32].

Bouchard et al., in 2015, performed a retrospective cohort study comparing outcomes, complications, and need for revision after TAA between obese and nonobese patients. They defined obesity as a BMI >30 kg/m$^2$ and also included morbidly obese patients in this cohort (BMI >40 kg/m$^2$). Outcome measures, including the Ankle Osteoarthritis Scale (AOS) and Short-Form 36 (SF-36), were performed at least 2 years postoperatively. In contrast to the Werner et al. study, they found no statistically significant difference between patient outcome scores, complication rate, and revision rate between the two groups. They concluded that TAA is a viable treatment option for obese patients with end-stage ankle osteoarthritis [33].

Sansoti et al. performed a systematic review in 2018, which evaluated the effects of obesity on TAA [34]. They specifically looked at the requirement for surgical revision of the TAA implant in obese patients with a BMI greater than 30 kg/m$^2$. They included four studies that met their inclusion criteria, including the aforementioned study by Bouchard et al., for a total of 400 implants. Of the 400 included implants, approximately 17.8% developed a complication requiring a revision surgical procedure. The most commonly performed revision procedures were revision of the metallic components and ankle gutter debridement. A total of 4 out of 400 required conversion to ankle arthrodesis. In a meta-analysis performed by Zaidi et al. in 2013, they found an overall complication rate of 13.5% for all patients undergoing TAA regardless of BMI [35]. The results of this systematic review and meta-analysis may suggest a slightly higher complication rate in obese patients undergoing TAA. A clear limitation to both studies is the inclusion of implants that are no longer available on the market due to excessively high revision rates.

Although many studies have highlighted the risks of obesity in TAA patients, it is noteworthy that BMI risks have a "J-shaped" distribution. The Althoff study found that although a BMI >30 kg/m$^2$ had higher odds of infection compared to normal BMI (OR 1.49; $P = 0.034$), they also found that being underweight was even more detrimental, BMI <19 kg/m$^2$ (OR 3.35; $P = 0.013$) [17]. Clearly, the role of nutritional status is more complex and bears more consideration in optimizing outcomes.

After a thorough evaluation of the literature, there is no clear definitive association of obesity with risk for revision total ankle replacement surgery, and as a result, no clear guideline has been established for performing TAA on obese patients.

## Tobacco Use

Tobacco use is a known risk factor for musculoskeletal surgery. It negatively impacts bone and soft tissue healing. Lampley and co-workers retrospectively stratified outcomes of 642 TAA patients into nonsmokers, former smokers, and active smokers. They found a statistically significant increased risk of wound breakdown in active smokers compared to nonsmokers undergoing total ankle replacements. They concluded active cigarette smokers undergoing TAA had a significantly higher risk for wound complications and thus worse outcome scores [36].

Other studies have not been able to identify increased complications related to a smoking history. Patton's investigation examined risk factors for total ankle replacement infection and found no significant difference between infected and uninfected groups with respect to tobacco use [37]. A subsequent study by Gross et al. in 2017 retrospectively compared TAAs that developed wound complications requiring surgical intervention (cases) versus TAAs that did not experience reoperation for wound complications (controls). Of the 762 total ankle replacements, 49 needed operative procedures to treat wound healing complications (cases). They found that there was no statistically significant difference in smoking history between cases (smoking history = 46.2%) and controls (smoking history = 40.4%), $P = 0.5$ [38].

It is possible that the Patton and Gross studies were underpowered to detect a statistically significant difference in smoking. The possibility of classification bias also exists as a history of smoking may be less relevant compared to an active tobacco user. Both the Patton and Gross studies are in stark contrast to the majority of studies which assess for tobacco including the Althoff 2018 study of 6,977 TAAs which found that both tobacco use (OR 1.59; $P = 0.002$) and chronic lung disease (OR 1.37; $P = 0.022$) were significant risk factors for periprosthetic joint infections [17].

Although a specific dose-response relationship for smoking and complications has not been described in the setting of TAA, we can draw guidance from other literature. A cohort of 396 patients found an overall nonunion rate of 18.2% in individuals smoking more than 10 cigarettes per day. The nonunion rate was 9.8% smoking <10 cigarettes per day and 8.9% in nonsmokers (odds ratio [OR] 2.01, $P < 0.016$) [39]. Whalen and colleagues looked at a smaller cohort of 57 consecutive TAAs [40]. Overall, they reported a 28% wound complication rate. They identified a smoking history of greater than 12 pack years as high risk for wound complications.

The nicotine concentration varies from product to product, and higher concentrations are potentially more harmful. Surgeons should be aware that cigarettes contain between 1.1 and 1.8 mg of nicotine. A pack of cigarettes has at least 22 mg of nicotine. Chewing tobacco contains 88 mg per can, and a loose leaf pouch contains 144 mg of nicotine [41]. Consuming smokeless tobacco is the equivalent of smoking between four and six packs of cigarettes. Patients are often unaware of these equivalencies and fail to appreciate the potential impact on their surgical outcomes. Overall, current evidence strongly supports that active tobacco use increases the risk of wound complications and infection in TAA patients. Unfortunately, data does not conclusively link a history of smoking with complication rates. All TAA candidates should be urged to cease nicotine containing products prior to surgery.

## Deformity

According to Dodd and Daniels, approximately 50% or more of patients presenting with severe ankle arthritis have some level of deformity. Post-traumatic arthritis, the most common cause of severe ankle arthritis, can often present with intra-articular deformities such as malleolar dysplasia and talar tilting, resulting in coronal plane malalignment. It is estimated that more than 75% of patients with deformity require an ancillary procedure with TAA in order to obtain a properly aligned foot and ankle [42].

When determining whether a patient is an appropriate candidate for TAA, asymmetric ankle joint deformity is an important consideration. In order to prevent malalignment of the implant and ultimately early failure, the deformity must be adequately assessed prior to correction. Assessment of ankle malalignment should first be performed clinically. Flexibility and stability of the hindfoot complex should be closely examined. Rigid hindfoot deformities may require additional corrective procedures, such as a calcaneal osteotomy, cuneiform osteotomy, and/or arthrodesis of one or more joints. A Coleman block test may be utilized to determine if there is a forefoot component in varus deformities [42, 43].

Radiographic assessment of ankle malalignment is necessary for evaluation of the deformity's center of rotation of angulation (CORA), as well as for preoperative planning. Weight-bearing anteroposterior radiographs are used to determine the tibiotalar angle (TTA), which is the angle formed by the longitudinal axis of the tibia and the line perpendicular to the talar dome. This angle evaluates intra-articular talar tilt in the coronal plane and is commonly used to determine the degree of coronal plane ankle varus and valgus. Normal values for this angle range from zero to five degrees [44, 45]. Anterior extrusion of the talus or anterior prolithesis can be identified with a lateral view of the ankle (Fig. 13.1). Additional radiographic views may be useful in further characterizing a patient's deformity, such as the Saltzman view, calcaneal axial, or long leg views [43, 46].

Knupp et al. described a technique for measuring the amount of talar tilt within the ankle joint. Using this method, they were able to classify asymmetric ankle joints as congruent or incongruent. Less than or equal to 4 degrees of tilt was defined

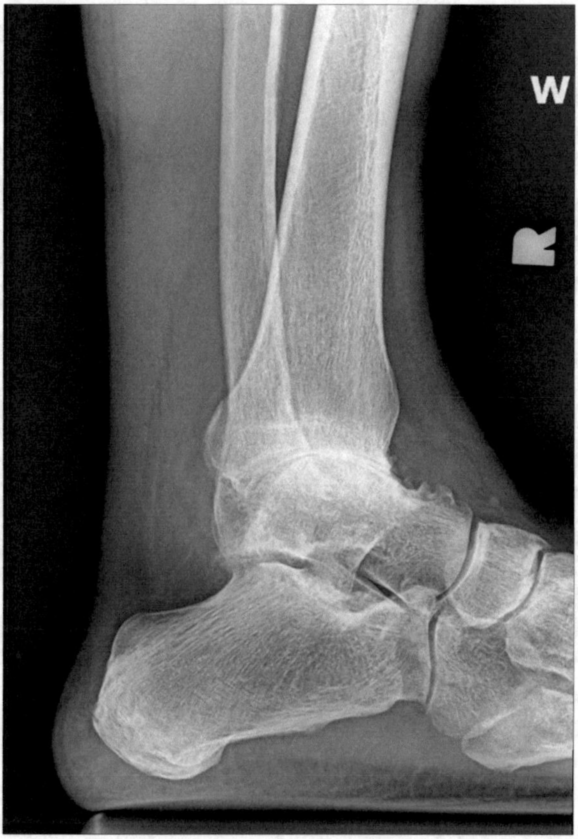


**Fig. 13.1** *Deformity*. Lateral radiograph demonstrating the concept of anterior prolithesis (anterior extrusion of the talus on the tibia), a type of deformity that should be identified when considering TAA

as a congruent ankle joint (type I), while greater than 4 degrees was considered incongruent (type II) (Fig. 13.2). Based on these definitions, they were able to propose a complicated algorithm for guiding treatment in correcting varus and valgus deformities of the ankle using supramalleolar osteotomies (SMO), as well as other ancillary procedures as dictated by the patient's individual deformity [46, 47]. When deconstructed to simpler terms, as described in a review by Brigido et al., congruent ankles may require soft tissue balancing procedures only, while incongruent ankles may need a combination of soft tissue and osteotomy procedures in order to achieve neutral alignment [48].

Classically, a contraindication to total ankle replacement is severe varus or valgus deformity, with severe usually being defined as greater than 15 degrees. With the advent of newer primary implants including an intramedullary tibial implant well suited for revisions and large coronal plane deformities greater than 15 degrees, experienced surgeons are considering more patients today for TAA than ever before.

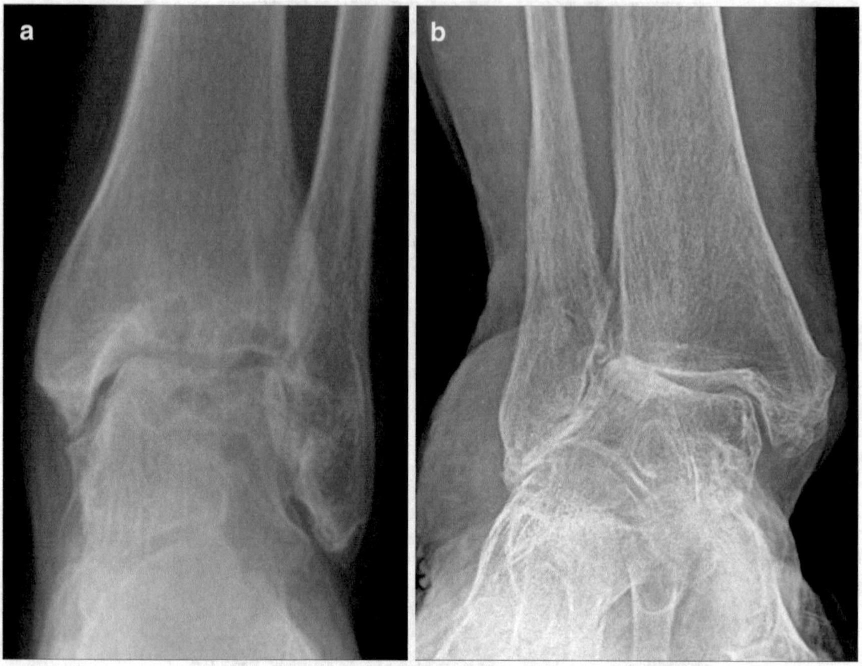


**Fig. 13.2** *Deformity*. (**a**) Example of a congruent ankle joint in which no talar tilt is noted. (**b**) Example of an incongruent ankle joint where there is obvious talar tilt in valgus and bony contact

Severe varus deformities are often amenable to single-stage correction combining TAA with various boney and soft tissue procedures (Fig. 13.3). However, valgus deformities with adequate deltoid integrity are often staged. The patient with a severe valgus deformity or stage IV posterior tibial tendon dysfunction with an attenuated deep deltoid ligament is often a poor candidate for TAA. These patients often receive a highly stable stemmed intramedullary tibial component with a flat cut talar component, though a chamfer cut talar component has also been found to be a feasible alternative, as will be discussed more in a later section (Fig. 13.4).

While we concede that greater deformities present greater challenges to correction efforts, the paradigm is not supported by the recent literature [49, 50]. In a prospective observational study by Queen et al., no significant difference in clinical outcomes following TAA was seen between patients with severe varus or valgus deformity compared to those with neutral alignment [44]. Sung et al. performed a similar comparative series in patients with varus deformity, with the first group containing patients with preoperative varus deformity greater than 20 degrees and the second group containing patients with varus deformity less than 20 degrees [45]. They found, at short-term follow-up after TAA, there was no statistically significant difference in clinical outcomes between the two groups.

Deformity correction is an important consideration for preoperative planning for patient's undergoing TAA, as correcting to neutral or as close to neutral as possible

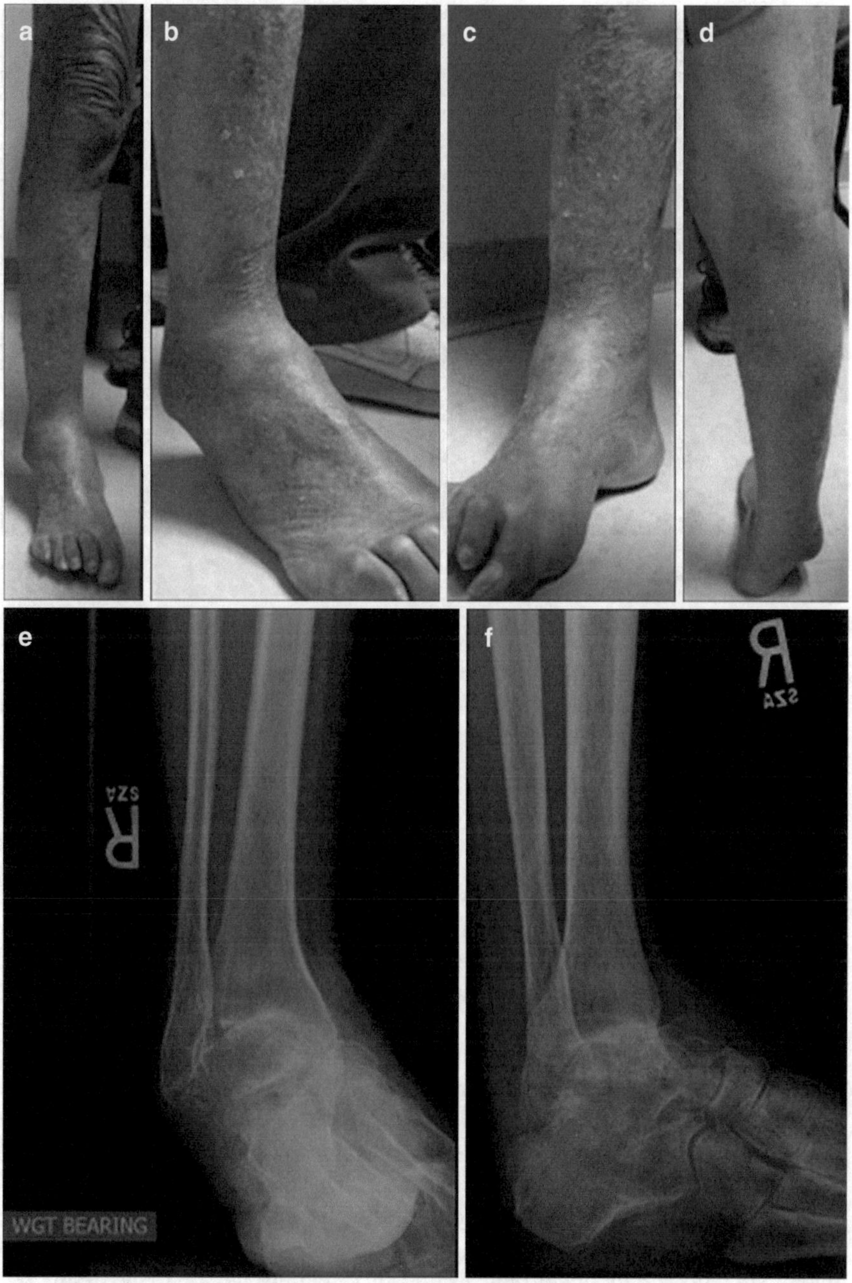


**Fig. 13.3** *Deformity*. 86-year-old healthy male with BMI = 23 kg/m$^2$ and 35 degree incongruent varus deformity. Failed three locked ankle AFO braces molded in varus (**a**–**f**). Three years post TAA (**g**, **h**). *Note intramedullary tibial component combined with flat cut talar component*

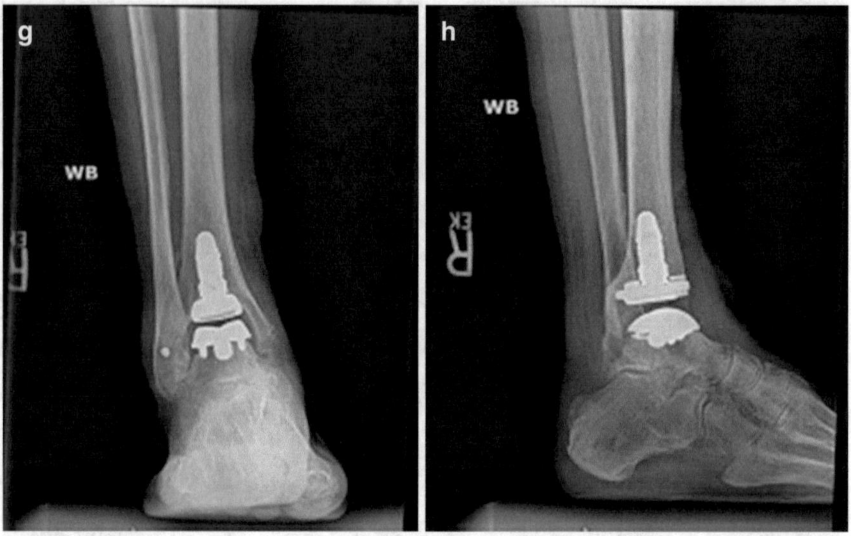


**Fig. 13.3** (continued)

can help prevent early implant failure. However, there are currently no strict guidelines regarding appropriate procedure selection for varus and valgus deformities in patients with ankle arthritis undergoing TAA. Further, it is beyond the scope of this chapter to describe concomitant procedures in detail.

## *Types of Implants*

The first generation of TAA implants were developed in the 1970s. These early attempts were composed of a concave polyethylene tibial component and a convex metal talar component. The talar component was made of cobalt chrome alloy, and both the talar and tibial components were fixated with cement. These implants were developed using the same principles as those for other total joint replacements; thus the use of cement fixation was preferred due to the added stability seen in total hip and knee replacements [51]. These devices came in both constrained and unconstrained designs. Constrained implants were developed for a simple hinge joint and restricted motion to ankle flexion and extension. This led to loosening as a result of inability to dissipate rotational forces produced at the ankle joint during ambulation. On the other end of the spectrum, unconstrained implants allowed excessive amounts of motion at the ankle joint, resulting in instability and soft tissue strain [52].

Both of the early TAA implant designs ignored the unique biomechanical characteristics of the ankle joint and, as a result, were associated with high failure rates. Complications with the first-generation TAA implants included prosthetic loosening, wide osteolysis, subsidence, and mechanical failure [51]. The next phase of

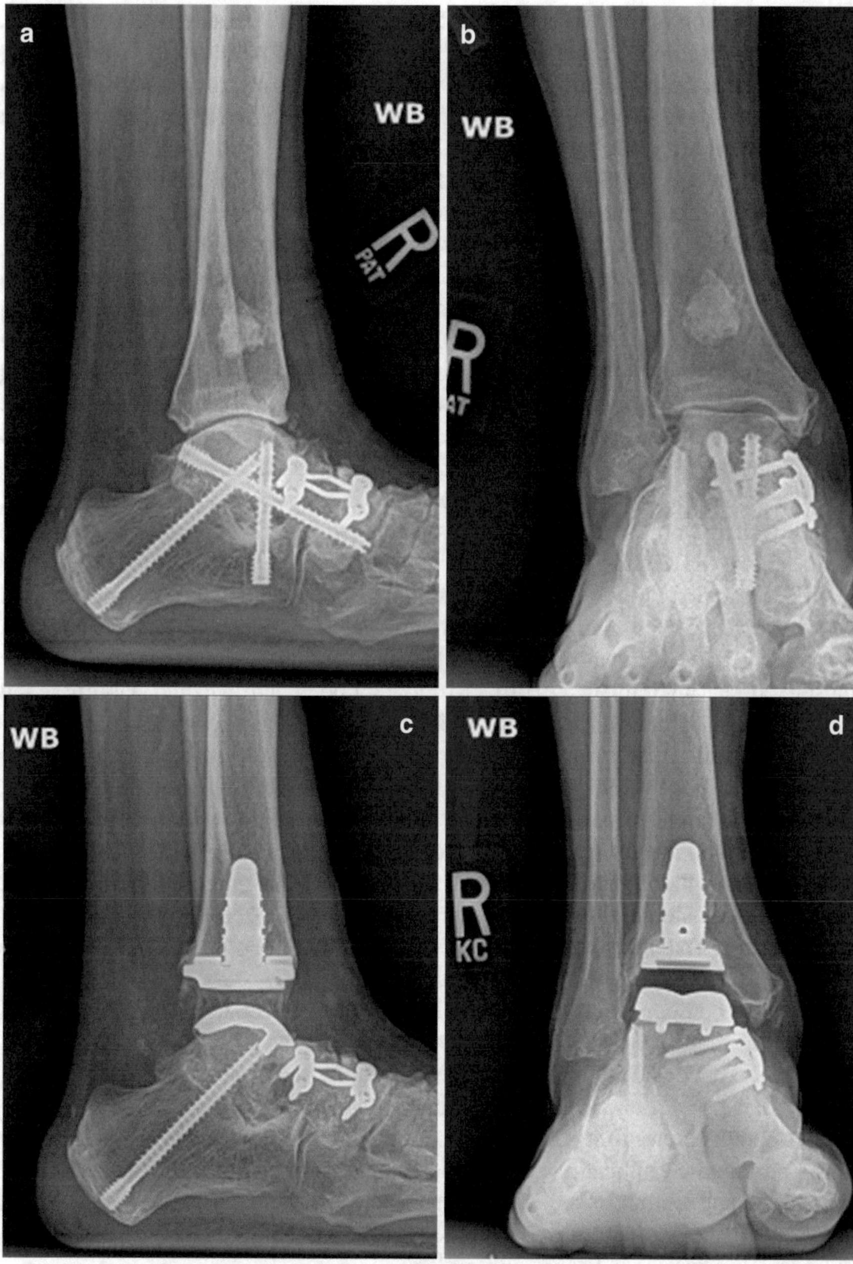


**Fig. 13.4** *Deformity*. 76-year-old healthy male, BMI = 31 kg/m$^2$. Incongruent valgus with residual 10-degree deformity 8 months post first-stage medial double arthrodesis and deltoid plication (**a**, **b**). Six months post TAA (**c**, **d**). *Note intramedullary tibial component combined with chamfer cut – resurfacing talar dome component*

implants, starting in the 1980s and continuing with small variations to present day, used a semiconstrained approach in order to accommodate rotational forces at the ankle while providing stability. In addition, these devices improved on prior designs by preserving bone stock, allowing for cementless application, and including porous coating to encourage biological fixation [52].

There have been significant evolutions to the design of total ankle implants over the past four decades; however, the basic components of the design have remained relatively stable. This includes a tibial component, a talar component, and a polyethylene interface component. By convention, present-day TAA implants are divided into either fixed-bearing (two component) implants or mobile-bearing (three component) implants. The fixed-bearing implants are unique in the fact that the polyethylene central component is locked into the tibial tray of the implant. Mobile-bearing implants allow the polyethylene component to float within the joint between the metallic tibial and talar components. In theory, the mobile-bearing implant allows for triplanar movement, which allows for a more natural, anatomic motion at the ankle joint. Currently in the United States, there is only one mobile-bearing implant that is available on the market and FDA approved, the Scandinavian Total Ankle Replacement (STAR) [53].

In general, tibial trays are unique in design to each implant. One example of this is the type of material used. The tibial component of mobile-bearing TAA implants is typically made of cobalt-chrome alloy, while titanium is the metal of choice for most fixed-bearing implants. In order to allow for bony ingrowth and stability of the implant, the proximal surface of the tibial tray typically has a porous coating consisting of titanium plasma spray. Titanium has been found to be bioinert and osteoconductive to promote bony ingrowth acting as a biologic form of fixation. Chrome alloy tends to remain separate from the surrounding bone by a thin layer of collagen [54]. Tibial trays also utilize different fixation components to penetrate the tibia for stabilization without increasing stress shielding of the implant. These different options include stemmed prosthesis (Inbone II, Invision), keel (Salto Talaris, Salto XT), barrel (STAR), cage and peg (Vantage), multiple peg (Infinity), peg and fin (cadence), and fixation rails (trabecular metal).

The talar component of the implant is composed of cobalt chrome alloy in all implants available in the United States. Similar to the tibial tray, the interface between the bone and the implant is typically composed of porous titanium plasma spray. Later-generation implants advocate for less bony resection of the talus with greater contact area of the talar component in order to prevent subsidence, which was a common complication of earlier implants [52]. The type of talar cuts performed for application of the talar component varies with the type of implant but includes anatomic, flattop, and chamfer. This will be discussed further in the "Surgical Techniques & Pearls" subsection.

The polyethylene central component in both fixed- and mobile-bearing devices is composed of ultrahigh-molecular-weight polyethylene (UHMWPE) or highly cross-linked polyethylene spacer (HXLPE). This component in modern TAA implants acts as a "meniscus" within the prosthesis to allow for smooth and congruent motion [53].

## Fixed- vs. Mobile-Bearing Devices

Modern convention separates TAA implants in fixed- and mobile-bearing devices, each with its proposed advantages. The major benefit of mobile-bearing prostheses, as previously alluded to, is greater distribution of load through the ankle joint leading to decreased wear of the polyethylene component and therefore longer lifespan of the implant. Proponents of fixed-bearing implants appreciate its ability to increase ankle motion, while also providing stability and decreasing strain on soft tissue structures [51–53].

Gaudot et al. evaluated the difference in short-term outcomes between mobile-bearing and fixed-bearing implants. Both implant designs showed significant improvement in the postoperative AOFAS score compared to the preoperative score after a mean follow-up of 2 years. There was no statistically significant difference appreciated between the two implants. A secondary measure evaluated complications associated with the implants. They found a rate of subluxation between the tibial component and polyethylene insert of 18% for the mobile-bearing implants. In addition, a significantly higher incidence of radiolucent lines surrounding the tibial component was reported in the mobile-bearing implant (39%) compared to the fixed-bearing implant (12%) [55].

Another study from 2014, by Queen et al., investigated functional outcomes in 90 patients after TAA with 49 receiving a mobile-bearing implant (STAR) and 41 receiving a fixed-bearing implant (Salto Talaris). They compared functional outcomes and gait analysis as well as patient-reported outcomes at three time points – preoperatively, 1-year postoperatively, and 2 years postoperatively. The fixed-bearing group showed greater improvements in ground reactive forces and ankle moment, while the mobile-bearing group had greater improvements in patient-reported pain outcomes. Ultimately, they found few significant differences between the two implant types across time, and all outcomes showed improved or maintained function following TAA. This study did not assess complications and was limited by its relatively short follow-up and lack of randomization into the implant groups [56].

## FDA-Approved Implants

The following list and subsequent table contain the current FDA-approved implants available (Table 13.1).

### Mobile Bearing

1. Scandinavian Total Ankle Replacement (STAR)

### Fixed-Bearing Implants

1. Inbone II
2. Salto Talaris
3. Trabecular metal
4. Infinity

**Table 13.1** Implants currently in use and available on the market with Food and Drug Administration (FDA) approval in the United States

| Implant | Manufacturer | Design | Year available in the United States |
|---|---|---|---|
| Scandinavian Total Ankle Replacement (STAR) | Stryker (Kalamazoo, MI) | Mobile bearing | 1999 |
| Inbone II | Wright Medical (Arlington, TN) | Fixed bearing | 2005 |
| Salto Talaris | Integra (Plainsboro, NJ) | Fixed bearing | 2006 |
| Trabecular metal | Zimmer Biomet (Warsaw, IN) | Fixed bearing | 2013 |
| Infinity | Wright Medical (Arlington, TN) | Fixed bearing | 2014 |
| Cadence | Integra (Plainsboro, NJ) | Fixed bearing | 2016 |
| Vantage | Exactech (Gainesville, FL) | Fixed bearing | 2016 |
| Salto XT | Integra (Plainsboro, NJ) | Fixed bearing | 2018 |
| Invision | Wright Medical (Arlington, TN) | Fixed bearing | 2018 |

5. Cadence
6. Vantage

**Revision Implants**

1. Salto XT
2. Invision

Over time, various iterations of implants have been introduced and modified. The convention is to designate these as generations. Generations of implants are based on the chronological order of the development of the implant as well as advancements in technique and implant design. Although the concept of classification by generation is widely accepted, some controversy exists, because there is a preference to be considered in a more contemporary generation. Many implants in earlier generations have undergone multiple iterations of improvements within the implant itself. For instance, the STAR implant is currently utilizing its fourth version of the implant in the United States, which is the only generation approved by the FDA. For organizational expediency, implants that were considered new versions with small improvements of previous implants or implants designed for revision were included in the same generation. In order to be considered a different generation, significant advancement of technology and/or technique was required (Table 13.2) [57].

**Table 13.2** Generation of implants currently available on the market in the United States based on chronological release and advancement of technologies associated with the implant

| **Second-generation implants** | |
|---|---|
| STAR | Stryker |
| Third-generation implants | |
| Inbone II | Wright |
| Salto Talaris | Integra |
| Salto XT | Integra |
| Trabecular metal | Zimmer |
| Invision | Wright |
| Fourth-generation implants | |
| Infinity | Wright |
| Vantage | Exactech |
| Cadence | Integra |

## Navigation Guidance

One of the most significant advancements in the fourth-generation implants has been the introduction of navigational guidance. In any joint replacement surgery, and particularly in the ankle joint, proper positioning and alignment of implants are critical for proper weight transfer and kinematics. As a result, systems have been devised utilizing preoperative computed tomography (CT) to produce patient-specific guides. This so-called navigation is theorized to provide more accurate and reproducible implant alignment and, as a result, reduce the rate of implant failure [58, 59].

The first preoperative computer-assisted guidance system developed specifically for the ankle was the PROPHECY Preoperative Navigation System, which was released in 2012. It is intended for use with the Inbone II Total Ankle System and the Infinity Total Ankle System (Wright Medical Technology, Inc., Memphis, TN). A hip-to-foot or knee-to-foot CT scan of the patient is performed preoperatively. From these images, a custom alignment guide is created for both the tibial and talar components of the implant. These custom guides reduce the amount of necessary intraoperative instrumentation and steps, which results in reduced operative time [59, 60].

The benefit of using computed navigation guidance in total knee arthroplasty is controversial, with recent outcomes demonstrating minimal clinical improvement over conventional techniques [61, 62]. Recent studies suggest that the unique biomechanical properties of the ankle do benefit from this guidance. In one study by Hsu et al., preoperative patient-specific guides were able to predict tibia component size in 100% of Inbone II cases and 92% of Infinity cases. The talar component sizing with the guides seemed to be less accurate with correct predictions in 76% of Inbone II cases and 46% in Infinity cases. Further, radiographic alignment of all postoperative TAA cases was within three degrees of the predicted preoperative CT scan-derived plans [63].

A retrospective comparative study by Daigre et al. using the Inbone II demonstrated similar results to that of Hsu et al. [64]. The implant size was correctly predicted in 98% of cases for the tibial component and 80% of cases for the talar component. The radiographic postoperative position of the tibial component was within three degrees of the preoperative plan in 79.5% of their 44 patients. Talar component postoperative position was not reported. Finally, a cadaveric study by Berlet et al. concluded that final Inbone II implant position using preoperative image-derived patient-specific guides was accurate and reproducible with less than two degrees of deviation from the preoperative plan [65].

While results regarding the accuracy and reproducibility with preoperative patient-specific navigation are promising thus far, questions regarding this technology still remain. For instance, long-term follow-up using this technology is needed to assess whether there is improvement in implant longevity and reduction in need for revision due to malalignment. Further, the cost-benefit of using a navigation system in TAA has not been studied. Therefore, further studies examining long-term outcomes need to be performed to fully understand the benefits of using patient-specific navigation guidance in TAA.

## *Surgical Technique and Pearls*

### Approach

An anterior approach is typically used for most total ankle replacement implants. A 10–14 cm longitudinal incision is centered on the anterior aspect of the ankle and carried down to the subcutaneous layer (Fig. 13.5). Nerves and tendons should be identified and protected with gentle retraction. The incision is then taken down to capsule, which provides adequate exposure of the ankle joint [3]. The anterior approach for TAA has many advantages, including level and ease of exposure. However, wound-healing issues are a commonly cited complication with this approach, with reported rates as high as 40% [16, 66, 67].

Alternatively, a lateral transfibular approach can be utilized with the Zimmer Trabecular Metal Total Ankle prosthesis. This approach necessitates a lateral skin incision measuring 8–15 cm along the lateral malleolus that curves toward the sinus tarsi. Unlike the anterior approach, which exposes the ankle through soft tissue dissection alone, the lateral approach also requires that an oblique lateral malleolar osteotomy be performed [66–68]. Theoretically, the lateral transfibular approach allows comparable or even improved visualization over the anterior approach. This approach also eliminates the risk of damaging the important anterior neurovascular structures but puts other structures at risk, such as the sural nerve and peroneal tendons. Further, it is purported to allow for less bone resection, but whether this is a result of the lateral approach itself or due to the curved design of the Zimmer implant remains to be seen.

Supporters of the lateral approach claim that its incision is more ideally placed in terms of preserving blood supply and adhering to the principle of angiosomes, which theoretically should decrease the incidence of wound dehiscence compared to the anterior incision. However, in a recent study by Useulli et al., no significant

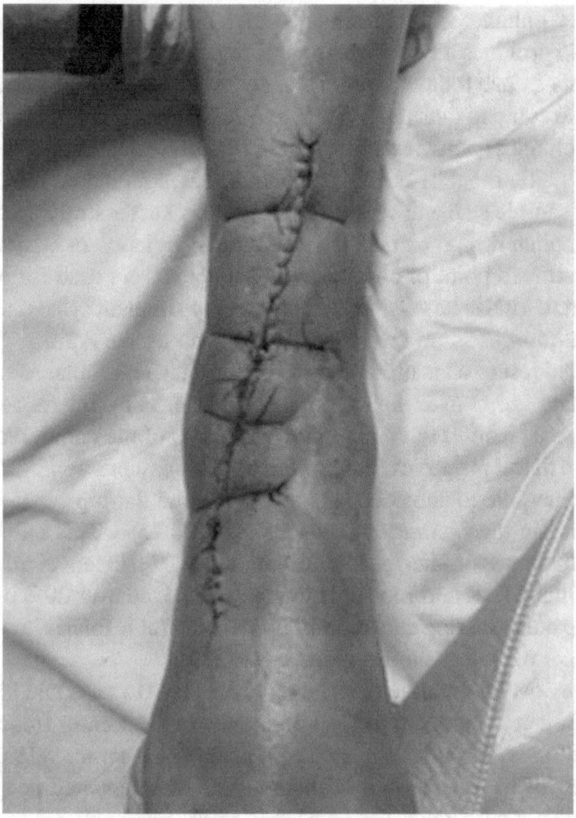

**Fig. 13.5** *Approach.* Anterior approach for TAA consisting of a 10–14 cm longitudinal incision

difference was found between the anterior and lateral approach in the frequency of superficial and deep wound infections within 1 year after TAA [67].

While the lateral transfibular approach has notable theoretical benefits over the anterior approach, review of the literature shows that it is, in practice, a safe and effective technique for TAA [66–69]. However, it is not without its disadvantages, particularly the significantly longer operating times required with this approach [67]. While uncommon, there is the added risk of delayed union, nonunion, and malunion of the fibular osteotomy not present in an uncomplicated anterior approach [66–69].

## Bone Resection

Insertion of the implants requires bone cuts in the tibia and talus. The amount of resection needed is often dictated by the type of implant being used, as well as the presence and degree of varus or valgus deformity. It is generally accepted that minimizing bony resection and maintaining the natural architecture of the bony surface is preferred to enhance joint mechanics and thereby increase longevity of the implant. It also provides a better substrate if revision is ever necessary [58, 70].

All implants in use today claim that they are bone sparing; however, only one study has made comparisons [70]. Goetz and colleagues observed significant differences in the volume of bony resection required for implantation between four different implants, with the STAR and Inbone II having greater resection. Despite limitations of sample size and cadaveric limbs, they successfully demonstrated that variation in implant design can lead to measurable variation in bony resection.

An oft-mentioned point of contention is the type of cut used for the talar dome, flat or contoured. This is largely dependent upon the implant system used. The more traditional flat-top cut is utilized in implants such as the Agility, Inbone II, and STAR. A curved resection is utilized with the Zimmer Trabecular Metal Total Ankle to accommodate the convex talar component. The Salto Talaris and the Infinity implants utilize a chamfer cut technique. Advocates of the contoured cuts, such as chamfer, argue that it preserves more of the original osseous architecture and therefore is less vulnerable to subsidence compared to the flat-top cut [58]. The rate of talar subsidence in the literature ranges from 1% to 15%. This rate has decreased over time with the use of later-generation implants [71]. Goetz et al. found that the flat-top cut of the STAR and Inbone II implants removed over 20% of the talar volume, while the bone-sparing cuts of the Zimmer and Salto Talaris implants removed 15% and 13% of the talar volume, respectively [70].

The relative novelty of ankle replacement compared to knee and hip arthroplasty makes it more open to innovation. The complexity of these cases frequently requires adaptive solutions. As mentioned before, patients with a severe valgus deformity or stage IV posterior tibial tendon dysfunction with an attenuated deep deltoid ligament are often poor candidates for TAA. In the past, these patients would be treated with a highly stable, stemmed intramedullary tibial component with a flat cut talar component or even told that TAA was not possible. In the past year, the author (PB) has adapted the standardized technique to be more inclusive. By combining the enhanced stability of an intramedullary tibia component with the chamfer cut talar component, greater osseous stability is possible (Fig. 13.4). This technique reduces the talar resection by at least 0.5 cm, which may reduce the risk of talar subsidence relative to the flat-top talar component. Thus far, ten patients have been treated with this modular interchange which was made possible with the use of CT planned preoperative guidance. There has not been an increase in operative time nor has the expected coronal and sagittal plane alignment of less than three degrees from the guidance report been sacrificed. Thus the technological advancements can build upon one another to expand the potential candidates for care.

## *Complications*

As with any surgical intervention, complications are a constant source of patient morbidity and surgeon frustration. The following sections define a range of complications and their incidence. In order to achieve this objective, the authors performed a meta-analysis of available literature spanning from 2013 to 2018. Sixteen studies, with 2,467 TAAs performed, met the desired selection criteria and were considered for part of the analysis [72]. These results were frequently compared to two other studies, performed by Gadd et al. and Glazebrook et al. [73, 74]. We believe the variability in outcomes is largely due to the evidence base utilized during different samples and implant generations. Glazebrook's team drew data from studies between 1997 and 2007 and, similar to our own investigation, used a collective assessment study design to report outcomes. In contrast, Gadd and colleagues used their own ankle replacement database for surgeries performed between 1995 and 2010. It is believed that since Knabel's data is taken from studies published between 2013 and 2018, the data is more reflective of more recent implant iterations [72].

## Wound Healing

Wound healing complications associated with the incision are not uncommon following TAA. As discussed in "Approach" above, the incision itself is vulnerable to compromised healing. Delayed wound healing or even frank wound dehiscence are poorly defined within the literature. The incidence has been reported to be as high as 12% according to one study by Criswell and colleagues [75]. The pooled data taken from 16 studies found that the mean incidence rate was 5% [72]. In that same summary, most patients responded well to simple wound care, while 1.4% needed some kind of soft tissue flap or graft to achieve closure (Fig. 13.6).

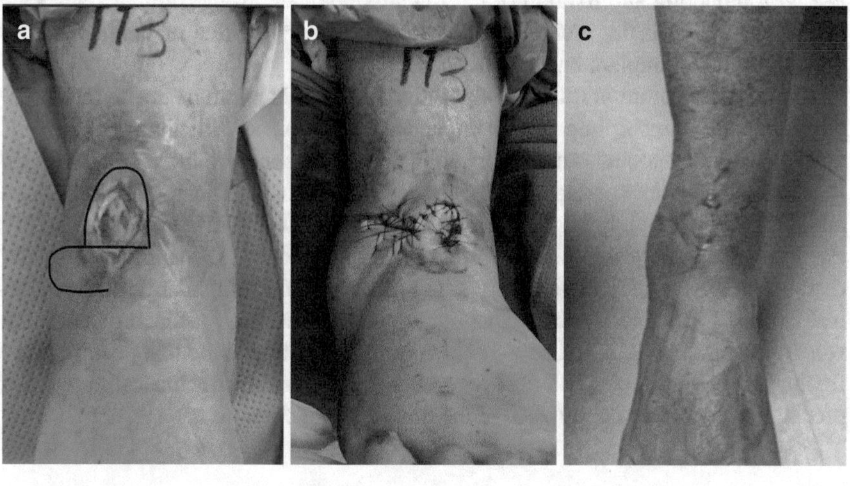


**Fig. 13.6** *Wound healing*. (**a**) Dehiscence of anterior ankle incision at 10 weeks status post TAA that was subsequently treated with a rotational flap. (**b**) Immediate postoperative photo of the rotational flap. (**c**) Well-healed incision at 9 months status post rotational flap and 1-year status post TAA

## Infection

A closely related complication is infection, either superficial or deep. A recent meta-analysis showed that mean infection rate in elective foot and ankle surgeries was 2.5% [76]. They further found that the presence of wound dehiscence increased the relative risk of infection by 21 [95% CI (9.96, 32.84)]. Kessler et al. reported on this phenomenon in a small case-control study of ankle replacements [77]. They found that the odds of periprosthetic ankle infection were 15.38 [95% CI (2.91, 81.34] times that of the controls in the setting of wound dehiscence. Limiting the discussion to TAA, superficial infection rates have been noted as high as 3.6% in one study of 249 implants [78]. Our pooled analysis found that TAA carried a 2% risk of superficial infection. The highest rate of deep infection reported was 30.7% in a small sample of 26 patients. The collective data indicates that the actual incidence of deep infection is approximately 1.2%. The pooled incidence of any infection is 1.9% [72].

## Fracture

TAA is vulnerable to two types of fracture. The first is intraoperative fracture and is largely the result of technical errors. The preparation of the recipient site is difficult and precise. Saw blade excursion can inadvertently take more bone than desired resulting in a stress riser through the malleolus. Our summary of data found that the mean incidence is 5.5% [72]. Glazebrook designated this as a low-grade complication occurring 8.1% of the time, infrequently resulting in TAA failure [74]. This complication is usually evident at the time of surgery and reasonably easy to manage with reduction and fixation of the fractured element. Some surgeons advocate prophylactically placing guide wires for fixation of the medial malleolus prior to making the tibial implant cuts in osteoporotic bone.

Slightly less common is the postoperative fracture. This can be due to instability of the implant or resorption of peri-implant bone combined with abnormal loading. Once the patient becomes ambulatory, the remodeling bone and increased forces led to fracture in a variety of anatomic locations. Glazebrook's systematic review found an incidence of 2%, but that led to implant failure in 16.7% of affected cases [74]. Early recognition is essential, prior to implant migration. Treatment involves standard internal fixation. Our summary suggests that the mean incidence in the literature is 3.1% [72]. Gadd reported that both intraoperative and postoperative fracture were uncommon with less than a 5% incidence [73]. They found that postoperative fracture had a far greater risk of revision than intraoperative fracture, with revision procedures occurring nearly 70% of the time in those cases.

## Osteolysis

The greatest concern with all joint replacements is the eventual loss of fixation from one or both of the metallic components. Osteolysis, or loss of bone, when associated with a total joint prosthesis, is synonymous with the term periprosthetic lucency.

Over time, the question remains as to how long, or if ever, will the radiolucencies progress to subsidence or aseptic loosening. The difficulty in clinical practice is how and when to correlate the radiographic findings with recommending surgical intervention. In the 2004 study by Knecht et al., relevant osteolysis was defined as an area >2 mm [79] (Fig. 13.7).

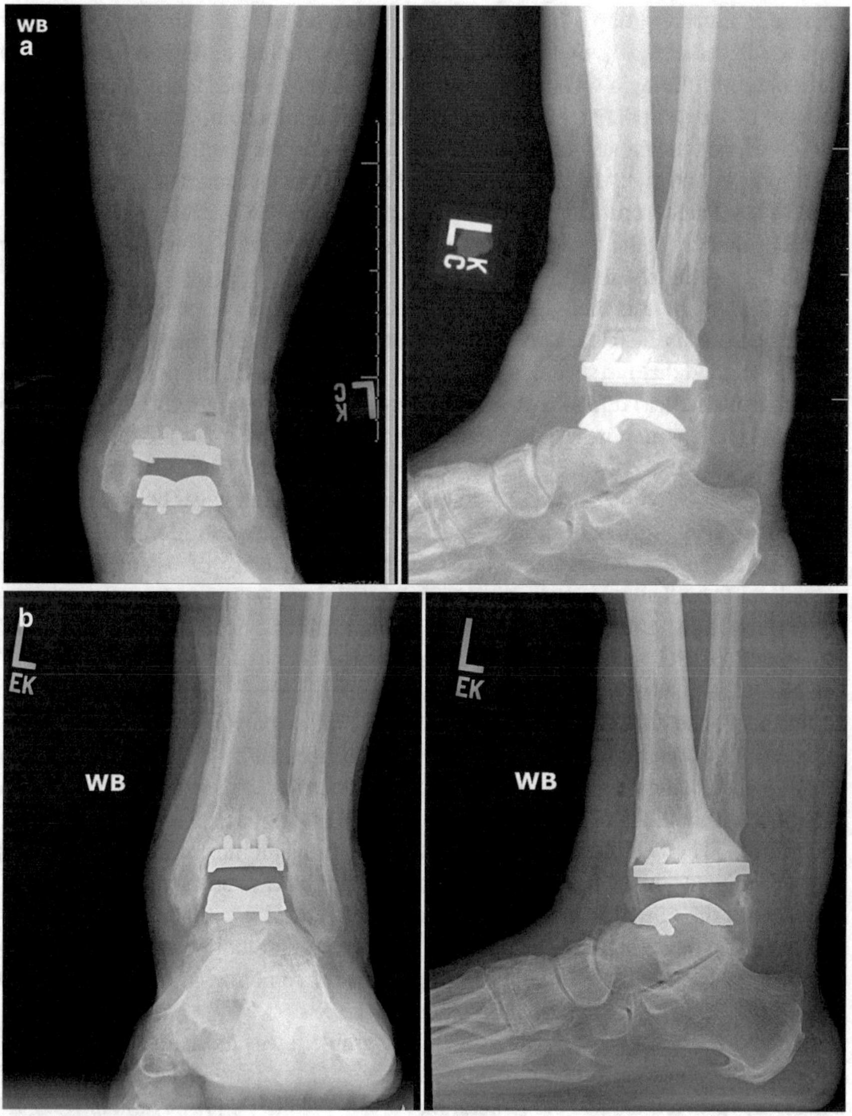


**Fig. 13.7** *Osteolysis*. (**a**) 60-year-old male 1-year post-op showing no zone of radiolucency. (**b**) At the 2-year postoperative evaluation, the patient has approximately 2 mm of radiolucency at the tibial component. Although the patient is asymptomatic, the patient will be monitored every 6 months for signs of progression

Treatment for this issue has largely relied on debridement and bone grafting to prevent progression and instability. A major roadblock to prevention has been the unclear mechanism of action, but several etiologies have been explored. One theory is that metal wear particles or particulate debris from degradation of the polyethylene insert results in an excessive inflammatory response. In 2018, Schipper et al. compared pathology samples from 57 fixed-bearing ankle prostheses with osteolysis and a mean in vivo longevity of 6.0 (range 0–15) years, compared to non-prosthetic control group of 11 samples of tissue taken at the time of a primary implant placement [80]. Seventy percent of the specimens in the osteolysis group were obtained during a revision procedure with the remainder taken during a bone grafting of the periphery of the intact undisturbed component. They observed that the osteolytic specimens were associated with inflammatory infiltrates composed of macrophages and giant cells which were not seen in the osteoarthritic control specimens. They found a correlation with abundant implant wear particles and inflammation. The authors concluded that future efforts should prioritize fabrication of wear resistant polyethylene inserts [80].

Another hypothesis thought to mediate osteolysis is the presence of a host reaction to necrotic tissue, bone ischemia, hydrostatic pressure, and micromotion. Koivu et al. concluded that the severe inflammatory reaction seen in the periprosthetic tissues of explants was due to a chronic, persistent foreign body reaction to necrotic tissue [81]. Other authors also analyzed pathology samples of periprosthetic tissues after explantation of the Ankle Evolutive System (AES), manufactured by Transysteme, (Nimes, France). Although this implant has never been available in the United States, it has been heavily studied in the European literature [82, 83]. This second-generation implant had an increased incidence of osteolysis. In the investigation by Koivu et al., they determined that there was an acute inflammatory event through increased expression of proinflammatory cytokines. The cascade of the RANKL/OPG pathway led to nuclear factor kappa B ligand stimulation of osteoclasts, ultimately causing osteolysis.

Further concern for the role of micromotion in the osteolytic process of TAA was explored by Sopher et al. in 2017 [84]. They utilized finite-element modeling to quantify the smallest amount of micromotion occurring at the implant-bone interface of either the tibial or talar component in three implant designs (BOX, Mobility, and Salto). They concluded that initial component malalignment had a significant role on implant loosening but that implant seating was even more critical. They emphasized the importance of complete seating of implant components with minimal to no gapping with the bone interface to prevent micromotion and implant loosening. They found this more relevant to prevent micromotion-mediated osteolysis than implant design or slight malalignment [84].

With regard to incidence of osteolysis, the problem was more ubiquitous in earlier designs compared to contemporary implants. One of the highest incidence of osteolysis involved the second generation Agility prosthesis [79]. Another second-generation implant, the STAR, is still widely used in spite of reports of as high as a 39% incidence of osteolysis [85, 86]. The pooled data from newer generations by Knabel reported that these cystic changes were evident in 3.5% of all cases [72].

Vigilance is key to identify these radiographic signs prior to progression. Surgeons often schedule patients for a biannual or an annual visit to monitor for early radiographic changes [87].

### Subsidence

Kopp and colleagues defined subsidence as implant migration or position change of either the tibial or talar component by ≥5 mm [88]. Hintermann used slightly different thresholds for the tibial and talar components [89]. They stated that talar component positional changes were meaningful when ≥5 mm or 5 degrees. That threshold is lower in the tibia, where changes of ≥2 mm or 2 degrees were considered significant. The underlying cause is due to lack of osseous integration or implant stability that leads to migration. The talar implant is more frequently the site of subsidence, although the introduction of chamfer cut talar preparation has been designed to reduce this risk [79]. Glazebrook et al. reported a subsidence rate of 10.7%, and that 32% went on to implant failure as a result [74]. Gadd et al. found that <1% of patients developed this complication, but when present, 100% of patients required some form of revision [73]. Our meta-analysis found that the incidence of subsidence was 3% and that survivorship was 92.6% [9, 72].

### Aseptic Loosening

This complication is defined as the absence of osseous ingrowth or ongrowth with either the tibial or talar component. It can also be the result of mechanical loading or osseous resorption after implantation. Radiographically, this is seen as ≥2 mm of lucency around the implants [90]. In some instances the lucency is surrounded by a sclerotic rim. The presence of this complication predisposes the implants to instability and subsidence, failure of cement when present, and fracture. Gadd et al. reported that this complication occurred only 3–4% of the time but typically led to a > 80% revision rate [73]. Glazebrook et al. determined that the incidence was 8.7% and led to failure in 70.3% of cases [74]. Knabel and colleagues found an incidence more similar to the Gadd et al. study with a mean rate of 3% [72].

### Heterotopic Ossification

More commonly referred to as "bone spurs" by patients and lay people, heterotopic ossification (HO) is postoperative, peri-prosthetic bone growth with no known etiology [91]. Although several luminaries have posited that it is associated with under-coverage of the prepared joint surface by the implant, termed undersizing, confirmation has been elusive. Another popular theory is that malalignment of the mechanical axis leads to soft tissue traction and that predisposes extra-osseous bone formation [92, 93]. A comprehensive study by

Manegold and co-investigators found that after 1 year, 86.4% of their patients developed HO [91]. As these patients were followed out to 3 years, the prevalence rate increased to 99%, simultaneously the severity was also observed to worsen. They investigated further and found that localization could occur in single or multiple sites. After 3 years, posterior gutter ossification occurred in 98.9% of patients, followed by lateral (54.5%), anterior (26.1%), and finally medial (22.7%). Only 13.7% of cases suffered from undersizing of the implants. They did find weak correlations between implant alignment and early ossification, but this correlation diminished by final follow-up. The lower rate of anterior HO may have been lower in this study due to the closed implant design. Another study reported a prevalence of 50% after 18 months in implants with a mismatch between the size of the tibial component and anteroposterior tibial depth dimensions [94]. Knabel et al. found that the mean incidence rate was 10.6% which may be reflective of inconsistent definitions used by different investigators and variable follow-up [72].

## Implant Failure

This final complication is primarily concerned with the structural failure of any of the implant components. Failure is largely the result of wear, and there are five major mechanisms of wear: adhesion, abrasion, third body, corrosion, and fatigue [95]. These mechanisms impart physical changes to the implants leaving both microscopic and macroscopic signs. This includes signs of abrasive wear that can be seen as scratching, burnishing, abrasion, pitting, and delamination to name a few. A superficial trail imprinted on the material surface is considered a scratch. Burnished materials have a shiny surface attributed to excessive rubbing and may be seen in areas where machine marks have disappeared. Abrasions are often seen as a shredded or tufted appearance. Points within the material surface are seen as pitting. And, delamination is when a thin layer of one surface separates from the deeper layers. A 2019 article by Currier and colleagues explanted 70 TAAs after a median in vivo time of 4.5 years [96]. Forty-one percent of the metallic implants were available for analysis, while 97% of the polyethylene components were available. They rated wear and fatigue of the polyethylene implants and found that burnishing followed by abrasion were the two most common signs of wear. Fatigue, represented by cracking and delamination, was also commonly observed after explantation. In fact, every polyethylene analyzed showed evidence of one of these modes of damage. Of these removals, 14.2% were associated with a fractured polyethylene insert. Knabel et al. found that the pooled polyethylene exchange rate was 3.1% [72].

Failure of the metallic portions is the most consequential to patients. Unlike polyethylene inserts which are relatively interchangeable, the loss of the metallic interfaces mean that revision will involve additional bone loss and reintegration with the bone. Glazebrook et al. reported that the implant failure rate was 5% in their pooled analysis [74]. This is higher than the ~2% reported by Gadd et al. [73].

When implant failure was present, ~80% of patients required a revision surgery. Knabel found that the mean implant failure rate was 2.4% in more recent literature [72].

## *Outcomes*

### Survivorship

Every patient that is treated with a joint replacement will eventually ask the question "How long will it last?" or what proportion of joint replacements are still present and unmodified after several years? Patients and physicians want to know how long implants will last and what the probability is that they will require a revision or replacement of the implant. Zaidi et al. performed a meta-analysis in 2013 looking at rates of complications as well as survivorship of replacements. The mean follow-up for the study was 8.2 years, with a reported survivorship of 89% at 10 years. They further delineated survivorship between registry and non-registry studies and calculated that the 10-year survivorship was 72.6% for registry-based studies and 88.7% for non-registry-based investigations [35].

A meta-analysis was performed evaluating the survivorship of total ankle implants in 2019, focused on contemporary publications after 2013. The hypothesis was that more recent publications would include more contemporary joint replacement techniques. The results showed an overall survivorship of 93% when evaluating over 1,900 implants after a mean follow up of 63.6 months. The authors attempted to determine if implant type had a relevant impact on survivorship. Mobile-bearing implant survivorship was 89.4% compared to fixed-bearing implant survivorship of 95.6%, although an interesting trend, no statistically significant difference was detected. A highly plausible partial explanation for this trend would be that the implant with the longest follow-up (Scandinavian Total Ankle Replacement) is a mobile-bearing implant and therefore imparts an exposure bias to that analysis. Their analysis indicated that there was a correlation between the duration of follow-up and implant failure rate. Ultimately, the authors concluded that the longer an implant remains in vivo, the more likely it was to fail. Regardless of implant type, a meta-regression analysis of the data revealed that patients with higher preoperative functional scores had an association with superior survivorship ($P = 0.00115$). Unfortunately, the available data did not allow for exploration of functional thresholds [9].

### Revision Rates

Overall survivorship was discussed in the preceding section, while this section is concerned with when the implants need to be revised. Longevity is important to any joint replacement system, and the benchmark, for decades, has been knee replacements. In order to appropriately place ankle replacements within the revision hierarchy, a baseline context is necessary. A large systematic review was performed looking at a wide spectrum of joint arthroplasties as reported by national registers [97]. Longevity was based upon the observed component years, which was defined as a joint that is at risk for revision from the time it is inserted until the time of a revision or the patient expires. They considered 1,107,886 primary implants, with 495,978 total revisions. They found that the mean total hip replacement rate was 1.29 revisions per 100 observed component years. They extrapolated this to a 5-year revision rate of 6.45% and a 10-year revision rate of 12.9%. Total knee replacements had a revision rate that corresponds to 6.3% after 5 years and 12.6% after 10 years. The mean shoulder replacement revision rate was translated to a revision rate of 6.95% and 13.9% at 5 and 10 years, respectively. Elbow replacements had the highest revision rate, with 5.08 per 100 observed component years. The sample for ankle replacements was relatively small, with 3 registries comprising 1,225 implants. The mean revision rate was 3.29 per 100 observed component years, which is calculated as a 16.45% revision rate after 5 years. The crude rate was 19.9% for all ankle replacements. It is noteworthy that these registries followed cases from 1993 to 2007 with a mean follow-up of 6.05 years [97].

Gadd et al. in 2014 retrospectively reviewed the Sheffield foot and ankle TAA database from 1995 to 2010 [73]. Although they found that 24.5% suffered some kind of complication, only 17% went on to a revision. The mean time to revision was 635 days or 1.73 years. Of the patients requiring revision, 33% (5.6% of all ankle replacements) needed a component exchange of the ankle replacement implant. Sixty-one percent required a conversion to ankle arthrodesis, and 5% underwent below-knee amputations. Knabel found that the poly exchange rate was 3.1% and metal implant revision rate was 6.4% [72]. Collectively, only 2.1% of patients went on to a revision with fusion. This is important because as generations of ankle replacement implants evolve, the revision rates have improved. Labek cites that regulatory institutions like the National Institute for Health and Care Excellence (NICE) demand a maximum revision rate of 10% after 10 years for hips and knees [97]. The technology and procedure are well established in these anatomic locations, while corresponding ankle replacement technology continues to undergo more significant contemporary changes. The 10-year, 10% revision rate is a worthy aspiration but remains out of reach for many hip and knee registries as well.

## Summary

Total ankle arthroplasties have yet to reach the ubiquitous implantation rates of knee and hip replacements, but acceptance has widened as the technology and techniques continue to evolve. The TAA evidence base remains relatively small, but the past decade has seen a massive increase in related publications. Very little high-level clinical evidence exists, and most of the knowledge base is collected from level 3 and 4 studies. Many traditional surgical risk factors apply to TAAs as well. One of the most critical is preoperative deformity, specifically relative to frontal plane alignments. Even these tolerances have increased over the past decade when the appropriate concomitant procedures are performed. There are a variety of complications that are unique to major joint replacement, and TAA is no exception. The frequency of complications has decreased in the literature as our understanding of patient selection becomes more optimized. Not only have complication rates diminished, but a corresponding improvement in overall implant survivorship has also been observed. As stated in the beginning, much contemporary literature heavily cites a systematic review of last generation's ankle implants. Further research with a focus on clinical efficacy is needed for today's technological strides.

## References

1. Malik AT, Noordin S. The top 50 most-cited articles on Total Ankle Arthroplasty: a bibliometric analysis. Orthop Rev (Pavia). 2018;10(1):7498.
2. Haddad SL, Coetzee JC, Estok R, Fahrbach K, Banel D, Nalysnyk LJ. Intermediate and long-term outcomes of total ankle arthroplasty and ankle arthrodesis. A systematic review of the literature. Bone Joint Surg Am. 2007;89(9):1899–905.
3. Reeves CL, Shane AM, Vazales R. Current concepts regarding total ankle replacement as a viable treatment option for advanced ankle arthritis: what you need to know. Clin Podiatr Med Surg. 2017;34(4):515–27.
4. Steck JK, Anderson JB. Total ankle arthroplasty: indications and avoiding complications. Clin Podiatr Med Surg. 2009;26:303–24.
5. Saltzman CL, Salamon ML, Blanchard GM, et al. Epidemiology of ankle arthritis: report of a consecutive series of 639 patients from a tertiary orthopaedic center. Iowa Orthop J. 2005;25:44–6.
6. Glazebrook M, Daniels T, Younger A, Foote CJ, Penner M, Wing K, Lau J, Leighton R, Dunbar M. Comparison of health-related quality of life between patients with end-stage ankle and hip arthrosis. J Bone Joint Surg Am. 2008;90(3):499–505.
7. Spirt AA, Assal M, Hansen ST Jr. Complications and failure after total ankle arthroplasty. J Bone Joint Surg Am. 2004;86-A(6):1172–8.
8. Demetracopoulos CA, Adams SB Jr, Queen RM, DeOrio JK, Nunley JA 2nd, Easley ME. Effect of age on outcomes in total ankle arthroplasty. Foot Ankle Int. 2015;36(8):871–80.
9. McKenna BJ, Cook J, Cook EA, Crafton J, Knabel M, Swenson E, Miner S, Manning E, Basile P. Total ankle arthroplasty survivorship: a meta-analysis. J Foot Ankle Surg. Under Review.
10. Somayaji R, Barnabe C, Martin L. Risk factors for infection following total joint arthroplasty in rheumatoid arthritis. Open Rheumatol J. 2013;7:119–24.
11. Grennan DM, Gray J, Loudon J, Fear S. Methotrexate and early postoperative complications in patients with rheumatoid arthritis undergoing elective orthopaedic surgery. Ann Rheum Dis. 2001;60(3):214–7.
12. Giles JT, Bartlett SJ, Gelber AC, et al. Tumor necrosis factor inhibitor therapy and risk of serious postoperative orthopedic infection in rheumatoid arthritis. Arthritis Rheum. 2006;55(2):333–7.
13. den Broeder AA, Creemers MC, Fransen J, et al. Risk factors for surgical site infections and other complications in elective surgery in patients with rheumatoid arthritis with special attention for anti-tumor necrosis factor: a large retrospective study. J Rheumatol. 2007;34(4):689–95.
14. Hazlewood D, Winfield J. Biological therapy in the management of inflammatory arthritis with particular reference to orthopedic surgery. Curr Orthop. 2007;21(5):358–63.
15. Pedersen E, Pinsker E, Younger AS, Penner MJ, Wing KJ, Dryden PJ, Glazebrook M, Daniels TR. Outcome of total ankle arthroplasty in patients with rheumatoid arthritis and noninflam-

matory arthritis. A multicenter cohort study comparing clinical outcome and safety. J Bone Joint Surg Am. 2014;96(21):1768–75.
16. Raikin SM, Kane J, Ciminiello ME. Risk factors for incision-healing complications following total ankle arthroplasty. J Bone Joint Surg Am. 2010;92(12):2150–5.
17. Althoff A, Cancienne JM, Cooper MT, Werner BC. Patient-related risk factors for periprosthetic ankle joint infection: an analysis of 6977 total ankle arthroplasties. J Foot Ankle Surg. 2018;57(2):269–72.
18. Wukich DK, Lowery NJ, McMillan RL, Frykberg RG. Postoperative infection rates in foot and ankle surgery: a comparison of patients with and without diabetes mellitus. J Bone Joint Surg Am. 2010;92(2):287–95.
19. Wukich DK, McMillen RL, Lowery NJ, Frykberg RG. Surgical site infections after foot and ankle surgery: a comparison of patients with and without diabetes. Diabetes Care. 2011;34(10):2211–3.
20. Wukich DK, Crim BE, Frykberg RG, Rosario BL. Neuropathy and poorly controlled diabetes increase the rate of surgical site infection after foot and ankle surgery. J Bone Joint Surg Am. 2014;96(10):832–9.
21. Courtney PM, Boniello AJ, Berger RA. Complications following outpatient total joint arthroplasty: an analysis of a national database. J Arthroplast. 2017;32(5):1426–30.
22. Schipper ON, Jiang JJ, Chen L, Koh J, Toolan BC. Effect of diabetes mellitus on perioperative complications and hospital outcomes after ankle arthrodesis and total ankle arthroplasty. Foot Ankle Int. 2015;36(3):258–67.
23. Gross CE, Green CL, DeOrio JK, Easley M, Adams S, Nunley JA 2nd. Impact of diabetes on outcome of total ankle replacement. Foot Ankle Int. 2015;36(10):1144–9.
24. Cancienne JM, Werner BC, Browne JA. Is there a threshold value of hemoglobin A1c that predicts risk of infection following primary total hip arthroplasty? J Arthroplast. 2017;32(9S):S236–40.
25. Parvizi J, Marrs J, Morrey BF. Total knee arthroplasty for neuropathic (Charcot) joints. Clin Orthop Relat Res. 2003;(416):145–50.
26. Yasin MN, Charalambous CP, Mills SP, Phaltankar PM, Nutton RW. Early failure of a knee replacement in a neuropathic joint: a case report. Acta Orthop Belg. 2011;77:132–6.
27. Tibbo ME, Chalmers BP, Berry DJ, Pagnano MW, Lewallen DG, Abdel MP. Primary total knee arthroplasty in patients with neuropathic (Charcot) arthropathy: contemporary results. J Arthroplast. 2018;33(9):2815–20.
28. Chalmers BP, Tibbo ME, Trousdale RT, Lewallen DG, Berry DJ, Abdel MP. Primary total hip arthroplasty for charcot arthropathy is associated with high complications but improved clinical outcomes. J Arthroplast. 2018;33(9):2912–8.
29. James WP. WHO recognition of the global obesity epidemic. Int J Obes. 2008;32(suppl 7):S120–6.
30. Boyce L, Prasad A, Barrett M, Dawson-Bowling S, Millington S, Hanna SA, Achan P. The outcomes of total knee arthroplasty in morbidly obese patients: a systematic review of the literature. Arch Orthop Trauma Surg. 2019;139(4):553–60.
31. Deakin AH, Iyayi-Igbinovia A, Love GJ. A comparison of outcomes in morbidly obese, obese and non-obese patients undergoing primary total knee and total hip arthroplasty. Surgeon. 2018;16(1):40–5.
32. Werner BC, Tyrrell Burrus M, Looney AM, Park JS, Perumal V, Truitt CM. Obesity is associated with increased complications after operative management of end-stage ankle arthritis. Foot Ankle Int. 2015;36(8):863–70.
33. Bouchard MR, Amin A, Pinsker E, Khan R, Deda E, Daniels T. The impact of obesity on the outcome of total ankle replacement. J Bone Joint Surg. 2015;97(11):904–10.
34. Sansosti LE, Van JC, Meyr AJ. Effect of obesity on total ankle arthroplasty: a systematic review of postoperative complications requiring surgical revision. J Foot Ankle Surg. 2018;57(2):353–6.

35. Zaidi R, Cro S, Gurusamy K, Siva N, Macgregor A, Henricson A, Goldberg A. The outcome of total ankle replacement: a systematic review and meta-analysis. Bone Joint J. 2013;95-B(11):1500–7.
36. Lampley A, Gross CE, Green CL, DeOrio JK, Easley M, Adams S, Nunley JA 2nd. Association of cigarette use and complication rates and outcomes following total ankle arthroplasty. Foot Ankle Int. 2016;37(10):1052–9.
37. Patton D, Kiewiet N, Brage M. Infected total ankle arthroplasty: risk factors and treatment options. Foot Ankle Int. 2015;36(6):626–34.
38. Gross CE, Hamid KS, Green C, Easley ME, DeOrio JK, Nunley JA. Operative wound complications following total ankle arthroplasty. Foot Ankle Int. 2017;38(4):360–6.
39. Andersen T, Christensen FB, Laursen M, Høy K, Hansen ES, Bünger C. Smoking as a predictor of negative outcome in lumbar spinal fusion. Spine (Phila Pa 1976). 2001;26(23):2623–8.
40. Whalen JL, Spelsberg SC, Murray P. Wound breakdown after total ankle arthroplasty. Foot Ankle Int. 2010;31(4):301–5.
41. Essenmacher CA. Nicotine content in tobacco products. Session 3031 Handout. 2012. https://sntc.medicine.ufl.edu/Content/Webinars/SupportingDocs/3031-Essenmacher_-_Handout_1.pdf. Accessed 24 Feb 2019.
42. Dodd A, Daniels TR. Total ankle replacement in the presence of talar varus or valgus deformities. Foot Ankle Clin. 2017;22(2):277–300.
43. Knupp M, Bolliger L, Hintermann B. Treatment of posttraumatic varus ankle deformity with supramalleolar osteotomy. Foot Ankle Clin. 2012;17(1):95–102.
44. Queen RM, Adams SB Jr, Viens NA, Friend JK, Easley ME, Deorio JK, Nunley JA. Differences in outcomes following total ankle replacement in patients with neutral alignment compared with tibiotalar joint malalignment. J Bone Joint Surg Am. 2013;95(21):1927–34.
45. Sung KS, Ahn J, Lee KH, Chun TH. Short-term results of total ankle arthroplasty for end-stage ankle arthritis with severe varus deformity. Foot Ankle Int. 2014;35(3):225–31.
46. Knupp M, Stufkens SA, Bolliger L, Barg A, Hintermann B. Classification and treatment of supramalleolar deformities. Foot Ankle Int. 2011;32(11):1023–31.
47. Knupp M. The use of osteotomies in the treatment of asymmetric ankle joint arthritis. Foot Ankle Int. 2017;38(2):220–9.
48. Brigido SA, Carrington SC, Protzman NM. Complex total ankle arthroplasty. Clin Podiatr Med Surg. 2017;34(4):529–39.
49. Shock RP, Christensen JC, Schuberth JM. Total ankle replacement in the varus ankle. J Foot Ankle Surg. 2011;50(1):5–10.
50. Tan KJ, Myerson MS. Planning correction of the varus ankle deformity with ankle replacement. Foot Ankle Clin. 2011;17(1):103–15.
51. Valderrbano V, Müller AM, Henninger HB. Mobile- and fixed-bearing total ankle prosthesis: is there really a difference? Foot Ankle Clin. 2012;17:565–85.
52. Bonasia DE, Dettoni F, Femino JE, Phisitkul P, Germano M, Amendola A. Total ankle replacement: why, when and how? Iowa Orthop J. 2010;30:119–30.
53. Gougoulias N, Maffulli N. History of total ankle replacement. Clin Podiatr Med Surg. 2013;30:1–20.
54. Ochsner PE. Osteointegration of orthopaedic devices. Semin Immunopathol. 2011;33(3):245–56.
55. Gaudot F, Colombier J, Bonnin M, Judet T. A controlled, comparative study of a fixed-bearing versus mobile- bearing ankle arthroplasty. Foot Ankle Int. 2014;35(2):131–40.
56. Queen RM, Sparling TL, Butler RJ, Adams SB Jr, DeOrio JK, Easley ME, Nunley JA. Patient-reported outcomes, function, and gait mechanics after fixed and mobile-bearing total ankle replacement. J Bone Joint Surg Am. 2014;96:987–93.
57. Brandao RA, Prissel MA, Hyer CF. Current and emerging insights on total ankle replacement. Podiatry Today. 2018;31(4):36–43.
58. Bibbo C. Controversies in total ankle replacement. Clin Podiatr Med Surg. 2013;30(1):21–34.

59. Reb CW, Berlet GC. Experience with navigation in total ankle arthroplasty. Is it worth the cost? Foot Ankle Clin. 2017;22(1):455–63.
60. Waly FJ, Yeo NE, Penner MJ. Computed navigation guidance for ankle replacement in the setting of ankle deformity. Clin Podiatr Med Surg. 2018;35(1):85–94.
61. Kosse NM, Heesterbeek PJC, Schimmel JJP, van Hellemondt GG, Wymenga AB, Defoort KC. Stability and alignment do not improve by using patient-specific instrumentation in total knee arthroplasty: a randomized controlled trial. Knee Surg Sports Traumatol Arthrosc. 2018;26(6):1792–9.
62. Van Leeuwen JAMJ, Snorrason F, Röhrl SM. No radiological and clinical advantages with patient-specific positioning guides in total knee replacement. Acta Orthop. 2018;89(1):89–94.
63. Hsu AR, Davis WH, Cohen BE, Jones CP, Ellington JK, Anderson RB. Radiographic outcomes of preoperative CT scan-derived patient-specific total ankle arthroplasty. Foot Ankle Int. 2015;36(10):1163–9.
64. Daigre J, Berlet G, Van Dyke B, Peterson KS, Santrock R. Accuracy and reproducibility using patient-specific instrumentation in total ankle arthroplasty. Foot Ankle Int. 2017;38(4):412–8.
65. Berlet GC, Penner MJ, Lancianese S, Stemniski PM, Obert RM. Total ankle arthroplasty accuracy and reproducibility using preoperative CT scan-derived, patient-specific guides. Foot Ankle Int. 2014;35(7):665–76.
66. Barg A, Bettin CC, Burstein AH, Saltzman CL, Gililland J. Early clinical and radiographic outcomes of trabecular metal total ankle replacement using a transfibular approach. J Bone Joint Surg Am. 2018;100(6):505–15.
67. Usuelli FG, Indino C, Maccario C, Manzi L, Liuni FM, Vulcano E. Infections in primary total ankle replacement: anterior approach versus lateral transfibular approach. Foot Ankle Surg. 2017;25:19. pii: S1268-7731(17)30790-7.
68. Usuelli FG, D'Ambrosi R, Manzi L, Maccario C, Indino C. Treatment of ankle osteoarthritis with total ankle replacement through a lateral transfibular approach. J Vis Exp. 2018;(131):56396.
69. Tan EW, Maccario C, Talusan PG, Schon LC. Early complications and secondary procedures in transfibular total ankle replacement. Foot Ankle Int. 2016;37(8):835–41.
70. Goetz JE, Rungprai C, Tennant JN, Huber E, Uribe B, Femino J, Phisitkul P, Amendola A. Variable volumes of resected bone resulting from different total ankle arthroplasty systems. Foot Ankle Int. 2016;37(8):898–904.
71. Li SY, Myerson MS. Management of talar component subsidence. Foot Ankle Clin. 2017;22(2):361–89.
72. Knabel M, Cook JJ, Basile P, McKenna B, Cook EA. Complication risk stratification for revision surgery following total ankle replacement. Poster presented at ACFAS Annual Scientific Conference 2019.
73. Gadd RJ, Barwick TW, Paling E, Davies MB, Blundell CM. Assessment of a three-grade classification of complications in total ankle replacement. Foot Ankle Int. 2014;35(5):434–7.
74. Glazebrook MA, Arsenault K, Dunbar M. Evidence-based classification of complications in total ankle arthroplasty. Foot Ankle Int. 2009;30(10):945–9.
75. Criswell B, Hunt K, Kim T, Chou L, Haskell A. Association of short-term complications with procedures through separate incisions during total ankle replacement. Foot Ankle Int. 2016;37(10):1060–4.
76. Manning E, Millonig K, McKenna BJ, Cook JJ, Cook EA. Meta-analysis of surgical site infections in elective foot and ankle surgery. Manuscript presented at ACFAS Annual Scientific Conference 2019.
77. Kessler B, Sendi P, Graber P, Knupp M, Zwicky L, Hintermann B, Zimmerli W. Risk factors for periprosthetic ankle joint infection: a case-control study. J Bone Joint Surg Am. 2012;94(20):1871–6.
78. Lewis JS Jr, Green CL, Adams SB Jr, Easley ME, DeOrio JK, Nunley JA. Comparison of first- and second-generation fixed-bearing total ankle arthroplasty using a modular intramedullary tibial component. Foot Ankle Int. 2015;36(8):881–90.

79. Knecht SI, Estin M, Callaghan JJ, et al. The Agility total ankle arthroplasty. Seven to sixteen-year follow up. J Bone Joint Surg Am. 2004;86(6):1161–71.
80. Schipper ON, Haddad SL, Fullam S, Pourzal R, Wimmer MA. Wear characteristics of conventional ultrahigh-molecular-weight polyethylene versus highly cross-linked polyethylene in total ankle arthroplasty. Foot Ankle Int. 2018;39(11):1335–44.
81. Koivu H, Mackiewicz Z, Takakubo Y, Trokovic N, Pajarinen J, Konttinen YT. RANKL in the osteolysis of AES total ankle replacement implants. Bone. 2012;51(3):546–52.
82. Rodriguez D, Bevernage BD, Maldague P, Deleu PA, Tribak K, Leemrijse T. Medium term follow-up of the AES ankle prosthesis: high rate of asymptomatic osteolysis. Foot Ankle Surg. 2010;16(2):54–60.
83. Kokkonen A, Ikävalko M, Tiihonen R, Kautiainen H, Belt EA. High rate of osteolytic lesions in medium-term followup after the AES total ankle replacement. Foot Ankle Int. 2011;32(2):168–75.
84. Sopher RS, Amis AA, Calder JD, Jeffers JRT. Total ankle replacement design and positioning affect implant-bone micromotion and bone strains. Med Eng Phys. 2017;42:80–90.
85. Brunner S, Barg A, Knupp M, Zwicky L, Kapron AL, Valderrabano V, Hintermann B. The Scandinavian total ankle replacement: long-term, eleven to fifteen-year, survivorship analysis of the prosthesis in seventy-two consecutive patients. J Bone Joint Surg Am. 2013;95(8):711–8.
86. Henricson A, Carlsson Å. Survival analysis of the single- and double-coated STAR ankle up to 20 Years: long-term follow-up of 324 cases from the Swedish Ankle Registry. Foot Ankle Int. 2015;36(10):1156–60.
87. Palanca A, Mann RA, Mann JA, Haskell A. Scandinavian total ankle replacement: 15-year follow-up. Foot Ankle Int. 2018;39(2):135–42.
88. Kopp FJ, Patel MM, Deland JT, O'Malley MJ. Total ankle arthroplasty with the Agility prosthesis: clinical and radiographic evaluation. Foot Ankle Int. 2006;27:97–103.
89. Hintermann B, Valderrabano V, Dereymaeker G, Dick W. The HINTEGRA ankle: rationale and short-term results of 122 consecutive ankles. Clin Orthop Relat Res. 2004;424:57–68.
90. Kim DR, Choi YS, Potter HG, Ae L, Chun KY, Jung YY, Kim JS, Young KW. Total ankle arthroplasty: an imaging overview. Korean J Radiol. 2016;17(3):413–23.
91. Manegold S, Springer A, Landvoigt K, Tsitsilonis S. Heterotopic ossification after total ankle replacement: the role of prosthesis alignment. Foot Ankle Surg. 2017;23(2):122–7.
92. Rogers J, Shepstone L, Dieppe P. Bone formers: osteophyte and enthesophyte formation are positively associated. Ann Rheum Dis. 1997;56(2):85–90.
93. Hayeri MR, Trudell DJ, Resnick D. Anterior ankle impingement and talar bony outgrowths: osteophyte or enthesophyte? Paleopathologic and cadaveric study with imaging correlation. Am J Roentgenol. 2009;193(4):W334–8.
94. King CM, Schuberth JM, Christensen JC, Swanstrom KM. Relationship of alignment and tibial cortical coverage to hypertrophic bone formation in Salto Talaris® total ankle arthroplasty. J Foot Ankle Surg. 2013;52(3):355–9.
95. American Academy of Orthopedic Surgeons. Implant wear in total joint replacement. 2001. http://people.unica.it/pau/files/2014/12/AAOS2001-WearinImplants.pdf. Accessed 9 Apr 2019.
96. Currier BH, Hecht PJ, Nunley JA, Mayor MB, Currier JH, Van Citters DW. Analysis of failed ankle arthroplasty components. Foot Ankle Int. 2019;40(2):131–8.
97. Labek G, Thaler M, Janda W, Agreiter M, Stöckl B. Revision rates after total joint replacement: cumulative results from worldwide joint register datasets. J Bone Joint Surg (Br). 2011;93(3):293–7.

# Index




D. E. Tower (ed.), *Evidence-Based Podiatry*,
https://doi.org/10.1007/978-3-030-50853-1

Printed in the United States
by Baker & Taylor Publisher Services